Staphylococcal Infections

Guest Editors

RACHEL J. GORWITZ, MD, MPH
JOHN A. JERNIGAN, MD, MS

INFECTIOUS DISEASE CLINICS OF NORTH AMERICA

www.id.theclinics.com

Consulting Editor
ROBERT C. MOELLERING, Jr, MD

March 2009 • Volume 23 • Number 1

SAUNDERS an imprint of ELSEVIER, Inc.

W.B. SAUNDERS COMPANY
A Division of Elsevier Inc.
1600 John F. Kennedy Blvd., Suite 1800, Philadelphia, PA 19103-2899.
http://www.theclinics.com
INFECTIOUS DISEASE CLINICS OF NORTH AMERICA Volume 23, Number 1
March 2009 ISSN 0891–5520, ISBN-10: 1-4377-0491-3, ISBN-13: 978-1-4377-0491-4
Editor: Barbara Cohen-Kligerman

Photocopying
Single photocopies of single articles may be made for personal use as allowed by national copyright laws. Permission of the Publisher and payment of a fee is required for all other photocopying, including multiple or systematic copying, copying for advertising or promotional purposes, resale, and all forms of document delivery. Special rates are available for educational institutions that wish to make photocopies for non-profit educational classroom use. For information on how to seek permission visit www.elsevier.com/permissions or call: (+44) 1865 843830 (UK)/(+1) 215 239 3804 (USA).

Derivative Works
Subscribers may reproduce tables of contents or prepare lists of articles including abstracts for internal circulation within their institutions. Permission of the Publisher is required for resale or distribution outside the institution. Permission of the Publisher is required for all other derivative works, including compilations and translations (please consult www.elsevier.com/permissions).

Electronic Storage or Usage
Permission of the Publisher is required to store or use electronically any material contained in this journal, including any article or part of an article (please consult www.elsevier.com/permissions). Except as outlined above, no part of this publication may be reproduced, stored in a retrieval system or transmitted in any form or by any means, electronic, mechanical, photocopying, recording or otherwise, without prior written permission of the Publisher.

Notice
No responsibility is assumed by the Publisher for any injury and/or damage to persons or property as a matter of products liability, negligence or otherwise, or from any use or operation of any methods, products, instructions or ideas contained in the material herein. Because of rapid advances in the medical sciences, in particular, independent verification of diagnoses and drug dosages should be made.

Although all advertising material is expected to conform to ethical (medical) standards, inclusion in this publication does not constitute a guarantee or endorsement of the quality or value of such product or of the claims made of it by its manufacturer.

Infectious Disease Clinics of North America (ISSN 0891–5520) is published in March, June, September, and December (For Post Office use only: volume 23 issue 1 of 4) by Elsevier Inc., 360 Park Avenue South, New York, NY 10010-1710. Business and Editorial Offices: 1600 John F. Kennedy Blvd., Suite 1800, Philadelphia, PA 19103-2899. Customer Service Office: 6277 Sea Harbor Drive, Orlando, FL 32887-4800. Periodicals postage paid at New York, NY and additional mailing offices. Subscription prices are $218.00 per year for US individuals, $366.00 per year for US institutions, $109.00 per year for US students, $257.00 per year for Canadian individuals, $453.00 per year for Canadian institutions, $307.00 per year for international individuals, $453.00 per year for international institutions, and $151.00 per year for Canadian and international students. To receive student rate, orders must be accompanied by name of affiliated institution, date of term, and the *signature* of program/residency coordinator on institution letterhead. Orders will be billed at individual rate until proof of status is received. Foreign air speed delivery is included in all *Clinics* subscription prices. All prices are subject to change without notice. **POSTMASTER:** Send address changes to *Infectious Disease Clinics of North America,* Elsevier Periodicals Customer Service, 11830 Westline Industrial Drive, St. Louis, MO 63146. **Customer Service: 1-800-654-2452 (US). From outside of the US, call 1-314-453-7041. Fax: 1-314-453-5170. E-mail: JournalsCustomerService-usa@elsevier.com (print support) or JournalsOnlineSupport-usa@elsevier.com (online support).**

Infectious Disease Clinics of North America is also published in Spanish by Editorial Inter-Médica, Junin 917, 1er A 1113, Buenos Aires, Argentina.

Reprints. For copies of 100 or more, of articles in this publication, please contact the Commercial Reprints Department, Elsevier Inc., 360 Park Avenue South, New York, New York 10010-1710. Tel. (212) 633-3812, Fax: (212) 462-1935, email: reprints@elsevier.com.

Infectious Disease Clinics of North America is covered in *MEDLINE/PubMed (Index Medicus), Current Contents/Clinical Medicine, Science Citation Alert, SCISEARCH,* and *Research Alert.*

Printed and bound in the United Kingdom
Transferred to Digital Print 2011

Contributors

GUEST EDITORS

RACHEL J. GORWITZ, MD, MPH
Division of Healthcare Quality Promotion, Centers for Disease Control and Prevention, Atlanta, Georgia

JOHN A. JERNIGAN, MD, MS
Division of Healthcare Quality Promotion, Centers for Disease Control and Prevention, Atlanta, Georgia

AUTHORS

DEVERICK J. ANDERSON, MD, MPH
Assistant Professor of Medicine, Division of Infectious Diseases, Duke University Medical Center, Durham, North Carolina

NICK DANEMAN, MD
Departments of Medicine and Microbiology and the Division of Infectious Diseases, Sunnybrook Health Sciences Centre, Toronto, Ontario, Canada

FRANK R. DELEO, PhD
Acting Chief and Senior Investigator, Laboratory of Human Bacterial Pathogenesis, Rocky Mountain Laboratories, National Institute of Allergy and Infectious Diseases, National Institutes of Health, Hamilton, Montana

BINH AN DIEP, PhD
Adjunct Instructor, Division of Infectious Diseases, Department of Medicine, University of California, San Francisco, San Francisco, California

PAUL D. FEY, PhD
Associate Professor, Department of Pathology and Microbiology; Department of Internal Medicine, University of Nebraska Medical Center, Omaha, Nebraska

HOWARD S. GOLD, MD
Assistant Professor of Medicine, Harvard Medical School, Division of Infectious Diseases; and Medical Director of Antimicrobial Management, Silverman Institute for Health Care Quality and Safety, Beth Israel Deaconess Medical Center, Boston, Massachusetts

SHELDON L. KAPLAN, MD
Department of Pediatrics, Baylor College of Medicine, Texas Children's Hospital, Infectious Disease Service, Houston, Texas

KEITH S. KAYE, MD, MPH
Professor of Medicine, Corporate Director, Infection Prevention, Epidemiology and Antimicrobial Stewardship, Wayne State University Health Center, Detroit, Michigan

JEAN C. LEE, PhD
Associate Professor, Channing Laboratory, Department of Medicine, Brigham and Women's Hospital and Harvard Medical School, Boston, Massachusetts

LOREN G. MILLER, MD, MPH
Division of Infectious Diseases, Director, Infection Control Program, Harbor-UCLA Medical Center, Torrance; Los Angeles Biomedical Research Institute at Harbor-UCLA Medical Center, Los Angeles; and the David Geffen School of Medicine at the University of California, Los Angeles, Los Angeles, California

MICHAEL OTTO, PhD
Senior Investigator, Laboratory of Human Bacterial Pathogenesis, Rocky Mountain Laboratories, National Institute of Allergy and Infectious Diseases, National Institutes of Health, Hamilton, Montana

SATISH K. PILLAI, MD
Instructor of Medicine, Harvard Medical School, Division of Infectious Diseases, Beth Israel Deaconess Medical Center, Boston, Massachusetts

KATHIE L. ROGERS, PhD
Research Associate, Department of Pathology and Microbiology, University of Nebraska Medical Center, Omaha, Nebraska

NAOMI L. RUFF, PhD
RuffDraft Communications, Duluth, Minnesota

MARK E. RUPP, MD
Professor, Department of Internal Medicine, University of Nebraska Medical Center, Omaha, Nebraska

ADAM C. SCHAFFER, MD
Instructor, Department of Medicine, Brigham and Women's Hospital and Harvard Medical School, Boston, Massachusetts

HENRY R. SHINEFIELD, MD
Clinical Professor of Pediatrics, University of California, San Francisco, San Francisco, California

ANDREW E. SIMOR, MD
Professor, Department of Medicine, University of Toronto; Department of Laboratory Medicine and Pathobiology, University of Toronto; and Chief, Department of Microbiology and the Division of Infectious Diseases, Sunnybrook Health Sciences Centre, Toronto, Ontario, Canada

Contents

Henry R. Shinefield and Naomi L. Ruff

Staphylococcus aureus is an unusually successful and adaptive human pathogen that can cause epidemics of invasive disease despite its frequent carriage as a commensal. Over the past 100 years and more, *S aureus* has caused cycles of outbreaks in hospitals and the community and has developed resistance to every antibiotic used against it, yet the exact mechanisms leading to epidemics of virulent disease are not fully understood. Approaches such as bacterial interference have been effective in interrupting outbreaks, but to better prevent staphylococcal disease, we will need to be vigilant about environmental factors that facilitate its spread. Even more importantly, we need to understand more about the mechanisms that lead to its virulence and transmission. With such information, it may be possible to develop a vaccine that will prevent both endemic and epidemic staphylococcal disease.

Frank R. DeLeo, Binh An Diep, and Michael Otto

Staphylococcus aureus is the most abundant cause of bacterial infections in the United States. As such, the pathogen has devised means to circumvent destruction by the innate immune system. Neutrophils are a critical component of innate immunity and the primary cellular defense against *S aureus* infections. This article reviews human neutrophil function in the context of *S aureus* virulence mechanisms and provides an overview of community-associated methicillin-resistant *S aureus* pathogenicity.

Loren G. Miller and Sheldon L. Kaplan

Staphylococcus aureus is a common human pathogen. *S aureus* infections most commonly clinically manifest as skin infections. There has been much interest in *S aureus* infections in the community over the past decade because of the rise of community-associated methicillin-resistant *S aureus* (CA-MRSA) infections, which have emerged globally over a relatively short period of time. In contrast to health care-associated methicillin resistant *S aureus* (HA-MRSA), circulating strains of CA-MRSA have characteristic pathogenesis, strain characteristics, epidemiology, and clinical manifestations that are distinct from HA-MRSA. In fact, CA-MRSA probably behaves more like community-associated methicillin-sensitive *S aureus* (MSSA). This article reviews current knowledge of the epidemiology and clinical manifestations of community-associated *S aureus* and CA-MRSA infections.

Staphylococcus aureus is the leading cause of surgical site infections (SSI) in the United States. In particular, SSI caused by methicillin-resistant *Staphylococcus aureus* (MRSA) has emerged as a devastating complication, leading to increased mortality rates, increased length of hospitalization, and increased costs. Proven strategies for prevention of SSI caused by *S aureus* include addressing modifiable risk factors and correct choice and timing of antimicrobial prophylaxis. Other strategies, including decolonization and the use of vancomycin, remain controversial.

Coagulase-negative staphylococci (CNS) are differentiated from the closely related but more virulent *Staphylococcus aureus* by their inability to produce free coagulase. Currently, there are over 40 recognized species of CNS. These organisms typically reside on healthy human skin and mucus membranes, rarely cause disease, and are most frequently encountered by clinicians as contaminants of microbiological cultures. However, CNS have been increasingly recognized to cause clinically significant infections. The conversion of the CNS from symbiont to human pathogen has been a direct reflection of the use of indwelling medical devices. This article deals with the clinical syndromes, epidemiology, prevention, and management of infections caused by this unique group of organisms.

These are interesting times in the treatment of infections caused by *Staphylococcus aureus*, with shifting epidemiology of antibiotic resistance; changing prevalence of clinical syndromes (probably reflecting changes in virulence of circulating strains); and the recent availability of a variety of new agents with activity against multidrug-resistant gram-positive cocci. The abundance of riches in new drugs for the multidrug-resistant gram-positive space is timely, and these agents show great potential, but as yet have incompletely tested durability and comparative efficacy. This article reviews the advantages and disadvantages of a variety of antistaphylococcal agents by providing basic information including mechanism of action; mechanisms of resistance; clinical use (including dosing for and data supporting common indications); drug toxicities; and major drug interactions.

> Decolonization may be defined as treatment to eradicate *Staphylococcus aureus* or methicillin-resistant *S aureus* (MRSA) carriage. Potential benefits of decolonization include decreased risk of subsequent staphylococcal infection and prevention of staphylococcal transmission to reduce endemic rates of infection or manage outbreaks. This article reviews available data regarding various proposed treatment regimens for eradicating staphylococcal carriage and the effectiveness of decolonization for infection prevention and as an infection control measure.

> *Staphylococcus aureus* is an important pathogen in the hospital and in the community, and it is increasingly resistant to multiple antibiotics. A nonantimicrobial approach to controlling *S aureus* is needed. The most extensively tested vaccine against *S aureus*, which is a capsular polysaccharide-based vaccine known as StaphVAX, showed promise in an initial phase 3 trial, but was found to be ineffective in a confirmatory trial, leading to its development being halted. Likewise, a human IgG preparation known as INH-A21 (Veronate) with elevated levels of antibodies to the staphylococcal surface adhesins ClfA and SdrG made it into phase 3 testing, where it failed to show a clinical benefit. Several novel antigens are being tested for potential inclusion in a staphylococcal vaccine, including cell wall-anchored adhesin proteins and exotoxins. Given the multiple and sometimes redundant virulence factors of *S aureus* that enable it to be such a crafty pathogen, if a vaccine is to prove effective, it will have to be multicomponent, incorporating several surface proteins, toxoids, and surface polysaccharides.

VISIT THE CLINICS ONLINE!

Access your subscription at:
www.theclinics.com

Preface

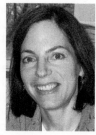 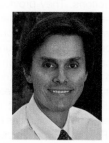

Rachel J. Gorwitz, MD, MPH   John A. Jernigan, MD, MS
Guest Editors

Staphylococci are both common human commensals and one of the leading causes of infection in humans. *Staphylococcus aureus* in particular, although persistently or intermittently colonizing most humans without incident, is a major cause of morbidity and mortality. Staphylococcal infections encompass a spectrum from relatively mild localized infections to rapidly fatal invasive infections. Before the antibiotic era, invasive staphylococcal infections were frequently fatal. The introduction of penicillin in the 1940s significantly improved the prognosis of these infections; however, staphylococci have proved to be adept at developing mechanisms to resist being killed by antimicrobial agents. Methicillin-resistant *S aureus* (MRSA), which possesses an altered penicillin-binding protein conferring resistance to all β-lactam antimicrobial agents except the recently developed ceftobiprole, was described shortly after the introduction of methicillin in the early 1960s. Throughout the subsequent decades, MRSA became an increasingly important cause of infection in hospitalized patients and remains a leading cause of health care–associated infections. In the 1990s, new strains of MRSA emerged as a cause of infection among otherwise healthy people in the general community, adding to the overall burden of community-associated *S aureus* infections.

With this issue of *Infectious Disease Clinics of North America*, we have been privileged to work with contributors who have generously shared their expertise in the areas of staphylococcal epidemiology and pathogenesis and the management and prevention of staphylococcal infections. The issue begins with an article by Drs. Shinefield and Ruff offering a historical perspective on staphylococcal infections and insight about how history can inform current efforts to prevent and control staphylococcal infections. Drs. Shinefield and Ruff point out that, despite all that has been learned thus far about staphylococcal disease, there is still an urgent need to understand more about the mechanisms of virulence and transmission that turn a common commensal organism into one that is highly pathogenic. To that end, Drs. DeLeo, Diep, and Otto present an overview of host defense and pathogenesis in *S aureus* infections, reviewing human neutrophil function in the context of *S aureus* virulence mechanisms and exploring the role of a number of virulence factors in the pathogenicity of community MRSA strains.

Infect Dis Clin N Am 23 (2009) ix–x
doi:10.1016/j.idc.2008.11.001
0891-5520/08/$ – see front matter © 2009 Elsevier Inc. All rights reserved.

Drs. Anderson and Kaye point out that surgical site infection remains a leading cause of morbidity and mortality in modern health care, with S aureus being the most common cause of these infections. They provide a thorough summary of the epidemiology, diagnosis, pathogenesis, and clinical management of S aureus surgical site infections, and both proven and controversial prevention strategies. Although S aureus has long been a common cause of community-associated infections, the recent emergence of MRSA as a community pathogen has altered the epidemiology of these infections. Drs. Miller and Kaplan describe the changing epidemiology and clinical manifestations of community-associated S aureus infections in adults and children and discuss implications for clinical management. Coagulase-negative staphylococci are most frequently encountered by clinicians as contaminants of microbiologic cultures; however, as Drs. Rogers, Fey, and Rupp indicate, coagulase-negative staphylococci have been increasingly recognized to cause clinically significant infections in patients with indwelling medical devices. In their article, they describe the epidemiology, clinical spectrum, and pathogenesis of coagulase-negative staphylococci infections, and discuss current and future prevention and management strategies.

The constantly evolving resistance of S aureus to antimicrobial agents and the increasing transmission and prevalence of resistant strains (notably MRSA) in both health care and community settings have presented challenges for the treatment of S aureus infections. Drs. Gold and Pillai provide a comprehensive review of available antistaphylococcal agents, including mechanisms of action and resistance, clinical use, and drug toxicities and interactions. Preventing staphylococcal infections in the first place is the ideal solution. The elimination or suppression of S aureus colonization (known as "decolonization") is one potential means of preventing S aureus infections. In their article, Drs. Simor and Daneman explore the evidence supporting S aureus decolonization as a prevention strategy in both health care and community settings. Development of an effective S aureus vaccine would provide the ultimate prevention strategy; however, efforts so far have been unsuccessful. In the final article of this issue, Drs. Schaffer and Lee describe the challenges in developing staphylococcal vaccines and immunotherapies, summarize trials completed to date, and outline considerations to be taken into account in vaccine development.

The articles in this issue cover some of the most important and sometimes controversial issues in the pathogenesis, prevention, and management of staphylococcal infections. They offer thorough reviews of established prevention and control strategies and provide a framework for considering the potential advantages and disadvantages of less established interventions. It is our hope that the reader finds these articles as informative and useful as we have.

Rachel J. Gorwitz, MD, MPH

John A. Jernigan, MD, MS
Division of Healthcare Quality Promotion
Centers for Disease Control and Prevention, MS A-35
1600 Clifton Road NE
Atlanta, GA 30333, USA

E-mail addresses:
RGorwitz@cdc.gov (R.J. Gorwitz)
JJernigan@cdc.gov (J.A. Jernigan)

Staphylococcal Infections: A Historical Perspective

Henry R. Shinefield, MD[a],*, Naomi L. Ruff, PhD[b]

KEYWORDS

- *Staphylococcal aureus* • MRSA • Epidemic • Virulence
- Hygiene • Antibiotic resistance • Bacterial interference

Staphylococcus aureus, a gram-positive, coagulase-positive bacterium, is among the most successful of human pathogens. Asymptomatic colonization by *S aureus* of the skin and mucosa, particularly the anterior nares, is extremely common, with about 20% of the population carrying *S aureus* chronically and 60% intermittently.[1] In addition to its frequent carriage as a commensal, *S aureus* is also the leading cause of bloodstream, lower respiratory tract, and skin and soft tissue infections worldwide.[2]

Despite its prevalence, much remains to be learned about how *S aureus* causes disease. Staphylococcal disease tends to appear in cycles of frequent outbreaks followed by quieter periods. Epidemic strains appear, sometimes leading to outbreaks worldwide, and then fade away again. Virulence is determined by various bacterial factors that control attachment, penetration, and evasion,[3,4] which presumably combine with host and environmental factors to promote transmission or invasion. Although we have learned much about the genetics and microbiology of staphylococci over the past few decades, we still do not fully understand what triggers a normally commensal organism to become invasive. Yet some aspects of staphylococcal disease remain constant: the emergence of new strains, their spread within hospitals and the community, the development of antibiotic resistance, and the need to remain vigilant against this pervasive organism.

STAPHYLOCOCCAL OUTBREAKS AND THE IMPORTANCE OF HANDS TO TRANSMISSION

Although staphylococci were first implicated in disease in 1880, when Alexander Ogston[5] linked them to abscesses, neonatal diseases such as pemphigus neonatorum (now known as scalded skin syndrome) were described as early as the 1700s. Newborns readily acquire staphylococci in the nares, throat, and umbilicus,[6,7] and the strains acquired shortly after birth may form part of the normal flora or may lead

[a] University of California in San Francisco, San Francisco, CA, USA
[b] RuffDraft Communications, 1211 Kenwood Avenue, Duluth, MN 55811, USA
* Corresponding author.
E-mail address: Henryshinefield@aol.com (H.R. Shinefield).

Infect Dis Clin N Am 23 (2009) 1–15
doi:10.1016/j.idc.2008.10.007
0891-5520/08/$ – see front matter © 2009 Elsevier Inc. All rights reserved.

id.theclinics.com

to disease of various types, such as furuncles, mastitis, scalded skin syndrome, and bacteremia. Some level of staphylococcal disease is probably always present in nurseries,[8] most often causing minor skin infections, but hospital neonatal wards have also been frequent and recurring sites of outbreaks. The first nursery epidemic reported in the United States occurred in 1889,[9] and subsequent outbreaks occurred throughout the 1900s.[10–19]

Staphylococcal outbreaks among adults are also common in hospitals, particularly in burn or surgical units,[20–22] where the presence of deep wounds and medical devices such as catheters provide environments conducive to the growth of staphylococci. The incidence of nosocomial staphylococcal disease has increased in recent decades, in part because of the increased use of intravascular devices[23] and the higher prevalence of immunodeficiencies.

What causes the shift from endemic to epidemic disease is not clear, but one prerequisite is that the organism be readily transmitted. Bacterial and environmental factors appear to contribute to the rapid spread of staphylococci through a hospital ward. Despite the presence of many staphylococcal strains within the same hospital, only a few become epidemic, suggesting that differences in the bacteria themselves contribute to their virulence. Although some outbreaks caused by staphylococci of the same phage type are associated with more severe disease than others,[12,24] small genetic changes have been shown to have large effects on virulence.[25] The persistence of staphylococci in the environment, their carriage by health care workers, and lapses in adherence to, or effectiveness of, aseptic techniques appear to be critical contributors to the maintenance, if not the onset, of outbreaks. The movement of infected patients from one hospital to another has also been linked to the spread of epidemic strains.[26,27]

Although nasal carriage of S aureus is frequent, airborne spread is not a common route of transmission;[28] however, nasal staphylococci can be distributed well by infants or adults who have respiratory infections.[29,30] Fomites are another potential source of cross-contamination. Infected patients readily contaminate their local environments,[20,31] and methicillin-resistant S aureus (MRSA) can survive for weeks on fabrics and plastics.[32] Staphylococci can also be spread throughout the hospital environment through the collection of contaminated waste or laundry.[33]

Mostly importantly, staphylococci are readily transmitted to the hands or gloves of health care workers from patients[34] or environmental sources.[21] The most common route of transmission has, in fact, proved to be the hands of health care workers, as first demonstrated by Wolinsky[28] in 1960. When infants were intentionally housed near an index infant known to carry a defined type of staphylococcus, the exposed infants obtained not the strain of the index infant, but that of the nurse caring for them. Exposure to the nurse's hands alone, even during a single session, was sufficient for transmission, whereas hours of exposure to the nurse in the same room but without direct contact did not result in transmission. Many subsequent reports have confirmed that health care workers are frequent carriers of epidemic and nonepidemic strains of staphylococci on the hands and in the nasopharynx[16,35,36] and have shown that their hands are major routes for the spread of staphylococci to adults and newborns.[15,26,36,37] Unfortunately, these repeated confirmations over several decades attest to the difficulty in stopping this route of transmission.

For the hands of health care workers to be a major source of staphylococcal transmission, several events must occur:[38] the worker must acquire the bacteria by touching the skin of a patient or a surface where the bacteria have been shed; the organisms must survive for some period; hand hygiene must be inadequate, perhaps because it is not performed properly, or at all, or is performed with an inappropriate agent; and the worker must then transfer the bacteria by touching another patient or a surface that the patient subsequently touches. Although aseptic methods were introduced in the nineteenth century, consistent application has proved challenging. In his 1880 studies linking micrococci (staphylococci) to abscesses, Ogston[5] noted that laxity in the application of aseptic technique allows micrococci to enter incisions and wounds where, once present, they are difficult to remove. In the mid–twentieth century, Williams[8] and Barber[39] noted an overreliance on antibiotics rather than aseptic technique to prevent infection, as did Wise and colleagues[16] in their later review of the period. Supporting a correlation between hygiene and decreased transmission, countries such as the Netherlands and Denmark, which enforce strict infection control measures, have much lower rates of MRSA infection than countries that do not.[40]

Despite the evidence that proper hygiene can reduce the spread of bacteria, hand hygiene continues to be poor in hospitals, in part because of real or perceived barriers to strict compliance with hygiene protocols.[41] The introduction of new guidelines in 2002 aimed to address some of these issues;[38] unfortunately, although widely implemented at the administrative level in hospitals, the guidelines have had little apparent effect on the actual performance of hand hygiene in clinical practice.[42]

Institutional implementation of changes that have a lasting effect on good hand hygiene practices will be needed to substantially reduce the incidence of nosocomial outbreaks of staphylococcal disease. Sustained educational efforts in the community may also be needed to reduce the spread outside of the hospital setting.

BACTERIAL INTERFERENCE THEN AND NOW

Once a staphylococcal outbreak has begun, it can be difficult to interrupt. In nurseries, approaches taken to prevent newborns from acquiring staphylococci have included the use of antimicrobials in staff, infants, and mothers; air purification; removal of carriers from contact with the infants; and emphasis on aseptic technique. However, no approach has been universally successful. Given the frequency and persistence of staphylococcal carriage,[6] the difficulty in identifying a source of transmission in all outbreaks,[43,44] and the fact that fewer than 10 bacteria are needed to colonize the umbilicus of a newborn,[45] completely stopping the spread of staphylococci within hospitals is likely to be impossible.

From the 1940s to the 1960s, the penicillin-resistant strain of phage type 52/52A/80/81 (commonly referred to as 80/81) was a major cause of staphylococcal disease throughout the world,[8,12,46,47] including epidemics originating in adult hospital wards (particularly surgical wards)[48–50] and nurseries.[7,12,16,24,51] The strain was first identified in Australia in 1953 in newborns and nursing mothers, but quickly also became associated with severe lesions in adults and recurring bouts of furunculosis among hospital staff.[52] By the late 1950s, epidemics of 80/81 disease were occurring worldwide.

Asymptomatic carriage of the epidemic-strain staphylococci was an important component of these outbreaks. Acquisition of 80/81 in the nursery often did not cause disease until weeks after discharge,[6,7,12,53] delaying the identification of outbreaks until long after they had begun. Instead, the staphylococci were carried into the home as a sort of "stealth weapon," where they had the potential to cause disaster for the infant, the mother, and the rest of the family. Many colonized, but otherwise healthy, infants developed severe sepsis, meningitis, or pneumonia, in addition to diseases of the skin. Colonized infants also transmitted the staphylococci to their mothers during nursing,[54] resulting in mastitis and the development of severe breast abscesses in the mother and the return of staphylococci to the infant through the infected breast milk.[47,54] Other family members subsequently became colonized, leading to recurrent disease that "ping-ponged" through the household for months, or even years.[53,55] As a result, mothers of infants colonized with 80/81 were instructed not to breastfeed and family life often underwent severe disruption. Hospital function and the lives of health care workers were also disrupted when colonized staff identified as the sources of 80/81 outbreaks in nurseries and adult wards were removed from their duties to prevent further spread.[48,50]

In the early 1960s, it was observed that neonates colonized with a staphylococcal strain not associated with disease were at much lower risk for acquiring type 80/81 and therefore of developing staphylococcal disease.[45] From this observation, a series of experiments was developed to test whether deliberate colonization with an avirulent strain, 502A, could prevent colonization with type 80/81 and thereby interrupt outbreaks,[7,24,45,51,56] a practice that came to be known as bacterial interference. The noses or umbilici of infants were successfully inoculated with 502A during epidemics in four locations in the United States; inoculation was more likely to be successful if no other staphylococci were present, supporting the idea that one strain can interfere with colonization by another. After successful inoculation, 502A was carried in the nose for several months, and the acquisition of 80/81 and the incidence of staphylococcal lesions were significantly lower in inoculated than in uninoculated infants. Bacterial interference was also used successfully in adults who had recurrent infections, some caused by strains other than 80/81,[57] although adults first needed antibiotic treatment to clear the resident strains before inoculation with 502A would take.[58–61] Bacterial interference also interrupted chronic recurrences within families.[62,63]

The incidence of strain 80/81 declined throughout the 1960s, and by 1970, this type was rare, having been replaced by strains of other types, such as 84/85/6557.[46] The disappearance of 80/81 may have been due, in part, to selective pressure from the extensive use of antibiotics to which this strain was susceptible, such as the semisynthetic penicillins and tetracycline, and to the natural tendency of staphylococci to shift phage type because of lysogenization.[46] However, some evidence[64] now indicates that 80/81 has re-emerged in a new guise as a MRSA clone, SWP, after acquiring the SCC*mec* type IV cassette (see later discussion). After the epidemics caused by 80/81 ended, so did the use of bacterial interference. However, in 2004, the use of bacterial interference with strain 502A in adults who had recurrent disease was again reported.[65]

A NEW CYCLE OF NURSERY EPIDEMICS?

Recently, a new nursery-associated staphylococcal disease has emerged, coinciding with the spread of a new MRSA strain. Toxic shock syndrome, caused by the staphylococcal toxin TSST-1, had been known in adults since the 1920s;[3] notably, large outbreaks occurred in the United States in the early 1980s that were associated with the use of highly absorbent tampons during menstruation. Another form of disease caused by TSST-1, neonatal toxic shock syndrome–like exanthematous disease (NTED), first emerged in nurseries in Japan in the early 1990s, and the incidence increased throughout the decade.[66] Unlike the 80/81 epidemic, however, this outbreak is evident within the nursery, is limited to the skin, and is associated with good prognoses.

MRSA have also caused recent outbreaks of more "traditional" diseases, such as mastitis and bacteremia, in nurseries and neonatal intensive care units in the United States.[44,67] In 2002, eight women developed skin and soft-tissue MRSA disease (caused by a USA400 strain; see later discussion) after giving birth in the same hospital in New York during a 2-week period;[44] four of the eight had mastitis, which, in three cases, progressed to breast abscesses requiring surgical drainage. In a retrospective case-control study, the affected women were no more likely to have breastfed than unaffected controls, and none of their infants developed staphylococcal disease, leaving the route of transmission uncertain. More recently, 9 infants born in the same hospital and 10 women who gave birth there developed disease caused by a different MRSA strain (USA300);[68] 12 additional infants were found to be colonized, and two health care workers were identified as carriers. To date no indication exists that this sort of nursery outbreak of MRSA has become epidemic or is a source of pervasive "ping-pong" recurrences within families, as was so common with 80/81. However, cases of MRSA transmission between family members have been reported over the last decade,[69–71] making clear the continued need for vigilance against virulent strains both in hospitals and in the community.

ANTIBIOTICS: THE CYCLE OF USE AND RESISTANCE

Despite the successes of bacterial interference, the mainstay of staphylococcal control in the United States has been antibiotics, and nowhere are historical cycles more apparent than in the development of resistance to new antibiotics. Before the introduction of antibiotics in the 1940s, invasive staphylococcal infections were often fatal.[72] Penicillin greatly reduced the fatality rate,[73] but it was only a few years until the first penicillin-resistant staphylococci were reported.[74,75] By the late 1940s, penicillin use was common in hospitals, and penicillin-resistant strains began to outnumber susceptible strains.[76]

The resistance of these strains to penicillin was due to their production of penicillinase (also known as β-lactamase), and the increase in resistance spurred the development of semisynthetic penicillins, such as methicillin and oxacillin, that were active against penicillinase-producing staphylococci—for a while. In fact, the first strains resistant to methicillin were reported within just a year or 2 of its introduction, although it took longer for MRSA to become established in hospitals (25 to 30 years) than the few years it had taken penicillin-resistant strains.[77,78] Large urban hospitals were the first to report the frequent isolation of MRSA, followed by smaller community hospitals.[78] In the United States, the percentage of MRSA among S aureus isolates in hospitals rose from 2.4% in 1975 to 29% in 1991, by which time 79% of hospitals were reporting MRSA cases.[78] By 2003, 59.5% of S aureus isolated in intensive care units in the United States were methicillin resistant, an 11% increase over the previous 5 years.[79] Similar increases have been reported elsewhere, for example, in the United Kingdom.[80]

Vancomycin has remained effective against most staphylococci, possibly because it has been kept in reserve for use only against multidrug-resistant staphylococcal strains; however, diminished susceptibility and outright resistance to vancomycin have been reported.[81–84] Prolonged treatment of infections due to MRSA with two recently introduced drugs, linezolid and daptomycin, has led to the emergence of reduced susceptibility to these antibiotics as well.[84,85] Such resistant strains remain rare for now, but will need to be carefully monitored, and perhaps it is only a matter of time until resistance to these antibiotics becomes common.

This pattern of heavy antibiotic use providing selective pressure for the development of resistant strains has thus been repeated again and again. Conversely, however, limiting the use of antibiotics may limit the occurrence of resistant strains.[40,86,87] Often, surgical drainage of a superficial lesion is sufficient to clear the infection without the use of antibiotics;[88] in one study, 30% of staphylococcal soft tissue infections severe enough to require hospitalization resolved despite the use of an antibiotic to which the causative strain was resistant.[89]

FROM THE HOSPITAL TO THE COMMUNITY

Another recurring trend has been for staphylococcal disease with particular character-istics (such as antibiotic resistance) to occur first in hospital outbreaks, followed after a delay by increased incidence in the community.[77]

Although penicillin-resistant strains were common in hospitals by the late 1940s, community-acquired (CA) isolates remained susceptible for much longer. By the 1960s, however, many strains in the community were penicillin resistant,[46] and by the 1970s, most were resistant,[90–92] although penicillin continued to be recommended for use against these infections until the early 1970s. This shift to the community seemed to occur when the proportion of penicillin-resistant hospital-acquired (HA) strains reached about 50%.[77]

Similarly, throughout the 1970s, more than 97% of staphylococci isolated in the community were susceptible to methicillin,[91] despite the increasing rates of methicillin resistance in hospital strains.[78] MRSA-related disease that did arise in the community could usually be linked to a health care–related risk factor, such as recent hospitaliza-tion, other exposure to health care settings, or an implanted device, which suggests that the MRSA infections had a nosocomial origin, even if the disease onset was in the community.[93,94] Intravenous drug users were one of the few groups in the commu-nity to be considered at high risk for acquiring MRSA.[95] MRSA then began appearing in other defined groups without clear exposure to the health care system, including prisoners,[96] athletes,[97,98] and some Aboriginal Australian[99,100] and Native Ameri-can[101–103] communities. Although the reasons for MRSA emergence in these groups is not clear, possible commonalities include crowding, poor hygiene, socioeconomic factors, and extensive previous antibiotic use.[94,98,99] As in hospitals, fomites can be a source of contamination in the community.[97,101] Evidence also indicates that MRSA can be spread by sexual activity in heterosexuals[104] and men who have sex with men,[105] although it is not clear whether it is truly transmitted sexually or simply through the associated skin-to-skin contact.[106]

In the late 1990s, as the rate of nosocomial MRSA infection approached 50%, sporadic cases began to arise in the general community among previously healthy individuals who had no known risk factors;[107,108] by 2002, up to 20% of CA-MRSA isolates were obtained from individuals who did not have any of the traditional risk factors.[88] Because of the fre-quent delay between the acquisition of a strain and the emergence of disease, some un-certainty existed at first as to whether these "community-associated" infections had, in fact, been acquired in the hospital and subsequently transmitted to the community.[109] However, genetic and epidemiologic studies have made clear that these outbreaks were caused by different strains than those responsible for nosocomial infections.

The propensity for staphylococci to become resistant to antibiotics is, in part, a result of the nature of the staphylococcal genome, which contains many mobile elements that enable the reshuffling of genetic information among strains,[3] and the ability of bacterio-phage to introduce new genetic elements through lysogenization. The gene for penicil-linase is encoded on a plasmid, a small extrachromosomal genetic element that is easily transferred among bacteria. In contrast, resistance to methicillin is encoded by a staph-ylococcal cassette chromosome (SCC), which carries the *mecA* resistance gene.[110] A specific set of recombinases that enable the excision and reinsertion of SCC*mec* are necessary for the mobility of methicillin resistance, limiting its transfer among strains. Five general types of SCC*mec* (types I–V) have now been identified.

McDougal and colleagues[111] used pulsed-field electrophoresis typing to categorize almost 1000 MRSA and methicillin-susceptible *S aureus* (MSSA) strains. Two of the eight lineages identified, USA300 and USA400, were predominantly associated with community-onset disease and contained SCC*mec* type IV, whereas most of the others carried SCC*mec* types I to III and were associated with nosocomial infections, with USA100 being the type most frequently associated with HA-MRSA. SCC*mec* type IV is smaller than the other SCC*mec* alleles and therefore potentially more mobile,[112] in part because it is small enough to be transmitted by phage;[113] it was likely transferred from *Staphylococcus epidermidis* to *S aureus* sometime in the 1980s.[114] CA-MRSA has also been associated with the more recently identified SCC*mec* type V. These and other genetic differences between CA-MRSA and HA-MRSA, and genetic similarities between CA-MRSA and CA-MSSA, suggest that CA-MRSA did not derive from the introduction of HA-MRSA to the community, but rather arose from transfer of *mecA* to MSSA within the community, probably multiple times.[115–117]

Unlike the multidrug-resistant strains of MRSA found in hospitals, CA-MRSA strains tend to be susceptible to most antibiotics other than the β-lactams,[115] perhaps because of lower selection pressure in the community setting. CA-MRSA has also been associated with a disease profile more similar to that of CA-MSSA than HA-MRSA, with a high prevalence of skin and soft tissue infections and a lower (but still meaningful) incidence of invasive disease.[93,102,108,118] However, these soft tissue infections can be particularly aggressive and destructive; in particular, CA-MRSA have been associated with the unusual presentations of necrotizing skin lesions and pneumonia.[119–121]

The particular pattern of virulence and disease presentation of CA-MRSA has been linked to Panton-Valentine leukocidin (PVL),[115,119,122,123] a phage-borne toxin that has been associated with necrotic skin disease and pneumonia. PVL is commonly expressed in MRSA carrying SCC*mec* type IV, but it has also been isolated from skin infections and pneumonia caused by MSSA strains.[124,125] Animal studies have provided conflicting evidence regarding the contribution of PVL to virulence.[126,127] Thus, PVL may be critical for the particular soft tissue infections or pneumonias seen in recent years, but it is not entirely clear whether PVL is, itself, a virulence factor. Indeed, the role of PVL in the virulence of strain 80/81 was already under investigation more than 40 years ago, but at that time PVL was found with equal frequency in carriage- and disease-associated strains (H. Shinefield, unpublished data, 1962), suggesting that the presence of PVL alone is not sufficient for virulence.

It is possible that some change to PVL has enabled it to directly initiate at least some CA-MRSA disease. More likely, PVL is a marker that is coinherited with some additional virulence or fitness factor. Because epidemic MRSA strains share a genetic background with epidemic MSSA strains, some critical element may lie within the common genomic regions.[128] Furthermore, at least one widely distributed USA300 variant contains about 20 genes, in addition to PVL, that are not present in HA-MRSA strains of the USA500 and USA100 pulsed-field types, or even in the virulent, but less commonly encountered, CA-MRSA USA400 variants.[129] These USA300-specific genes include elements associated with resistance, virulence, and pathogenicity. Because USA400 isolates also produce the PVL toxin and other toxins not present in common HA-MRSA strains,[130] one of the factors unique to USA300 may hold the key to the ability of USA300 isolates to spread widely and cause disease in a wide range of hosts.

CURRENT STATUS AND SUMMARY

The epidemiology of staphylococcal infections is beginning to change again; strains generally associated with CA-MRSA (eg, USA300) are now showing up in nosocomial infections[44,67,68,131,132] and some health care–related strains are being acquired in the community.[133] Although CA-MRSA are generally more susceptible to non–β-lactam antibiotics than HA-MRSA, and may therefore be more easily treated at this time, it is not yet clear how quickly these strains will become resistant to multiple antibiotics, and their high virulence is of concern. What is apparent is that staphylococci have proved to be extremely adaptable, and we are unlikely to win the battle against them solely by developing new antibiotics, to which widespread resistance is almost certainly inevitable. Measures to prevent staphylococcal infections are more likely to be effective, and more consistent adherence to proper hygiene practices would be a good start. To make real progress in the prevention of staphylococcal disease, however, we urgently need to understand more about the mechanisms of virulence and transmission that turn a common commensal organism into one that is highly pathogenic. With such information, it may be possible to develop a vaccine that will prevent both endemic and epidemic staphylococcal disease.

REFERENCES

1. Kluytmans J, van Belkum A, Verbrugh H. Nasal carriage of Staphylococcus aureus: epidemiology, underlying mechanisms, and associated risks. Clin Microbiol Rev 1997;10:505–20.
2. Diekema DJ, Pfaller MA, Schmitz FJ, et al. Survey of infections due to Staphylococcus species: frequency of occurrence and antimicrobial susceptibility of isolates collected in the United States, Canada, Latin America, Europe, and the Western Pacific region for the sentry antimicrobial surveillance program, 1997–1999. Clin Infect Dis 2001;32(Suppl 2):S114–32.
3. Moreillon P, Que Y-A, Glauser M. Staphyloccocus aureus (including staphylococcal toxic shock). In: Mandell G, Bennett J, Dolin R, editors. Mandell, Douglas, and Bennett's principles and practices of infectious diseases. 6th edition. vol. 2. Philadelphia: Elsevier Churchill Livingstone; 2005. p. 2321–51.
4. Lowy FD. Staphylococcus aureus infections. N Engl J Med 1998;339:520–32.
5. Classics in infectious diseases. "On abscesses": Alexander Ogston (1844–1929). Rev Infect Dis 1984;6:122–8.
6. Hurst V. Staphylococcus aureus in the infant upper respiratory tract. I. Observations on hospital-born babies. J Hyg (Lond) 1957;55:299–312.
7. Shinefield HR, Boris M, Ribble JC, et al. Bacterial interference: its effect on nursery-acquired infection with Staphylococcus aureus. III. The Georgia epidemic. Am J Dis Child 1963;105:663–73.
8. Williams RE. Investigations of staphylococcal infection acquired in Great Britain's hospitals. Public Health Rep 1958;73:961–70.
9. Kilham EB. An epidemic of pemphigus neonatorum. Am J Obstet 1889;22:1039.
10. Call E. An epidemic of pemphigus neonatorum. Am J Obstet 1904;50:473.
11. Rulison E. Control of impetigo neonatorum. Advisability of a radical departure in obstetrical care. JAMA 1929;93:903.
12. Shaffer TE, Sylvester RF Jr, Baldwin JN, et al. Staphylococcal infections in newborn infants. II. Report of 19 epidemics caused by an identical strain of Staphylococcus pyogenes. Am J Public Health Nations Health 1957;47:990–4.
13. Gould JC, Cruikshank JD. Staphylococcal infection in general practice. Lancet 1957;273:1157–61.
14. Seidemann I, Eisenoff H. Rooming-in service in a medium-sized community hospital; report on four-and-one-half-years observation. N Y State J Med 1956;56:2533–6.

15. Nakashima AK, Allen JR, Martone WJ, et al. Epidemic bullous impetigo in a nursery due to a nasal carrier of Staphylococcus aureus: role of epidemiology and control measures. Infect Control 1984;5:326–31.
16. Wise RI, Ossman EA, Littlefield DR, et al. Personal reflections on nosocomial staphylococcal infections and the development of hospital surveillance. Rev Infect Dis 1989;11:1005–19.
17. Boyce JM, Garner JS, Twenge JA, et al. Nosocomial staphylococcal cervical lymphadenitis in infants: report of an outbreak. Pediatrics 1976;57:854–60.
18. Dancer SJ, Poston SM, East J, et al. An outbreak of pemphigus neonatorum. J Infect 1990;20:73–82.
19. Dancer SJ, Simmons NA, Poston SM, et al. Outbreak of staphylococcal scalded skin syndrome among neonates. J Infect 1988;16:87–103.
20. Shooter RA, Smith MA, Griffiths JD, et al. Spread of staphylococci in a surgical ward. Br Med J 1958;1:607–13.
21. Crossley K, Landesman B, Zaske D. An outbreak of infections caused by strains of Staphylococcus aureus resistant to methicillin and aminoglycosides. II. Epidemiologic studies. J Infect Dis 1979;139:280–7.
22. Boyce JM, Landry M, Deetz TR, et al. Epidemiologic studies of an outbreak of nosocomial methicillin-resistant Staphylococcus aureus infections. Infect Control 1981;2:110–6.
23. Steinberg JP, Clark CC, Hackman BO, et al. Nosocomial and community-acquired Staphylococcus aureus bacteremias from 1980 to 1993: impact of intravascular devices and methicillin resistance. Clin Infect Dis 1996;23:255–9.
24. Shinefield HR, Sutherland JM, Ribble JC, et al. Bacterial interference: its effect on nursery-acquired infection with Staphylococcus aureus. II. The Ohio epidemic. Am J Dis Child 1963;105:655–62.
25. Kennedy AD, Otto M, Braughton KR, et al. Epidemic community-associated methicillin-resistant Staphylococcus aureus: recent clonal expansion and diversification. Proc Natl Acad Sci U S A 2008;105:1327–32.
26. Bitar CM, Mayhall CG, Lamb VA, et al. Outbreak due to methicillin- and rifampin-resistant Staphylococcus aureus: epidemiology and eradication of the resistant strain from the hospital. Infect Control 1987;8:15–23.
27. Roman RS, Smith J, Walker M, et al. Rapid geographic spread of a methicillin-resistant Staphylococcus aureus strain. Clin Infect Dis 1997;25:698–705.
28. Wolinsky E, Lipsitz PJ, Mortimer EA Jr, et al. Acquisition of staphylococci by newborns. Direct versus indirect transmission. Lancet 1960;2:620–2.
29. Eichenwald HF, Kotsevalov O, Fasso LA, et al. Some effects of viral infection on aerial dissemination of staphylococci and on susceptibility to bacterial colonization. Bacteriol Rev 1961;25:274–81.
30. Sheretz RJ, Reagan DR, Hampton KD, et al. A cloud adult: the Staphylococcus aureus-virus interaction revisited. Ann Intern Med 1996;124:539–47.
31. Asoh N, Masaki H, Watanabe H, et al. Molecular characterization of the transmission between the colonization of methicillin-resistant Staphylococcus aureus to human and environmental contamination in geriatric long-term care wards. Intern Med 2005;44:41–5.
32. Neely AN, Maley MP. Survival of enterococci and staphylococci on hospital fabrics and plastic. J Clin Microbiol 2000;38:724–6.
33. Hurst V, Grossman M, Ingram FR, et al. Hospital laundry and refuse chutes as source of staphylococcic cross-infection. JAMA 1958;167:1223–9.
34. McBryde ES, Bradley LC, Whitby M, et al. An investigation of contact transmission of methicillin-resistant Staphylococcus aureus. J Hosp Infect 2004;58:104–8.

35. Lin YC, Lauderdale TL, Lin HM, et al. An outbreak of methicillin-resistant Staphylococcus aureus infection in patients of a pediatric intensive care unit and high carriage rate among health care workers. J Microbiol Immunol Infect 2007;40:325–34.

36. Cookson B, Peters B, Webster M, et al. Staff carriage of epidemic methicillin-resistant Staphylococcus aureus. J Clin Microbiol 1989;27:1471–6.

37. Mortimer EA Jr, Lipsitz PJ, Wolinsky E, et al. Transmission of staphylococci between newborns. Importance of the hands to personnel. Am J Dis Child 1962; 104:289–95.

38. Boyce JM, Pittet D. Guideline for hand hygiene in health-care settings. Recommendations of the Healthcare Infection Control Practices Advisory Committee and the HICPAC/SHEA/APIC/IDSA Hand Hygiene Task Force. Society for Healthcare Epidemiology of America/Association for Professionals in Infection Control/Infectious Diseases Society of America. MMWR Recomm Rep 2002;51:1–45.

39. Barber M. Hospital infection yesterday and today. J Clin Pathol 1961;14:2–10.

40. Boyce JM. Understanding and controlling methicillin-resistant Staphylococcus aureus infections. Infect Control Hosp Epidemiol 2002;23:485–7.

41. Pittet D. Improving compliance with hand hygiene in hospitals. Infect Control Hosp Epidemiol 2000;21:381–6.

42. Larson EL, Quiros D, Lin SX. Dissemination of the CDC's Hand Hygiene Guideline and impact on infection rates. Am J Infect Control 2007;35:666–75.

43. Back NA, Linnemann CC Jr, Pfaller MA, et al. Recurrent epidemics caused by a single strain of erythromycin-resistant Staphylococcus aureus. The importance of molecular epidemiology. JAMA 1993;270:1329–33.

44. Saiman L, O'Keefe M, Graham PL 3rd, et al. Hospital transmission of community-acquired methicillin-resistant Staphylococcus aureus among postpartum women. Clin Infect Dis 2003;37:1313–9.

45. Shinefield HR, Ribble JC, Boris M, et al. Bacterial interference: its effect on nursery-acquired infection with Staphylococcus aureus. I. Preliminary observations on artificial colonization of newborns. Am J Dis Child 1963;105:646–54.

46. Jessen O, Rosendal K, Bulow P, et al. Changing staphylococci and staphylococcal infections. A ten-year study of bacteria and cases of bacteremia. N Engl J Med 1969;281:627–35.

47. Rountree PM, Beard MA. Further observations on infection with phage type 80 staphylococci in Australia. Med J Aust 1958;45:789–95.

48. Nahmias AJ, Godwin JT, Updyke EL, et al. Postsurgical staphylococcic infections. Outbreak traced to an individual carrying phase strains 80/81 and 80/81/52/52A. JAMA 1960;174:1269–75.

49. Blair JE, Carr M. Staphylococci in hospital-acquired infections; types encountered in the United States. JAMA 1958;166:1192–6.

50. Ayliffe GA, Collins BJ. Wound infections acquired from a disperser of an unusual strain of Staphylococcus aureus. J Clin Pathol 1967;20:195–8.

51. Boris M, Shinefield HR, Ribble JC, et al. Bacterial interference: its effect on nursery-acquired infection with Staphylococcus aureus. IV. The Louisiana epidemic. Am J Dis Child 1963;105:674–82.

52. Rountree PM, Freeman BM. Infections caused by a particular phage type of Staphylococcus aureus. Med J Aust 1955;42:157–61.

53. Hurst V, Grossman M. The hospital nursery as a source of staphylococcal disease among families of newborn infants. N Engl J Med 1960;262:951–6.

54. Wysham DN, Mulhern ME, Navarre GC, et al. Staphylococcal infections in an obstetric unit. II. Epidemiologic studies of puerperal mastitis. N Engl J Med 1957; 257:304–6.

55. Nahmias AJ, Lepper MH, Hurst V, et al. Epidemiology and treatment of chronic staphylococcal infections in the household. Am J Public Health Nations Health 1962;52:1828–43.
56. Shinefield HR, Ribble JC, Eichenwald HF, et al. Bacterial interference: its effect on nursery-acquired infection with Staphylococcus aureus. V. An analysis and interpretation. Am J Dis Child 1963;105:683–8.
57. Strauss WG, Maibach HI, Shinefield HR, et al. Bacterial interference treatment of recurrent furunculosis. 2. Demonstration of the relationship of strain to pathogenicity. JAMA 1969;208:861–3.
58. Smith CC, Bird EL, Carey-Smith KA. Bacterial substitution for staphylococcal infection. N Z Med J 1968;67:407–9.
59. Steele RW. Recurrent staphylococcal infection in families. Arch Dermatol 1980; 116:189–90.
60. Shinefield HR, Ribble JC, Boris M, et al. Bacterial interference between strains of S. aureus. Ann N Y Acad Sci 1974;236:444–55.
61. Boris M, Sellers TF Jr, Eichenwald HF, et al. Bacterial interference; protection of adults against nasal Staphylococcus aureus infection after colonization with a heterologous S aureus strain. Am J Dis Child 1964;108:252–61.
62. Fine RN, Onslow JM, Erwin ML, et al. Bacterial interference in the treatment of recurrent staphylococcal infections in a family. J Pediatr 1967;70:548–53.
63. Boris M, Shinefield HR, Romano P, et al. Bacterial interference. Protection against recurrent intrafamilial staphylococcal disease. Am J Dis Child 1968; 115:521–9.
64. Robinson DA, Kearns AM, Holmes A, et al. Re-emergence of early pandemic Staphylococcus aureus as a community-acquired methicillin-resistant clone. Lancet 2005;365:1256–8.
65. Nouwen J, Fieren M, Snijders S, et al. Bacterial interference therapy with Staphylococcus aureus 502A for eradication of wild type S. aureus. Presented at: 44th ICAAC; Washington, DC: October 30-November 2, 2004.
66. Kikuchi K, Takahashi N, Piao C, et al. Molecular epidemiology of methicillin-resistant Staphylococcus aureus strains causing neonatal toxic shock syndrome-like exanthematous disease in neonatal and perinatal wards. J Clin Microbiol 2003; 41:3001–6.
67. Healy CM, Hulten KG, Palazzi DL, et al. Emergence of new strains of methicillin-resistant Staphylococcus aureus in a neonatal intensive care unit. Clin Infect Dis 2004;39:1460–6.
68. Graham PL III. Transmission of USA-300 Methicillin-resistant Staphylococcus aureus in a newborn nursery also affecting post-partum women [abstract]. Presented at: Society for Healthcare Epidemiology of America; Orlando, Florida: April 4–8, 2008.
69. L'Heriteau F, Lucet JC, Scanvic A, et al. Community-acquired methicillin-resistant Staphylococcus aureus and familial transmission. JAMA 1999;282:1038–309.
70. Gross-Schulman S, Dassey D, Mascola L, et al. Community-acquired methicillin-resistant Staphylococcus aureus. JAMA 1998;280:421–2.
71. Huijsdens XW, van Santen-Verheuvel MG, Spalburg E, et al. Multiple cases of familial transmission of community-acquired methicillin-resistant Staphylococcus aureus. J Clin Microbiol 2006;44:2994–6.
72. Skinner D, Keefer C. Significance of bacteremia caused by Staphylococcus aureus. A study of one hundred and twenty-two cases and a review of the literature concerned with experimental infection in animals. Arch Intern Med 1941;68:851–75.
73. Spink W, Hall W. Penicillin therapy at the University of Minnesota hospitals: 1942–1944. Ann Intern Med 1945;22:510–25.

74. Kirby WM. Extraction of a highly potent penicillin inactivator from penicillin resistant staphylococci. Science 1944;99:452–3.

75. Kirby WM. Properties of a penicillin inactivator extracted from penicillin-resistant staphylococci. J Clin Invest 1945;24:170–4.

76. Barber M, Rozwadowska-Dowzenko M. Infection by penicillin-resistant staphylococci. Lancet 1948;1:641–4.

77. Chambers HF. The changing epidemiology of Staphylococcus aureus? Emerging Infect Dis 2001;7:178–82.

78. Panlilio AL, Culver DH, Gaynes RP, et al. Methicillin-resistant Staphylococcus aureus in U.S. hospitals, 1975–1991. Infect Control Hosp Epidemiol 1992;13:582–6.

79. National Nosocomial Infections Surveillance (NNIS) system report, data summary from January 1992 through June 2004, issued October 2004. Am J Infect Control 2004;32:470–85.

80. Johnson AP, Pearson A, Duckworth G. Surveillance and epidemiology of MRSA bacteraemia in the UK. J Antimicrob Chemother 2005;56:455–62.

81. Centers for Disease Control and Prevention. Staphylococcus aureus with reduced susceptibility to vancomycin–Illinois, 1999. MMWR Morb Mortal Wkly Rep 2000;48:1165–7.

82. Centers for Disease Control and Prevention. Staphylococcus aureus resistant to vancomycin–United States, 2002. MMWR Morb Mortal Wkly Rep 2002;51:565–7.

83. Fridkin SK, Hageman J, McDougal LK, et al. Epidemiological and microbiological characterization of infections caused by Staphylococcus aureus with reduced susceptibility to vancomycin, United States, 1997–2001. Clin Infect Dis 2003;36:429–39.

84. Bennett JW, Murray CK, Holmes RL, et al. Diminished vancomycin and daptomycin susceptibility during prolonged bacteremia with methicillin-resistant Staphylococcus aureus. Diagn Microbiol Infect Dis 2008;60:437–40.

85. Hentschke M, Saager B, Horstkotte MA, et al. Emergence of linezolid resistance in a methicillin resistant Staphylococcus aureus strain. Infection 2008;36:85–7.

86. Rosendal K, Jessen O, Bentzon MW, et al. Antibiotic policy and spread of Staphylococcus aureus strains in Danish hospitals, 1969–1974. Acta Pathol Microbiol Scand [B] 1977;85:143–52.

87. Dunkle LM, Naqvi SH, McCallum R, et al. Eradication of epidemic methicillin-gentamicin-resistant Staphylococcus aureus in an intensive care nursery. Am J Med 1981;70:455–8.

88. Fridkin SK, Hageman JC, Morrison M, et al. Methicillin-resistant Staphylococcus aureus disease in three communities. N Engl J Med 2005;352:1436–44.

89. Young DM, Harris HW, Charlebois ED, et al. An epidemic of methicillin-resistant Staphylococcus aureus soft tissue infections among medically underserved patients. Arch Surg 2004;139:947–51.

90. Ross S, Rodriguez W, Controni G, et al. Staphylococcal susceptibility to penicillin G. The changing pattern among community strains. JAMA 1974;229:1075–7.

91. Hahn DL, Baker WA. Penicillin G susceptibility of "rural" Staphylococcus aureus. J Fam Pract 1980;11:43–6.

92. Hughes GB, Chidi CC, Macon WL. Staphylococci in community-acquired infections: increased resistance to penicillin. Ann Surg 1976;183:355–7.

93. Klevens RM, Morrison MA, Nadle J, et al. Invasive methicillin-resistant Staphylococcus aureus infections in the United States. JAMA 2007;298:1763–71.

94. Salgado CD, Farr BM, Calfee DP, et al. Community-acquired methicillin-resistant Staphylococcus aureus: a meta-analysis of prevalence and risk factors. Clin Infect Dis 2003;36:131–9.

95. Saravolatz LD, Markowitz N, Arking L, et al. Methicillin-resistant Staphylococcus aureus. Epidemiologic observations during a community-acquired outbreak. Ann Intern Med 1982;96:11–6.
96. Centers for disease control and prevention. Methicillin-resistant Staphylococcus aureus infections in correctional facilities–Georgia, California, and Texas, 2001–2003. MMWR Morb Mortal Wkly Rep 2003;52:992–6.
97. Centers for Disease Control and prevention. Methicillin-resistant Staphylococcus aureus infections among competitive sports participants–Colorado, Indiana, Pennsylvania, and Los Angeles County, 2000–2003. MMWR Morb Mortal Wkly Rep 2003;52:793–5.
98. Kazakova SV, Hageman JC, Matava M, et al. A clone of methicillin-resistant Staphylococcus aureus among professional football players. N Engl J Med 2005;352:468–75.
99. Maguire GP, Arthur AD, Boustead PJ, et al. Emerging epidemic of community-acquired methicillin-resistant Staphylococcus aureus infection in the Northern Territory. Med J Aust 1996;164:721–3.
100. O'Brien FG, Pearman JW, Gracey M, et al. Community strain of methicillin-resistant Staphylococcus aureus involved in a hospital outbreak. J Clin Microbiol 1999;37:2858–62.
101. Baggett HC, Hennessy TW, Rudolph K, et al. Community-onset methicillin-resistant Staphylococcus aureus associated with antibiotic use and the cytotoxin Panton-Valentine leukocidin during a furunculosis outbreak in rural Alaska. J Infect Dis 2004;189:1565–73.
102. Groom AV, Wolsey DH, Naimi TS, et al. Community-acquired methicillin-resistant Staphylococcus aureus in a rural American Indian community. JAMA 2001;286:1201–5.
103. Stemper ME, Shukla SK, Reed KD, et al. Emergence and spread of community-associated methicillin-resistant Staphylococcus aureus in rural Wisconsin, 1989–1999. J Clin Microbiol 2004;42:5673–80.
104. Cook HA, Furuya EY, Larson E, et al. Heterosexual transmission of community-associated methicillin-resistant Staphylococcus aureus. Clin Infect Dis 2007;44:410–3.
105. Diep BA, Chambers HF, Graber CJ, et al. Emergence of multidrug-resistant, community-associated, methicillin-resistant Staphylococcus aureus clone USA300 in men who have sex with men. Ann Intern Med 2008;148:249–57.
106. Gorwitz R, Fridkin SK, Workowski KA. More challenges in the prevention and management of community-associated, methicillin-resistant Staphylococcus aureus skin disease. Ann Intern Med 2008;148:310–2.
107. Centers for disease control and prevention. Four pediatric deaths from community-acquired methicillin-resistant Staphylococcus aureus–Minnesota and North Dakota, 1997–1999. MMWR Morb Mortal Wkly Rep 2000;48:707–10.
108. Herold BC, Immergluck LC, Maranan MC, et al. Community-acquired methicillin-resistant Staphylococcus aureus in children with no identified predisposing risk. JAMA 1998;279:593–8.
109. Boyce JM. Are the epidemiology and microbiology of methicillin-resistant Staphylococcus aureus changing? JAMA 1998;279:623–4.
110. Katayama Y, Ito T, Hiramatsu K. A new class of genetic element, staphylococcus cassette chromosome mec, encodes methicillin resistance in Staphylococcus aureus. Antimicrobial Agents Chemother 2000;44:1549–55.
111. McDougal LK, Steward CD, Killgore GE, et al. Pulsed-field gel electrophoresis typing of oxacillin-resistant Staphylococcus aureus isolates from the United States: establishing a national database. J Clin Microbiol 2003;41:5113–20.

112. Ma XX, Ito T, Tiensasitorn C, et al. Novel type of staphylococcal cassette chromosome mec identified in community-acquired methicillin-resistant Staphylococcus aureus strains. Antimicrob Agents Chemother 2002;46:1147–52.
113. Narita S, Kaneko J, Chiba J, et al. Phage conversion of Panton-Valentine leukocidin in Staphylococcus aureus: molecular analysis of a PVL-converting phage, phiSLT. Gene 2001;268:195–206.
114. Wisplinghoff H, Rosato AE, Enright MC, et al. Related clones containing SCCmec type IV predominate among clinically significant Staphylococcus epidermidis isolates. Antimicrob Agents Chemother 2003;47:3574–9.
115. Naimi TS, LeDell KH, Como-Sabetti K, et al. Comparison of community- and health care-associated methicillin-resistant Staphylococcus aureus infection. JAMA 2003;290:2976–84.
116. Miller LG, Perdreau-Remington F, Bayer AS, et al. Clinical and epidemiologic characteristics cannot distinguish community-associated methicillin-resistant Staphylococcus aureus infection from methicillin-susceptible S. aureus infection: a prospective investigation. Clin Infect Dis 2007;44:471–82.
117. Enright MC, Robinson DA, Randle G, et al. The evolutionary history of methicillin-resistant Staphylococcus aureus (MRSA). Proc Natl Acad Sci U S A 2002;99:7687–92.
118. Fridkin SK. Vancomycin-intermediate and -resistant Staphylococcus aureus: what the infectious disease specialist needs to know. Clin Infect Dis 2001;32:108–15.
119. Lina G, Piemont Y, Godail-Gamot F, et al. Involvement of Panton-Valentine leukocidin-producing Staphylococcus aureus in primary skin infections and pneumonia. Clin Infect Dis 1999;29:1128–32.
120. Miller LG, Perdreau-Remington F, Rieg G, et al. Necrotizing fasciitis caused by community-associated methicillin-resistant Staphylococcus aureus in Los Angeles. N Engl J Med 2005;352:1445–53.
121. Francis JS, Doherty MC, Lopatin U, et al. Severe community-onset pneumonia in healthy adults caused by methicillin-resistant Staphylococcus aureus carrying the Panton-Valentine leukocidin genes. Clin Infect Dis 2005;40:100–7.
122. Boyle-Vavra S, Daum RS. Community-acquired methicillin-resistant Staphylococcus aureus: the role of Panton-Valentine leukocidin. Lab Invest 2007;87:3–9.
123. Diep BA, Carleton HA, Chang RF, et al. Roles of 34 virulence genes in the evolution of hospital- and community-associated strains of methicillin-resistant Staphylococcus aureus. J Infect Dis 2006;193:1495–503.
124. Campbell SJ, Deshmukh HS, Nelson CL, et al. Genotypic characteristics of Staphylococcus aureus isolates from a multinational trial of complicated skin and skin structure infections. J Clin Microbiol 2008;46:678–84.
125. Gillet Y, Issartel B, Vanhems P, et al. Association between Staphylococcus aureus strains carrying gene for Panton-Valentine leukocidin and highly lethal necrotising pneumonia in young immunocompetent patients. Lancet 2002;359:753–9.
126. Labandeira-Rey M, Couzon F, Boisset S, et al. Staphylococcus aureus Panton-Valentine leukocidin causes necrotizing pneumonia. Science 2007;315:1130–3.
127. Voyich JM, Otto M, Mathema B, et al. Is Panton-Valentine leukocidin the major virulence determinant in community-associated methicillin-resistant Staphylococcus aureus disease? J Infect Dis 2006;194:1761–70.
128. de Lencastre H, Oliveira D, Tomasz A. Antibiotic resistant Staphylococcus aureus: a paradigm of adaptive power. Curr Opin Microbiol 2007;10:428–35.

129. Tenover FC, McDougal LK, Goering RV, et al. Characterization of a strain of community-associated methicillin-resistant Staphylococcus aureus widely disseminated in the United States. J Clin Microbiol 2006;44:108–18.
130. Baba T, Takeuchi F, Kuroda M, et al. Genome and virulence determinants of high virulence community-acquired MRSA. Lancet 2002;359:1819–27.
131. Klevens RM, Edwards JR, Tenover FC, et al. Changes in the epidemiology of methicillin-resistant Staphylococcus aureus in intensive care units in US hospitals, 1992–2003. Clin Infect Dis 2006;42:389–91.
132. Maree CL, Daum RS, Boyle-Vavra S, et al. Community-associated methicillin-resistant Staphylococcus aureus isolates causing healthcare-associated infections. Emerg Infect Dis 2007;13:236–42.
133. Klevens RM, Morrison MA, Fridkin SK, et al. Community-associated methicillin-resistant Staphylococcus aureus and healthcare risk factors. Emerg Infect Dis 2006;12:1991–3.

Host Defense and Pathogenesis in *Staphylococcus aureus* Infections

Frank R. DeLeo, PhD[a],*, Binh An Diep, PhD[b], Michael Otto, PhD[a]

KEYWORDS

- Staphylococcus • Neutrophil • Innate immunity • Virulence

Staphylococcus aureus has been a leading cause of human infections throughout history. From 1997 to 1999, *S aureus* was reported as the most abundant cause of bloodstream, skin and soft tissue, and lower respiratory tract infections in the United States, Canada, Europe, Latin America, and the Western Pacific.[1] The pathogen is the leading cause of hospital-associated infections in the United States,[2] and was associated with a remarkable economic burden of $14.5 billion in 2003.[3] A high percentage of hospital infections are caused by methicillin-resistant *S aureus* (MRSA).[4] Notably, there is a relatively high mortality rate (approximately 20%) associated with invasive MRSA infections, most of which are health care-associated.[5] This finding may be related in part to the prior health status of the patient, because these infections typically occur in individuals who have predisposing risk factors, such as those who have had surgery, or in patients who are immunocompromised or have granulocyte defects.

By comparison, community-associated (CA) *S aureus* causes infections in otherwise healthy individuals. Historically, CA *S aureus* infections almost always were caused by methicillin-susceptible *S aureus* (MSSA) rather than MRSA,[4] but this distribution has changed dramatically in the United States over the past 10 years.[6] Two reports in the late 1990s marked the beginning of a new era in MRSA epidemiology.[7,8] Isolates classified as pulsed-field gel electrophoresis type USA400 emerged as the prototype CA-MRSA genotype.[9,10] A complete genome sequence is available for MW2, a representative USA400 clinical isolate that caused fatal septicemia in 1998.[10] Although

This work was supported by the Intramural Program of the National Institute of Allergy and Infectious Diseases, National Institutes of Health.

[a] Laboratory of Human Bacterial Pathogenesis, Rocky Mountain Laboratories, National Institute of Allergy and Infectious Diseases, National Institutes of Health, 903 South 4th Street, Hamilton, MT 59840, USA

[b] Division of Infectious Diseases, Department of Medicine, University of California, San Francisco, 1001 Potrero Avenue, Building 30 Room 3300, San Francisco, CA 94110, USA

* Corresponding author.

E-mail address: fdeleo@niaid.nih.gov (F.R. DeLeo).

USA400 remained a significant cause of CA-MRSA infections through 2005,[11,12] it has been replaced almost completely by a genotype known as USA300,[6,13] which is now epidemic in the United States. The current CA-MRSA epidemic is caused by clonal emergence of USA300 isolates that have enhanced virulence or a hypervirulence phenotype.[14,15] Hypervirulence, defined here as the ability of CA-MRSA to cause widespread infections in otherwise healthy individuals, likely is related in part to the ability of USA300 and USA400 to circumvent killing by human polymorphonuclear leukocytes (PMNs) and cause rapid destruction of these host cells.[16,17]

In general, the ability of bacteria to cause disease in humans is caused by evasion of innate host defense, which includes resistance to antimicrobial peptides (AMPs) and killing by phagocytic leukocytes. Inasmuch as PMNs (also called neutrophils or granulocytes) constitute the greatest number of leukocytes in people, they are the primary cellular defense against S aureus infections. This article reviews critical components of neutrophil function as they relate to S aureus infection and staphylococcal virulence factors that contribute to immune evasion, including those produced by prominent CA-MRSA strains.

POLYMORPHONUCLEAR LEUKOCYTES IN THE INNATE IMMUNE RESPONSE
Neutrophil Recruitment, Chemotaxis, and Priming

A first step in the eradication of invading microorganisms is active recruitment of PMNs to the site of infection by chemotaxis.[18] This is a multistep process whereby neutrophils are mobilized from peripheral blood or bone marrow in response to host- and pathogen-derived chemotactic factors. Host molecules, such as interleukin-8 (IL-8, CXCL8), GROα (CXCL1), granulocyte chemotactic protein 2 (GCP2, CXCL6), and complement component C5a recruit neutrophils to the site of infection.

S aureus has been shown to elicit production of numerous chemotactic factors in vitro and in vivo. For example, S aureus lipoteichoic acid (LTA) and capsular polysaccharide induce production of IL-8 by peripheral blood monocytes[19] and epithelial and endothelial cells,[20] respectively. S aureus-activated endothelial cells produce IL-8 that promotes transmigration of neutrophils.[21] Freely secreted virulence molecules of S aureus, including toxic shock syndrome toxin-1 (TSST1), enterotoxin A (SEA), or enterotoxin B (SEB), also elicit production of IL-8 by human monocytic cells.[22] Recent studies have demonstrated that stimulation of CD4+ T-cells by S aureus capsular polysaccharide leads to production of chemokines that recruit neutrophils to the site of infection.[23,24] Further, S aureus cell surface components, primarily peptidoglycan (PGN), long have been known to elicit production of C5a,[25] a potent chemotactic molecule for PMNs. S aureus also produces molecules that directly recruit PMNs (eg, phenol soluble modulin-like peptides, PSMs).[26] Although the pathogen elicits a robust proinflammatory response, it generates several molecules that block chemotaxis, and these will be discussed (**Table 1**).

Many chemoattractants are priming agents (rather than activating agents) for neutrophils. Neutrophil priming first was described as the ability of a primary agonist, typically at substimulatory concentration, to enhance superoxide production elicited by a second stimulus.[27] Neutrophils can be primed for enhanced adhesion, phagocytosis, production of reactive oxygen species (ROS), cytokine secretion, leukotriene synthesis, degranulation, and bactericidal activity.[28] Many neutrophil priming agents are host-derived molecules such as cytokines, chemokines, and growth factors.[28] Cell–cell contact and adhesion also prime PMNs for enhanced function. Some bacteria-derived priming agents, such as S aureus LTA, are Toll-like receptor (TLR) agonists, and TLRs are components important to the pathogen-mediated priming process. There is

Table 1
Staphylococcus aureus molecules that contribute to immune evasion or alter host immune function

Gene(s)	Protein or Molecule	Function/Effect on Immune System
ahpC, ahpF	Alkyl hydroperoxide reductase subunits C and F, AhpC and AhpF	Promotes resistance to reactive oxygen species (ROS)
aur	Zinc metalloproteinase aureolysin, Aur	Degrades LL-37
cap5 or *cap8* genes	Capsular polysaccharide	Inhibits phagocytosis
katA	Catalase, KatA	Detoxifies hydrogen peroxide
chp	Chemotaxis inhibitory protein of *Staphylococcus aureus*, chemotaxis inhibitory protein of *S aureus*	Inhibits chemotaxis
clfA	Clumping factor A, ClfA	Inhibits phagocytosis, causes platelet activation
crtM, crtN	Carotenoid pigment, staphyloxanthin	Promotes resistance to ROS
dlt operon	Dlt operon, DltABCD	Promotes resistance to cationic antimicrobial peptides (AMPs) and group IIA phospholipase A_2
eap	Extracellular adherence protein, Eap	Inhibits leukocyte adhesion
ecb	Extracellular complement-binding protein, Ecb	Inhibits C5a generation
efb	Extracellular fibrinogen-binding protein, Efb	Inhibits C5a generation
fnbA, fnbB	Fibronectin-binding proteins A and B, FnbA and FnbB	Cause platelet activation
hla, hly	Alpha-hemolysin (α-hemolysin), Hla	Causes host cell lysis
hld	Delta-hemolysin, Hld	Causes host cell lysis
hlgA, hlgB, hlgC	Gamma-hemolysin subunits A, B, and C; HlgA, HlgB, HlgC; two-component leukocidin	Causes leukocyte and erythrocyte lysis
icaA, icaD, icaB, icaC, icaR	Polysaccharide intercellular adhesin, PIA	Resistance to cationic AMPs
isdA, isdB	Iron-regulated surface determinants of *S aureus*, IsdA and IsdB	Resistance to AMPs, skin fatty acids, and neutrophil ROS
lukS-PV, lukF-PV	Leukocidin S-PV and F-PV subunits; LukS/F-PV; PVL; two-component leukocidin	Causes phagocyte lysis
lukD, lukE	Leukocidin D and E; LukD and LukE; two-component leukocidin	Causes leukocyte lysis

(continued on next page)

Table 1
Staphylococcus aureus molecules that contribute to immune evasion or alter host immune function

Gene(s)	Protein or Molecule	Function/Effect on Immune System
mprF	Multiple peptide resistance factor, MprF	Promotes resistance to cationic AMPs
psm	Phenol-soluble modulin-like peptides, PSMs	Cause leukocyte lysis
sak	Staphylokinase	Inhibits host α-defensins
sbi	IgG-binding protein, Sbi	Sequesters host IgG
scn	Staphylococcal inhibitor of complement, SCIN	Inhibits complement
sea, seb, sec$_n$, sed, see, seg, seh, sei, sej, sek, sel, sep	Staphylococcal enterotoxins; SEA, SEB, SEC$_n$, SED, SEE, SEG, SEH, SEI, SEJ, SEK, SEL, and SEP	Activate T-cells
sodA, sodM	Superoxide dismutase, SodA, SodM	Promotes resistance to ROS
spa	Protein A	Sequesters host IgG, inhibits phagocytosis
ssl5	Staphylococcal superantigen-like 5, SSL5	Binds PSGL-1 and inhibits neutrophil rolling
ssl7	Staphylococcal superantigen-like 7, SSL7	Binds to C5a and IgA
tst	Toxic shock syndrome toxin-1, TSST1	Activates T-cells

Function of each molecule was determined based upon published studies. (Available at: PubMed, http://www.ncbi.nlm.nih.gov/sites/entrez/). See also the review by T.J. Foster.[57]

a distinction between primed neutrophils and those that are activated fully. Priming includes mobilization of secretory vesicles (and thus up-regulation of specific cell surface receptors, eg, CD11b/CD18) and secretion of cytokines, but fails to trigger release of azurophilic granules or elicit production of superoxide.[29] Importantly, chemotactic/priming agents ultimately promote efficient clearance of invading microorganisms.

Pathogen Recognition and Phagocytosis

Phagocytosis is a process whereby neutrophils bind and ingest invading microorganisms (**Fig. 1**). It is a critical step in the removal of bacteria during infection. Also, opsonophagocytosis is the means by which vaccines prevent bacterial disease. PMNs recognize many surface-bound or freely secreted molecules produced by bacteria, including PGN, lipoproteins, LTA, lipopolysaccharide (LPS), CpG-containing DNA, and flagellin. These conserved molecules, known as pathogen-associated molecular patterns (PAMPs), interact with pattern recognition receptors expressed on the neutrophil cell surface, including TLRs.[30] Neutrophil TLRs activate signal transduction pathways that prolong cell survival;[31] promote or enhance adhesion, phagocytosis, release of cytokines, chemokines, and ROS;[31,32] and trigger granule exocytosis,[33] thereby contributing to microbicidal activity. As an example of the importance of the TLRs in host defense, mice deficient in TLR2 are more susceptible to *S aureus* infection compared with wild-type mice.[34]

Peptidoglycan recognition protein (PGRP) is a secreted host protein that contributes to intracellular killing of gram-positive bacteria by neutrophils.[35] There are four

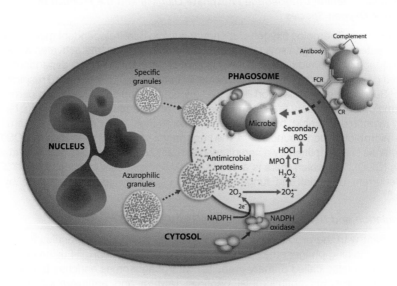

Fig. 1. Polymorphonuclear leukocytes phagocytosis and microbicidal activity. Bacteria are destroyed by NADPH oxidase-derived reactive oxygen species and antimicrobial proteins released from granules after phagocytosis by neutrophils. *Abbreviations:* CR, complement receptor; FCR, Fc receptor; MPO, myeloperoxidase. (*From* Quinn MT, Ammons MC, DeLeo FR. The expanding role of NADPH oxidases in health and disease: no longer just agents of death and destruction. Clin Sci (Lond) 2006:111(1):1–20; with permission.)

reported isoforms of PGRP in mammals, and neutrophils express PGRP-short (PGRP-S).[36] In contrast to TLRs, which promote recognition of bacteria, PGRP-S contributes directly to bactericidal activity.[35]

NOD-like receptors (NLRs) are cytoplasmic proteins that detect intracellular microbial components.[37] NOD2 senses muramyl dipeptide derived from *S aureus* PGN and ultimately promotes transcription of NF-κB target genes in the nucleus.[37] Phagocytosis also is facilitated by host pattern recognition molecules known as collectins, such as mannose-binding lectin, and these molecules are reviewed elsewhere.[38]

Although pattern recognition receptors are important for detection of microbes by phagocytes, the efficiency of phagocytosis (ie, uptake or ingestion) is enhanced if bacteria are opsonized with serum host proteins, such as complement or antibody. Complement-opsonized microbes are bound by complement surface receptors on PMNs, including C1qR, CD35 (CR1), CD11b/CD18 (CR3), and CD11c/CD18 (CR4). Antibody-coated microbes are recognized by PMN antibody-Fc receptors, namely CD16 (FcγRIIIb, IgG receptor), CD23 (FcεRI, IgE receptor), CD32 (FcγRIIa, IgG receptor), CD64 (FcγRI, IgG receptor), and CD89 (FcαR, IgA receptor). The concerted action of pattern recognition receptors/molecules and antibody and complement receptors promotes efficient phagocytosis of microbes (see **Fig. 1**).

NEUTROPHIL MICROBICIDAL ACTIVITY
Nicotinamide Adenine Dinucleotide Phosphate Oxidase and the Production of Reactive Oxygen Species

Human neutrophils employ oxygen-dependent and oxygen-independent mechanisms to kill ingested microorganisms. Phagocytosis of microorganisms activates a membrane-bound nicotinamide adenine dinucleotide phosphate (NADPH)-dependent oxidase that generates high levels of superoxide, a process traditionally called respiratory burst.[39] Superoxide anion is short-lived and dismutates rapidly to hydrogen peroxide and forms other secondary reactive products. These secondarily derived products, including hypochlorous acid, hydroxyl radical, chloramines, and singlet oxygen, are effective microbicidal compounds.[40–43] The importance of NADPH oxidase and ROS for host defense is exemplified by a hereditary disorder known as chronic granulomatous disease (CGD),[44] in which there is a defect in NADPH oxidase. Individuals with CGD have recurrent bacterial and fungal infections, especially infections caused by S aureus.[44]

Degranulation and Neutrophil Antimicrobial Peptides and Proteins

Concomitant with the production of ROS, neutrophil cytoplasmic granules fuse with bacteria-containing phagosomes, a process called degranulation.[45] Fusion of azurophilic granules (also called primary granules) with phagosomes enriches the vacuole lumen with numerous antimicrobial peptides (AMPs) and antimicrobial proteins, including α-defensins, cathepsins, proteinase-3, elastase, and azurocidin (see **Fig. 1**).[45,46] Neutrophil α-defensins comprise up to 50% of the protein in azurophilic granules and have potent antimicrobial activity.[47] Defensins are cationic polypeptides of 3 to 5 kDa that interact with negatively charged molecules at the pathogen surface and permeabilize bacterial membranes. Degranulation also enriches phagosomes with components of the specific granules, such as lactoferrin, further augmenting antimicrobial potential.[48]

Although killing of bacteria by neutrophils occurs primarily after phagocytosis, the process can be enhanced by extracellular molecules. For instance, group IIA phospholipase A_2 (gIIA-PLA$_2$), a small (approximately 14 kDa) cationic antimicrobial protein found in extracellular fluids, synergizes with the neutrophil NADPH oxidase to promote digestion of S aureus phospholipids.[49] More recently, studies by Corbin and colleagues[50] found that neutrophil calprotectin (S100A8/A9) inhibits S aureus growth by sequestering nutrient Mn^{2+} and Zn^{2+} within abscesses.

Neutrophil Extracellular Traps

Work by Brinkmann and colleagues[51] identified structures called neutrophil extracellular traps (NETs), composed of chromatin, histones, and azurophilic granule proteins, which have the capacity to kill bacteria, including S aureus. Whether these structures are produced by live cells or simply represent a byproduct of host cell lysis remains unclear. Uncontrolled release of granule proteins and other cytotoxic molecules into host tissues likely would be problematic for the resolution of the inflammatory response (**Fig. 2**). It is possible that formation of NETs is a relatively infrequent process, thus limiting host tissue damage. In any case, NETs have significant microbicidal activity toward numerous organisms, and further research is needed to better understand these interesting structures.

Neutrophil Apoptosis and the Resolution of Inflammation

Bacterial infections typically are accompanied by tremendous influx of neutrophils to the affected tissues. Although neutrophils kill most ingested microorganisms

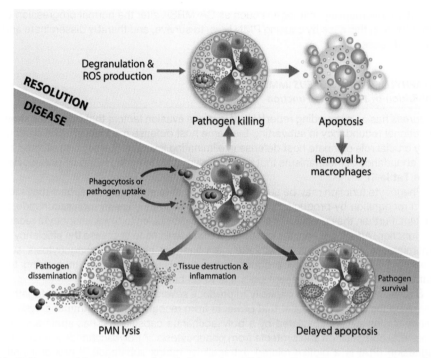

Fig. 2. Two possible outcomes of bacteria–neutrophil interaction. Phagocytosis of bacteria triggers production of reactive oxygen species and degranulation. These processes work collectively to kill ingested bacteria, after which neutrophils undergo apoptosis and are removed by macrophages. This process promotes healthy resolution of infection (*top panel*). Alternatively, bacterial pathogens cause neutrophil lysis or delay apoptosis, and thereby survive and cause disease (*bottom panel*). (*From* Quinn MT, Ammons MC, DeLeo FR. The expanding role of NADPH oxidases in health and disease: no longer just agents of death and destruction. Clin Sci (Lond) 2006:111(1):1–20; with permission.)

efficiently, host tissues can be damaged by the inadvertent release of cytotoxic components from PMNs. Thus, neutrophil turnover must be regulated highly during infection. To that end, normal turnover of aging neutrophils occurs by spontaneous apoptosis and in the absence of an activating agent.[52] On the other hand, neutrophil apoptosis is accelerated significantly following phagocytosis,[53,54] and this phenomenon appears critical to the resolution of the inflammatory response (see **Fig. 2**). Therefore, one might predict that bacterial pathogens have evolved mechanisms to exploit normal neutrophil turnover and apoptosis.

Indeed, bacterial pathogens have devised mechanisms to alter apoptosis and promote pathogenesis.[55,56] For example, USA300 and USA400 cause rapid PMN lysis and/or accelerate bacteria-induced apoptosis to the point of secondary lysis.[16,17] Although these strains produce cytolytic leukotoxins known to cause destruction of human neutrophils, the contribution (if any) of these toxins to PMN lysis after phagocytosis remains to be determined.[16] A model schematic based upon much of the published data suggests that there are two possible outcomes for neutrophil–bacteria interactions (see **Fig. 2**). On one hand, phagocytosis and killing of bacteria culminate with induction of neutrophil apoptosis (also called phagocytosis-induced cell death) and subsequent removal by macrophages, ultimately resulting in the resolution of infection. Alternatively, pathogens such as CA-MRSA alter the normal progression to apoptosis, in this case by causing PMN lysis, to survive, and thereby disseminate and cause disease.

STAPHYLOCOCCUS AUREUS IMMUNE EVASION
Inhibition of Phagocyte Function

S aureus has an astounding repertoire of immune evasion factors that frequently show functional redundancy in subverting the same host defense mechanism. The particularly crucial role of innate host defense in eliminating invading S aureus is reflected by the abundance of mechanisms that the bacterium uses to evade killing by phagocytes (see **Table 1**).[57]

Phagocyte function may be subverted at many different stages. S aureus may hide from recognition by producing protective coats, such as capsular polysaccharide or biofilm. Further, they produce or secrete specific molecules to block phagocyte receptor function. After ingestion, the bacteria use mechanisms to decrease the efficiency of antimicrobial mechanisms, which likely account for noted postphagocytosis survival.[17,58] Finally, they often produce toxins that lyse phagocytes, thus using the same kind of weapon that neutrophils use to kill bacteria.

S aureus strains have the capacity to produce several exopolymers, which together make up the camouflage coat that protects from recognition by the immune system. Many strains are encapsulated by a polysaccharide capsule that has strain-specific chemical composition and protects from phagocytosis.[59] Polysaccharide intercellular adhesion (PIA) is a biofilm-related extracellular matrix substance,[60] predominantly characterized in S epidermidis but produced by most S aureus strains, whose most important and unique feature is a positive net charge.[61] It has been shown to protect from neutrophil phagocytosis and AMPs.[62]

As described previously, receptors on the surface of neutrophils and other phagocytes play a key role in recognizing bacteria and secreted bacterial molecules, promoting phagocyte chemotaxis and activation. S aureus produces a molecule called CHIPS (chemotaxis inhibitory protein of S aureus) that blocks receptor-mediated recognition of formylated peptides,[63] which are PAMPs secreted by bacteria and central for phagocyte detection of bacterial invaders. Other secreted S aureus molecules block the complement system, thereby reducing phagocytosis after opsonization. The C3 convertase blocker SCIN (staphylococcal complement inhibitor) is but one of a series of S aureus factors with the task of inhibiting complement function.[64] In fact, complement inhibition is an excellent example of the functional redundancy of S aureus molecules interfering with the same immune defense mechanism (see **Table 1**).[65]

After being ingested, S aureus uses even more manifold weaponry of immune evasion molecules. Catalase and superoxide dismutase eliminate harmful ROS (see **Table 1**). ROS also trigger a broad response of S aureus to circumvent innate host defense mechanisms, which includes production of many toxins and mechanisms involved in the uptake of iron.[66] In addition, the characteristic yellow pigment of S aureus, a carotenoid pigment called staphyloxanthin, recently has been shown to play an additional, crucial role in protecting from ROS.[67] Moreover, S aureus secretes a series of proteins aimed at moderating the oxygen-independent killing mechanisms of the innate immune system, which include AMPs. First, relatively nonspecific proteases are released to digest any protein-based antimicrobial effector.[68] In addition, S aureus senses the presence of AMPs and reacts by up-regulation of mechanisms to interfere specifically with the activity of cationic AMPs, using a dedicated three-component AMP sensing system.[69,70] The regulated resistance mechanisms include D-alanylation of teichoic acids and incorporation of cationic phospholipid lysyl–phosphatidyl glycerol in the cytoplasmic membrane. These two mechanisms are aimed to reduce the negative net charge of the bacterial surface, thereby decreasing binding of cationic AMPs, and they are encoded by the dlt operon and the mprF locus, respectively.[71,72] Furthermore, expression of the VraFG transporter is increased upon AMP exposure.[70] VraFG has a demonstrated role in AMP resistance[69] and the putative task of removing AMPs from the cell or cytoplasmic membrane.

The immune evasion mechanisms described so far are rather passive, enabling the bacteria to hide from recognition or blocking receptors or effectors involved in the elimination of the bacteria. *S aureus,* however, also produces toxins that directly attack human white and red blood cells. These toxins include the large family of leukocidins and α-toxin (also known as α-hemolysin), recently discovered PSMs, and other hemolysins. The β-barrel structured leukocidins form pores almost exclusively in leukocytes, by means of a mechanism similar to that used by α-toxin.[73] Although the biochemical function of leukocidins—that is, lysis of leukocytes—has been clearly established, their role in *S aureus* virulence and the biological reason for the presence of many similar toxins are not understood. This is also true for Panton-Valentine leukocidin (PVL), in which there has been recent renewed interest because of its epidemiologic correlation with community-associated MRSA. Finally, PSMs are short, α-helical and amphipathic peptides that have the capacity to lyse human neutrophils.[26]

Moderating the Acquired Immune Response

Protein A is probably the best known *S aureus* protein because of its use in the laboratory for antibody purification, which is based on the interaction of protein A with the Fc part of IgG molecules.[74] During pathogenesis, this feature enables *S aureus* to sequester nonspecific antibodies on its surface, which protects efficiently from attacks by the innate and acquired immune systems.[75] Protein A also has a more specific role in the pathogenesis of airway infections by interacting with the tumor necrosis factor α receptor on airway epithelia.[76]

Potentiation of the Immune Response By Superantigenic Toxins

Potentiation or overstimulation of the immune response represents a way of interfering with the human immune system that is clearly opposite to the mechanisms described so far, but equally as effective. *S aureus* produces many superantigenic toxins, a class of secreted toxins that activate T-cells without the need for the presence of an antigen on an antigen-presenting cell (see **Table 1**).[77] Activation of T-cells by superantigenic toxins is accomplished by cross-linking the T-cell receptor with the major histocompatibility complex (MHC) class 2.[77] These toxins include the TSST, exfoliative toxins involved in staphylococcal scalded skin syndrome, and the staphylococcal enterotoxins (SEs).[78] Toxic shock syndrome (TSS) is a severe acute disease and may be of menstrual or nonmenstrual origin. Menstrual TSS is caused by *S aureus* colonization of tampons.[79] Nonmenstrual TSS also may be caused by enterotoxins, which, however have a more notorious role as the cause for *S aureus* food poisoning.[80]

COMMUNITY-ASSOCIATED METHICILLIN-RESISTANT *STAPHYLOCOCCUS AUREUS* VIRULENCE
Hospital-Associated Versus Community-Associated Methicillin-Resistant Staphylococcus aureus

Epidemiologically unassociated outbreaks of CA-MRSA have been reported throughout the world, but the epidemic caused by the clonally related USA300 strains in the

United States appears to be the most serious. Notably, CA-MRSA lineages differ markedly in genotypic and phenotypic characters from traditional hospital-associated MRSA lineages.[10,13,81]

Antibiotic Resistance Per Se Does Not Contribute to Virulence

The frequent reporting in the lay press of MRSA strains as superbugs reflects recognition of the unusually severe and difficult-to-treat infections caused by CA-MRSA strains. Experimental infections in mice indicate that CA-MRSA strains indeed cause more rapidly lethal infections when compared with traditional hospital-associated MRSA strains.[17] The attenuated virulence of hospital-associated MRSA strains in part is caused by the fitness cost associated with resistance to β-lactams and other antibiotics encoded by type I to III staphylococcal chromosomal cassette mec (SCCmec). A unique attribute of CA-MRSA strains is carriage of the type IV SCCmec, which is smaller in size and encodes resistance to only β-lactam class antibiotics. Notably, precise deletion of the entire resistance cassette does not impact virulence in a rabbit infection model.[82] This indicates that type IV SCCmec does not contribute to virulence and, more importantly, does not impose a biological fitness cost to CA-MRSA strains.

VIRULENCE FACTORS
Panton-Valentine Leukocidin

Association with community-associated methicillin-resistant Staphylococcus aureus and Panton-Valentine leukocidin as a toxin

The epidemiologic association between genetically diverse S aureus strains carrying the PVL genes (lukS-PV and lukF-PV, abbreviated as lukS/F-PV) and fatal necrotizing pneumonia renewed and intensified interest in understanding the biological role of this bicomponent cytolytic toxin.[83] Epidemiologic data alone, however, are insufficient to establish whether PVL directly contributes to widespread dissemination of CA-MRSA clones.[84,85] It is of interest that early studies led Woodin to conclude that PVL alone is not a very toxic substance,[86] as intravenous injection of PVL in rabbits resulted in granulocytopenia followed by a marked granulocytosis, and was not lethal.

Lessons Learned from Isogenic Community-Associated Methicillin-Resistant Staphylococcus aureus Luks/F-PV Deletion Mutants

Isogenic lukS/F-PV deletion mutants and wild-type parental strains of USA300 and USA400 were tested in mouse abscess and bacteremia models[16] to reproduce the most common clinical manifestations associated with CA-MRSA disease.[5,6] No significant differences between PVL-positive and PVL-negative strains were detected using these mouse models.[16] As the same mouse models have been used successfully to demonstrate the roles of other CA-MRSA virulence factors,[26] the null effect of PVL in these models strongly indicates that this toxin is not a major virulence factor of USA300 and USA400 strains.

Pneumonia is a rare disease caused by CA-MRSA.[5] Using purified toxin or a laboratory strain of S aureus that overproduced PVL, the toxin was shown to impact mouse survival in a model of pneumonia.[87] In contrast, when comparing isogenic strain pairs with and without lukS/F-PV in the USA300 and USA400 genotypes, or when overexpressing PVL in S aureus strain Newman, no significant contribution of PVL to lethal pneumonia was found.[88,89] Additionally, passive immunization with anti-PVL immune sera failed to protect mice against challenge with USA300 in the murine pneumonia model,[90] indicating that PVL is not necessary for the pathogenesis of pulmonary disease. Although future research on the biological relevance of PVL may be warranted, attributing enhanced CA-MRSA virulence to PVL alone ignores the possible contributions of numerous other determinants.

Does Panton-Valentine Leukocidin Have an Impact on Virulence By a Gene Regulatory Effect?

Recently, a pronounced global gene regulatory effect was attributed to PVL.[87] In that study, PVL appeared to up-regulate production of protein A, which was thought to be fundamental in causing the overwhelming inflammation and necrosis of the mouse lungs.[87,91] The apparent lack of confirmatory experiments by genetic complementation analysis, however, might have resulted in misinterpretation of the gene expression data and thus led to the model of PVL as a global regulator of gene expression.[87] Recently, the failure to replicate the regulatory effects of PVL in USA300 and USA400 indicated that PVL does not contribute to CA-MRSA virulence by means of a gene regulatory mechanism.[92]

Arginine Catabolic Mobile Element

The arginine catabolic mobile element (ACME) is a genetic feature of USA300[13] found infrequently in other *S aureus* strains (ACME-arcA has been detected in multilocus sequence types.[1,5,59,82,93–95] Deletion of ACME in USA300 attenuated pathogenicity in a rabbit bacteremia model, providing evidence that ACME contributes to pathogenesis.[82] Two gene clusters identified in ACME, *arc* and *opp-3*, may function as virulence determinants. As L-arginine is a substrate for nitric oxide production, depletion of L-arginine by the arginine deiminase system (*arc*) might inhibit nitric oxide production, a molecule used in both the innate and adaptive immune responses against bacterial infections.[96] L-arginine catabolism also could be important for ATP production and pH homeostasis on the acidic human skin. *opp-3* belongs to the ABC transporter family, members of which have various central physiologic functions. Thus, ACME may enhance growth, survival, and dissemination of USA300 during infection.

α-Toxin (α-Hemolysin, Hla)

α-toxin is a well-characterized pore forming cytolytic toxin that is similar in sequence and function to the leukocidins,[97] albeit it does not lyse neutrophils.[98] Recently, it was shown to be an essential virulence factor during *S aureus* pneumonia.[88] Immunization with inactivated α-toxin or passive transfer of anti-α-toxin antibodies also protected mice from lethal pneumonia.[90] Taken together, these studies indicate that α-toxin plays an essential role in pneumonia.

Phenol Soluble Modulin-Like Peptides

It has remained obscure which molecules are responsible for neutrophil lysis in vivo and the pronounced cytolytic activity associated with CA-MRSA. Recently, novel cytolytic peptides have been found in *S aureus*, the α-type PSMs, which are encoded in an operon on the genomes of all sequenced *S aureus* strains.[26] The α-helical and amphipathic α-type PSMs have pronounced in vitro and in vivo leukocidal activity, in addition to proinflammatory and chemotactic activities.[26] Whereas hospital-associated MRSA often lack PSM production or produces PSMs only at reduced levels, however, PSMs are expressed at considerable levels in CA-MRSA. Notably, overexpression of α-type PSMs in a prominent hospital-associated MRSA strain increased leukocidal activity to a level equal to that observed in CA-MRSA strains, indicating that expression of these peptides is the main cause for the extreme difference in cytolytic activity between CA-MRSA and hospital-associated MRSA and a possible major contributor to the pronounced pathogenic potential of CA-MRSA strains. In fact, a dramatic influence of the α-type PSMs on the virulence of CA-MRSA was demonstrated using mouse bacteremia and abscess models of infection.[26]

Role of Gene Expression and Regulation in Community-Associated Methicillin-Resistant Staphylococcus aureus Pathogenesis

The results obtained with the PSMs indicate that differential gene expression between CA-MRSA and HA-MRSA strains could explain differences in virulence. For example, as α-toxin and the PSMs, the only molecules described so far to impact virulence of CA-MRSA in a significant manner,[26,88] are under control of the global regulator agr, and there is strong expression of the agr regulatory molecule RNAIII in CA-MRSA strains, there may be a key role of this virulence regulator in CA-MRSA disease that remains to be investigated.[100]

Should Infection By Toxin-Producing Community-Associated Methicillin-Resistant Staphylococcus aureus Strains Impact How Patients are Treated?

CA-MRSA strains elaborate numerous exotoxins, including PVL, α-toxin, and PSMs, that could impact disease severity. Intravenous immunoglobulin (IVIg) could improve outcome of severe staphylococcal infections when used as an adjunct to appropriate antibiotic therapy because of the presence of neutralizing antitoxin antibodies. It remains to be determined whether PVL-specific antibodies in commercial IVIg provide any protective effect. In a mouse pneumonia model, passive transfer of anti-α-toxin antibodies—but not anti-PVL antibodies—protected against lethal pneumonia,[90] providing proof of principle that commercial IVIg could be effective adjunct therapy. Furthermore, inappropriate treatment of CA-MRSA infections with β-lactam antibiotics or ciprofloxacin that may induce bacterial SOS response in these toxin-producing strains could result in increased exotoxin production and disease severity. As such, it is reasonable to propose that clindamycin or linezolid could be beneficial in inhibiting protein synthesis and thus toxin production in CA-MRSA infections.[95] Nonetheless, the emergence of multidrug-resistant isolates of USA300 with resistance to clindamycin,[13,99] and the potential to acquire even more antibiotic resistance, present further complications in staphylococcal disease management.

SUMMARY

S aureus has been a major cause of human infections throughout history and today remains among the most abundant causes of bacterial infections. The pathogen has evolved numerous means to avoid destruction by the human innate immune system, including those that block almost all of the key antimicrobial functions of phagocytic leukocytes. CA-MRSA is especially adept at circumventing normal neutrophil function, which could explain in part the enhanced virulence phenotype of the most prominent CA-MRSA lineages. Future studies directed to better understand the interface between innate immunity, host infection susceptibility, and S aureus are critical for a comprehensive understanding of pathogenesis.

REFERENCES

1. Diekema DJ, Pfaller MA, Schmitz FJ, et al. Survey of infections due to *Staphylococcus* species: frequency of occurrence and antimicrobial susceptibility of isolates collected in the United States, Canada, Latin America, Europe, and the Western Pacific region for the SENTRY Antimicrobial Surveillance Program, 1997–1999. Clin Infect Dis 2001;32(Suppl 2):S114–32.

2. Styers D, Sheehan DJ, Hogan P, et al. Laboratory-based surveillance of current antimicrobial resistance patterns and trends among *Staphylococcus aureus*: 2005 status in the United States. Ann Clin Microbiol Antimicrob 2006;5:2.
3. Noskin GA, Rubin RJ, Schentag JJ, et al. National trends in *Staphylococcus aureus* infection rates: impact on economic burden and mortality over a 6-year period (1998–2003). Clin Infect Dis 2007;45(9):1132–40.
4. Chambers HF. The changing epidemiology of *Staphylococcus aureus*? Emerg Infect Dis 2001;7(2):178–82.
5. Klevens RM, Morrison MA, Nadle J, et al. Invasive methicillin-resistant *Staphylococcus aureus* infections in the United States. JAMA 2007;298(15):1763–71.
6. Moran GJ, Krishnadasan A, Gorwitz RJ, et al. Methicillin-resistant *S aureus* infections among patients in the emergency department. N Engl J Med 2006;355(7): 666–74.
7. Herold BC, Immergluck LC, Maranan MC, et al. Community-acquired methicillin-resistant *Staphylococcus aureus* in children with no identified predisposing risk. JAMA 1998;279(8):593–8.
8. From the Centers for Disease Control and Prevention. Four pediatric deaths from community-acquired methicillin-resistant *Staphylococcus aureus*—Minnesota and North Dakota, 1997–1999. JAMA 1999;282(12):1123–5.
9. McDougal LK, Steward CD, Killgore GE, et al. Pulsed-field gel electrophoresis typing of oxacillin-resistant *Staphylococcus aureus* isolates from the United States: establishing a national database. J Clin Microbiol 2003;41(11):5113–20.
10. Baba T, Takeuchi F, Kuroda M, et al. Genome and virulence determinants of high virulence community-acquired MRSA. Lancet 2002;359(9320):1819–27.
11. Adem PV, Montgomery CP, Husain AN, et al. *Staphylococcus aureus* sepsis and the Waterhouse-Friderichsen syndrome in children. N Engl J Med 2005;353(12): 1245–51.
12. King MD, Humphrey BJ, Wang YF, et al. Emergence of community-acquired methicillin-resistant *Staphylococcus aureus* USA 300 clone as the predominant cause of skin and soft-tissue infections. Ann Intern Med 2006;144(5):309–17.
13. Diep BA, Gill SR, Chang RF, et al. Complete genome sequence of USA300, an epidemic clone of community-acquired methicillin-resistant *Staphylococcus aureus*. Lancet 2006;367(9512):731–9.
14. Kennedy AD, Otto M, Braughton KR, et al. Epidemic community-associated methicillin-resistant *Staphylococcus aureus*: recent clonal expansion and diversification. Proc Natl Acad Sci U S A 2008;105(4):1327–32.
15. Diep BA, Sensabaugh GF, Somboona NS, et al. Widespread skin and soft-tissue infections due to two methicillin-resistant *Staphylococcus aureus* strains harboring the genes for Panton-Valentine leucocidin. J Clin Microbiol 2004;42(5):2080–4.
16. Voyich JM, Otto M, Mathema B, et al. Is Panton-Valentine leukocidin the major virulence determinant in community-associated methicillin-resistant *Staphylococcus aureus* disease? J Infect Dis 2006;194(12):1761–70.
17. Voyich JM, Braughton KR, Sturdevant DE, et al. Insights into mechanisms used by *Staphylococcus aureus* to avoid destruction by human neutrophils. J Immunol 2005;175(6):3907–19.
18. Cicchetti G, Allen PG, Glogauer M. Chemotactic signaling pathways in neutrophils: from receptor to actin assembly. Crit Rev Oral Biol Med 2002; 13(3):220–8.
19. Standiford TJ, Arenberg DA, Danforth JM, et al. Lipoteichoic acid induces secretion of interleukin-8 from human blood monocytes: a cellular and molecular analysis. Infect Immun 1994;62(1):119–25.

20. Soell M. Capsular polysaccharide types 5 and 8 of *Staphylococcus aureus* bind specifically to human epithelial (KB) cells, endothelial cells, and monocytes and induce release of cytokines. Infect Immun 1995;63(4):1380–6.
21. Yao L, Lowy FD, Berman JW. Interleukin-8 gene expression in *Staphylococcus aureus*-infected endothelial cells. Infect Immun 1996;64(8):3407–9.
22. Krakauer T. Interleukin-8 production by human monocytic cells in response to staphylococcal exotoxins is direct and independent of interleukin-1 and tumor necrosis factor-alpha. J Infect Dis 1998;178(2):573–7.
23. McLoughlin RM, Solinga RM, Rich J, et al. CD4+ T cells and CXC chemokines modulate the pathogenesis of *Staphylococcus aureus* wound infections. Proc Natl Acad Sci U S A 2006;103(27):10408–13.
24. Tzianabos AO, Wang JY, Lee JC. Structural rationale for the modulation of abscess formation by *Staphylococcus aureus* capsular polysaccharides. Proc Natl Acad Sci U S A 2001;98(16):9365–70.
25. Schmeling DJ, Peterson PK, Hammerschmidt DE, et al. Chemotaxigenesis by cell surface components of *Staphylococcus aureus*. Infect Immun 1979;26(1): 57–63.
26. Wang R, Braughton KR, Kretschmer D, et al. Identification of novel cytolytic peptides as key virulence determinants for community-associated MRSA. Nat Med 2007;13(12):1510–4.
27. McPhail LC, Clayton CC, Snyderman R. The NADPH oxidase of human polymorphonuclear leukocytes. Evidence for regulation by multiple signals. J Biol Chem 1984;259(9):5768–75.
28. Kobayashi SD, Voyich JM, Burlak C, et al. Neutrophils in the innate immune response. Arch Immunol Ther Exp (Warsz) 2005;53(6):505–17.
29. DeLeo FR, Renee J, Mccormick S, et al. Neutrophils exposed to bacterial lipopolysaccharide up-regulate NADPH oxidase assembly. J Clin Invest 1998; 101(2):455–63.
30. Akira S, Takeda K. Toll-like receptor signalling. Nat Rev Immunol 2004;4(7): 499–511.
31. Sabroe I, Prince LR, Jones EC, et al. Selective roles for toll-like receptor (TLR)2 and TLR4 in the regulation of neutrophil activation and life span. J Immunol 2003;170(10):5268–75.
32. Hayashi F, Means TK, Luster AD. Toll-like receptors stimulate human neutrophil function. Blood 2003;102(7):2660–9.
33. Lotz S, Aga E, Wilde I, et al. Highly purified lipoteichoic acid activates neutrophil granulocytes and delays their spontaneous apoptosis via CD14 and TLR2. J Leukoc Biol 2004;75(3):467–77.
34. Takeuchi O, Hoshino K, Akira S. Cutting edge: TLR2-deficient and MyD88-deficient mice are highly susceptible to *Staphylococcus aureus* infection. J Immunol 2000;165(10):5392–6.
35. Liu C, Gelius E, Liu G, et al. Mammalian peptidoglycan recognition protein binds peptidoglycan with high affinity, is expressed in neutrophils, and inhibits bacterial growth. J Biol Chem 2000;275(32):24490–9.
36. Liu C, Xu Z, Gupta D, et al. Peptidoglycan recognition proteins: a novel family of four human innate immunity pattern recognition molecules. J Biol Chem 2001; 276(37):34686–94.
37. Kanneganti TD, Lamkanfi M, Nunez G. Intracellular NOD-like receptors in host defense and disease. Immunity 2007;27(4):549–59.
38. Fujita T, Matsushita M, Endo Y. The lectin-complement pathway—its role in innate immunity and evolution. Immunol Rev 2004;198:185–202.

39. Quinn MT, Ammons MC, DeLeo FR. The expanding role of NADPH oxidases in health and disease: no longer just agents of death and destruction. Clin Sci (Lond) 2006;111(1):1–20.

40. Klebanoff SJ. Myeloperoxidase-halide-hydrogen peroxide antibacterial system. J Bacteriol 1968;95(6):2131–8.

41. Rosen H, Klebanoff SJ. Formation of singlet oxygen by the myeloperoxidase-mediated antimicrobial system. J Biol Chem 1977;252(14):4803–10.

42. Marcinkiewicz J. Neutrophil chloramines: missing links between innate and acquired immunity. Immunol Today 1997;18(12):577–80.

43. Klebanoff SJ. Myeloperoxidase: friend and foe. J Leukoc Biol 2005;77(5): 598–625.

44. Lekstrom-Himes JA, Gallin JI. Immunodeficiency diseases caused by defects in phagocytes. N Engl J Med 2000;343(23):1703–14.

45. Hirsch JG, Cohn ZA. Degranulation of polymorphonuclear leucocytes following phagocytosis of microorganisms. J Exp Med 1960;112:1005–14.

46. Faurschou M, Borregaard N. Neutrophil granules and secretory vesicles in inflammation. Microbes Infect 2003;5(14):1317–27.

47. Ganz T, Selsted ME, Szklarek D, et al. Defensins. Natural peptide antibiotics of human neutrophils. J Clin Invest 1985;76(4):1427–35.

48. Bellamy W, Takase M, Yamauchi K, et al. Identification of the bactericidal domain of lactoferrin. Biochim Biophys Acta 1992;1121(1–2):130–6.

49. Femling JK, Nauseef WM, Weiss JP. Synergy between extracellular group IIA phospholipase A2 and phagocyte NADPH oxidase in digestion of phospholipids of *Staphylococcus aureus* ingested by human neutrophils. J Immunol 2005; 175(7):4653–61.

50. Corbin BD, Seeley EH, Raab A, et al. Metal chelation and inhibition of bacterial growth in tissue abscesses. Science 2008;319(5865):962–5.

51. Brinkmann V, Reichard U, Goosmann C, et al. Neutrophil extracellular traps kill bacteria. Science 2004;303(5663):1532–5.

52. Savill JS, Wyllie AH, Henson JE, et al. Macrophage phagocytosis of aging neutrophils in inflammation. Programmed cell death in the neutrophil leads to its recognition by macrophages. J Clin Invest 1989;83(3):865–75.

53. Coxon A, Rieu P, Barkalow FJ, et al. A novel role for the β2 integrin CD11b/CD18 in neutrophil apoptosis: a homeostatic mechanism in inflammation. Immunity 1996;5(6):653–66.

54. Kobayashi SD, Voyich JM, Buhl CL, et al. Global changes in gene expression by human polymorphonuclear leukocytes during receptor-mediated phagocytosis: cell fate is regulated at the level of gene expression. Proc Natl Acad Sci U S A 2002;99(10):6901–6.

55. Urban CF, Lourido S, Zychlinsky A. How do microbes evade neutrophil killing? Cell Microbiol 2006;8:1687–96.

56. DeLeo FR. Modulation of phagocyte apoptosis by bacterial pathogens. Apoptosis 2004;9(4):399–413.

57. Foster TJ. Immune evasion by staphylococci. Nat Rev Microbiol 2005;3(12): 948–58.

58. Gresham HD, Lowrance JH, Caver TE, et al. Survival of *Staphylococcus aureus* inside neutrophils contributes to infection. J Immunol 2000;164(7):3713–22.

59. O'Riordan K, Lee JC. *Staphylococcus aureus* capsular polysaccharides. Clin Microbiol Rev 2004;17(1):218–34.

60. Mack D, Fischer W, Krokotsch A, et al. The intercellular adhesin involved in biofilm accumulation of *Staphylococcus epidermidis* is a linear beta-1,6-linked

glucosaminoglycan: purification and structural analysis. J Bacteriol 1996;178(1): 175–83.

61. Vuong C, Kocianova S, Voyich JM, et al. A crucial role for exopolysaccharide modification in bacterial biofilm formation, immune evasion, and virulence. J Biol Chem 2004;279(52):54881–6.

62. Vuong C, Voyich JM, Fischer ER, et al. Polysaccharide intercellular adhesin (PIA) protects *Staphylococcus epidermidis* against major components of the human innate immune system. Cell Microbiol 2004;6(3):269–75.

63. de Haas CJ, Veldkamp KE, Peschel A, et al. Chemotaxis inhibitory protein of *Staphylococcus aureus*, a bacterial anti-inflammatory agent. J Exp Med 2004; 199(5):687–95.

64. Rooijakkers SH, Ruyken M, Roos A, et al. Immune evasion by a staphylococcal complement inhibitor that acts on C3 convertases. Nat Immunol 2005;6(9): 920–7.

65. Jongerius I, Kohl J, Pandey MK, et al. Staphylococcal complement evasion by various convertase-blocking molecules. J Exp Med 2007;204(10):2461–71.

66. Palazzolo-Ballance AM, Reniere ML, Braughton KR, et al. Neutrophil microbi-cides induce a pathogen survival response in community-associated methicil-lin-resistant *Staphylococcus aureus*. J Immunol 2008;180(1):500–9.

67. Liu GY, Essex A, Buchanan JT, et al. *Staphylococcus aureus* golden pigment impairs neutrophil killing and promotes virulence through its antioxidant activity. J Exp Med 2005;202(2):209–15.

68. Sieprawska-Lupa M, Mydel P, Krawczyk K, et al. Degradation of human antimi-crobial peptide LL-37 by *Staphylococcus aureus*-derived proteinases. Antimi-crobial Agents Chemother 2004;48(12):4673–9.

69. Li M, Cha DJ, Lai Y, et al. The antimicrobial peptide-sensing system aps of *Staphylococcus aureus*. Mol Microbiol 2007;66(5):1136–47.

70. Li M, Lai Y, Villaruz AE, et al. Gram-positive three-component antimicrobial pep-tide-sensing system. Proc Natl Acad Sci U S A 2007;104(22):9469–74.

71. Peschel A, Jack RW, Otto M, et al. *Staphylococcus aureus* resistance to human defensins and evasion of neutrophil killing via the novel virulence factor MprF is based on modification of membrane lipids with l-lysine. J Exp Med 2001;193(9): 1067–76.

72. Peschel A, Otto M, Jack RW, et al. Inactivation of the dlt operon in *Staphylococ-cus aureus* confers sensitivity to defensins, protegrins, and other antimicrobial peptides. J Biol Chem 1999;274(13):8405–10.

73. Joubert O, Voegelin J, Guillet V, et al. Distinction between pore assembly by staphylococcal alpha-toxin versus leukotoxins. J Biomed Biotechnol 2007; 2007:25935.

74. Langone JJ. Protein A of *Staphylococcus aureus* and related immunoglobulin receptors produced by streptococci and pneumonococci. Adv Immunol 1982; 32:157–252.

75. Forsgren A, Nordstrom K. Protein A from *Staphylococcus aureus*: the biological significance of its reaction with IgG. Ann N Y Acad Sci 1974;236:252–66.

76. Gomez MI, Lee A, Reddy B, et al. *Staphylococcus aureus* protein A induces air-way epithelial inflammatory responses by activating TNFR1. Nat Med 2004; 10(8):842–8.

77. McCormick JK, Yarwood JM, Schlievert PM. Toxic shock syndrome and bacterial superantigens: an update. Annu Rev Microbiol 2001;55:77–104.

78. Dinges MM, Orwin PM, Schlievert PM. Exotoxins of *Staphylococcus aureus*. Clin Microbiol Rev 2000;13(1):16–34.

79. Bohach GA, Fast DJ, Nelson RD, et al. Staphylococcal and streptococcal pyrogenic toxins involved in toxic shock syndrome and related illnesses. Crit Rev Microbiol 1990;17(4):251–72.
80. Le LY, Baron F, Gautier M. *Staphylococcus aureus* and food poisoning. Genet Mol Res 2003;2(1):63–76.
81. Holden MT, Feil EJ, Lindsay JA, et al. Complete genomes of two clinical *Staphylococcus aureus* strains: evidence for the rapid evolution of virulence and drug resistance. Proc Natl Acad Sci U S A 2004;101(26):9786–91.
82. Diep BA, Stone GG, Basuino L, et al. The arginine catabolic mobile element and staphylococcal chromosomal cassette mec linkage: convergence of virulence and resistance in the USA300 clone of methicillin-resistant *Staphylococcus aureus*. J Infect Dis 2008;197(1):1523–30.
83. Gillet Y, Issartel B, Vanhems P, et al. Association between *Staphylococcus aureus* strains carrying gene for Panton-Valentine leukocidin and highly lethal necrotising pneumonia in young immunocompetent patients. Lancet 2002; 359(9308):753–9.
84. Chambers HF. Community-associated MRSA—resistance and virulence converge. N Engl J Med 2005;352(14):1485–7.
85. Rossney AS, Shore AC, Morgan PM, et al. The emergence and importation of diverse genotypes of methicillin-resistant *Staphylococcus aureus* (MRSA) harboring the Panton-Valentine leukocidin gene (pvl) reveal that pvl is a poor marker for community-acquired MRSA strains in Ireland. J Clin Microbiol 2007; 45(8):2554–63.
86. Woodin AM. Staphylococcal leukocidin. In: Montje T, Kadis S, Ajl S, editors. Microbial toxins (Bacterial protein toxins), vol. 3. New York and London: Academic Press, Incorporated; 1970. p. 327–55.
87. Labandeira-Rey M, Couzon F, Boisset S, et al. *Staphylococcus aureus* Panton-Valentine leukocidin causes necrotizing pneumonia. Science 2007;315(5815): 1130–3.
88. Bubeck Wardenburg J, Bae T, Otto M, et al. Poring over pores: alpha-hemolysin and Panton-Valentine leukocidin in *Staphylococcus aureus* pneumonia. Nat Med 2007;13(12):1405–6.
89. Bubeck Wardenburg J, Palazzolo-Ballance AM, Otto M, et al. Panton-Valentine leukocidin is not a virulence determinant in murine models of community-associated methicillin-resistant *Staphylococcus aureus* disease. J Infect Dis 2008;198(8):1166–70.
90. Bubeck Wardenburg J, Schneewind O. Vaccine protection against *Staphylococcus aureus* pneumonia. J Exp Med 2008;205(2):287–94.
91. Kahl BC, Peters G. Microbiology. Mayhem in the lung. Science 2007;315(5815): 1082–3.
92. Diep BA, Palazzolo-Ballance AM, Tattevin P, et al. Contribution of Panton-Valentine leukocidin in community-associated methicillin-resistant *Staphylococcus aureus* pathogenesis. PLoS ONE 2008;3(9):e3198.
93. Goering RV, McDougal LK, Fosheim GE, et al. Epidemiologic distribution of the arginine catabolic mobile element among selected methicillin-resistant and methicillin-susceptible *Staphylococcus aureus* isolates. J Clin Microbiol 2007; 45(6):1981–4.
94. Ellington MJ, Yearwood L, Ganner M, et al. Distribution of the ACME-arcA gene among methicillin-resistant *Staphylococcus aureus* from England and Wales. J Antimicrob Chemother 2008;61(1):73–7.

95. Stevens DL, Ma Y, Salmi DB, et al. Impact of antibiotics on expression of virulence-associated exotoxin genes in methicillin-sensitive and methicillin-resistant*Staphylococcus aureus*. J Infect Dis 2007;195(2):202–11.
96. Moncada S, Higgs A. The L-arginine-nitric oxide pathway. N Engl J Med 1993; 329(27):2002–12.
97. Bhakdi S, Tranum-Jensen J. Alpha-toxin of *Staphylococcus aureus*. Microbiol Rev 1991;55(4):733–51.
98. Valeva A, Walev I, Pinkernell M, et al. Transmembrane beta-barrel of staphylococcal alpha-toxin forms in sensitive but not in resistant cells. Proc Natl Acad Sci U S A 1997;94(21):11607–11.
99. Diep BA, Chambers HF, Graber CJ, et al. Emergence of multidrug-resistant, community-associated, methicillin-resistant *Staphylococcus aureus* clone USA300 in men who have sex with men. Ann Intern Med 2008;148(4):249–57.
100. Montgomery CP, Boyle-Vavra S, Adem PV, et al. Comparison of virulence in community-associated methicillin-resistant *Staphylococcus aureus* pulsotypes USA300 and USA400 in a rat model of pneumonia. J Infect Dis 2008;198(4): 561–70.

Staphylococcus aureus: A Community Pathogen

Loren G. Miller, MD, MPH[a,b,c,]*, Sheldon L. Kaplan, MD[d]

KEYWORDS

- *Staphylococcus aureus* • Methicillin-resistance • MRSA
- Epidemiology • Clinical syndromes • Community infections

Staphylococcus aureus is a common human pathogen that most commonly manifests clinically as skin infections. There has been much interest in *S aureus* infections in the community over the past decade because of the rise of community-associated methicillin-resistant *S aureus* (CA-MRSA) infections, which have emerged globally over a relatively short period of time. Despite the commonality of β-lactam resistance that commonly circulating strains have with health care–associated methicillin-resistant *Staphylococcus aureus* (HA-MRSA) strains, CA-MRSA isolates have distinct pathogenesis, epidemiology, and clinical manifestations that differ from those of HA-MRSA isolates. In fact, they probably behave more like community-associated methicillin-sensitive *S aureus* (MSSA) infections. This article reviews current knowledge of the epidemiology and clinical manifestations of *S aureus* and CA-MRSA infections.

EPIDEMIOLOGY OF COMMUNITY-ASSOCIATED *STAPHYLOCOCCUS AUREUS* AND METHICILLIN-RESISTANT *STAPHYLOCOCCUS AUREUS*
Defining Community-Associated Methicillin-Resistant Staphylococcus aureus

When categorizing *S aureus* and MRSA infections that originate in the community, terminology can be confusing and inconsistent. Most experts prefer "community-associated" to other terms found in the literature (eg, "community-acquired," "community-onset"). Many experts prefer the term "community-associated," as it

[a] Harbor-UCLA Medical Center, Division of Infectious Diseases, Infection Control Program, 1000 W. Carson Street, Box 466, Torrance CA 90509, USA
[b] Los Angeles Biomedical Research Institute at Harbor-UCLA Medical Center, Los Angeles, CA, USA
[c] David Geffen School of Medicine at the University of California, Los Angeles, CA, USA
[d] Department of Pediatrics, Baylor College of Medicine, Texas Children's Hospital MC3-2371, Infectious Disease Service, 6621 Fannin, Houston, TX 77030, USA
* Corresponding author. Harbor-UCLA Medical Center, Division of Infectious Diseases, Infection Control Program, 1000 W. Carson Street, Box 466, Torrance CA 90509.
E-mail address: Lgmiller@ucla.edu (L.G. Miller).

Infect Dis Clin N Am 23 (2009) 35–52
doi:10.1016/j.idc.2008.10.002
0891-5520/08/$ – see front matter
id.theclinics.com

describes the locale where the infection occurred (ie, a "community" setting of relatively healthy persons as opposed to a health care setting such as a hospital, dialysis clinic, or nursing home). "Community-associated" has also been used to describe the likely organism source (ie, the MRSA isolate causing infection was known to be the same as a strain circulating in the community).

Terminology aside, definitions of "community-associated" are inconsistent.[1,2] Epidemiologic definitions and strain-based (typically molecular) definitions are commonly used to distinguish CA-MRSA infections from HA-MRSA infections. From an epidemiologic perspective, a common definition of community-associated infection is that used by the Active Bacterial Core surveillance (ABC) program of the US Centers for Disease Control and Prevention (CDC).[3] For MRSA infections, this definition states that a community-associated infection occurs in a person without a history of prior MRSA infection or colonization and in which the MRSA culture was obtained in the outpatient setting or isolated within 48 hours of hospitalization. Additionally, the patient needs to lack exposures associated with HA-MRSA infections, such as recent (with recent defined as "in the prior 12 months") hospitalization, receipt of hemodialysis, residence in a chronic care facility, or presence of an indwelling catheter. Others definitions have been used, for example a modified ABC criteria in which prior hospitalization is excluded,[4] as many otherwise healthy community-dwelling persons with recurrent hospitalizations for MRSA would be categorized as HA-MRSA if they had a previous relatively recent hospitalization for a CA-MRSA infection.

From an organism standpoint, molecular characteristics are also used to categorize isolates as either community associated or health care associated. Much of this work on using molecular definitions has focused on MRSA infections, specifically distinguishing CA-MRSA and HA-MRSA strains using molecular tools. SCCmec (which stands for staphylococcal cassette chromosome mec) is a DNA cassette that is inserted in the chromosome of S aureus and confers resistance to β-lactams such as methicillin.[5] Typically CA-MRSA infections are caused by strains that carry SCCmec type IV element (or occasionally type V). HA-MRSA infections are typically caused by MRSA strains that contain SCCmec types I to III.[6] CA-MRSA isolates commonly carry genes encoding toxins such as lukS-PV/lukF-PV (which encode the Panton-Valentine leukocidin [PVL] toxin), sea, seb, sec, seh, and sek.[6] CA-MRSA strains also have distinct patterns of accessory gene regulators (agr, sar), which are operons that regulate virulence gene expression,[7,8] although the role of these toxins and regulators in virulence remains unclear or controversial. The SCCmec IV found in CA-MRSA isolates is also characterized by its smaller size and lack of genetic material conferring resistance to non–β-lactam antimicrobials.[9,10] CA-MRSA isolates are often susceptible to many non–β-lactam antimicrobials including trimethoprim-sulfamethoxazole, clindamycin, and tetracyclines.[11–13]

Based on definitions using pulsed field gel electrophoresis (PFGE), the predominant strain of CA-MRSA in the United States is the USA300 strain. This strain is associated with CA-MRSA infection in football players,[14] prisoners,[15] and nonoutbreak settings.[16] USA300 has also begun to appear globally.[16–19] The USA400 strain (also called the MW-2 strain) has been the cause of infection in the US Midwest,[20–22] although the USA300 strain appears to becoming increasingly common in this region. Other strains, such as USA700, USA800, USA1000, and USA1100 are epidemic or endemic in Asia, Australia, and Europe.[23–30] CA-MSSA strains, on the other hand, are typically very diverse from a molecular standpoint, with many strains circulating locally.[4]

In the early days of the CA-MRSA epidemic, molecular definitions were usually very reliable at distinguishing CA-MRSA from HA-MRSA infections. However, the use of a strictly molecular definition to distinguish CA-MRSA is increasingly problematic.

SCC*mec* type IV–containing MRSA strains are now well established causes of health care–associated infections,[13,31–33] such as surgical site infections,[34] bloodstream infections,[32] and infections in dialysis patients.[35] In one hospital in Los Angeles, SCC*mec* type IV–containing MRSA strains are now the most prevalent SCC*mec* type among HA-MRSA infections.[36] The blurring of molecular types in the health care setting suggests using a molecular definition has become obsolete. Nevertheless, epidemiologic definitions are imperfect; prevalence rates of CA-MRSA versus HA-MRSA vary dramatically depending on the definitions of "community-associated" that are used and the data sources used to determine community-associated status.[37,38]

The Scope of Staphylococcus aureus and Community-Associated Methicillin-Resistant Staphylococcus aureus Infections

Data on estimates of the burden of CA–*S aureus* infections are surprisingly few. During 2001 to 2003, approximately 11.6 million annual ambulatory care visits for skin and soft tissue infections occurred in the United States.[39] Many or most of these infections were presumed to be caused by *S aureus*, although there were no estimates quantifying the proportion of infections cultured and the number of these that were proven to be caused by *S aureus*. Until this century, the vast majority of ambulatory skin infections were caused by MSSA.

CA-MRSA infections were extremely rare until the 1990s.[13,40] During the first part of that decade, infections were noted in Australia in persons without "traditional" MRSA risk factors, such as hospitalization or other health care exposures.[41,42] During the later part of the decade, CA-MRSA infections were noted in the United States.[21,43,44] Retrospective investigations during the 1990s demonstrated 15-fold and 7-fold increases in the proportion of CA–*S aureus* isolates that were methicillin resistant among Native Americans in the rural Midwestern United States[44] and of hospitalized children in Chicago.[43] Similarly, a retrospective study from Texas found a 7-fold increase in the incidence of CA-MRSA infections from 1997 to 2000 relative to 1990 to 1996.[45] By the middle of the first decade of the twenty-first century, many centers in the United States have found that MRSA is responsible for over 50% of CA–*S aureus* infections.[4,46–50]

Besides apparently endemic infections, many outbreaks of CA-MRSA have been reported. These outbreaks typically affect populations of relatively healthy persons, including incarnated persons,[51–53] athletes participating in contact sports,[14,51] military personnel,[54,55] HIV-infected men who have sex with men (MSM),[56–58] and intravenous drug users.[2,49,59] CA-MRSA strains, based on molecular definitions, have also been noted to infect postpartum women.[60] CA-MRSA outbreaks and infections have been reported in North America, Europe, Australia, and Asia.[18,26,29,51,53,61–66]

Risk Factors and Transmission

There is there is a paucity of literature examining the epidemiology of CA–*S aureus* infections, especially skin infections,[67,68] Much data about the pathogenesis of CA–*S aureus* infections has been obtained from CA-MRSA outbreak investigations. These investigations commonly occur in relatively homogeneous patient populations, such as athletes on a sports team. In sports team outbreaks, infections are commonly associated with breaks in skin integrity, touching colonized or infected persons, and sharing of contaminated fomites (eg, towels, balms).[14,69,70] One outbreak of CA-MRSA among fencers occurred because fencers were sharing sensor wires under their clothes (to record when touched by an opponent's weapon) that were not routinely cleaned.[70] In an outbreak in remote Alaskan villages, contaminated fomites again appeared to play an important role. Many sauna benches in these villages were colonized with MRSA and were presumed to help fuel the spread of MRSA.[71]

These outbreaks have led to the development of a conceptual model of CA-MRSA transmission. This model, called the "Five Cs of CA-MRSA transmission" (**Box 1**),[3,72] suggests that MRSA infection results from a collection of risks: (1) Contact (with infected or colonized persons), (2) Cleanliness (or lack of optimal personal hygiene), (3) Compromised skin integrity, (4) Contaminated objects and surfaces and items, and (5) Crowded living conditions. A sixth "C" is often quoted, antibiotic capsules (and tablets, liquids, and so forth), as exposure to antibiotics may help drive the emergence of these drug-resistant pathogens.[14,71,73,74] Although it has been believed that another "C," nasal colonization, plays an important role in the development of *S aureus* and MRSA infections, the role of nasal colonization in CA-MRSA pathogenesis is much less certain. Data from CA-MRSA outbreaks suggest that skin-skin and skin-fomite contact represent important and common alternative routes of acquisition. CA-MRSA infections may not require a intermediate nasal colonization step before infection.[16]

Although the validity of the five (or six) Cs framework in epidemics appears relatively solid, the relative requirements of each of the Cs are unclear. Additionally, its validity in the development of endemic CA-MRSA (ie, non-outbreak) infections is less certain. Risk factors for CA-MRSA from population-based studies have been obtained from large databases that are unable to capture more detailed risk behaviors or exposures (eg, hygiene measures, recent incarceration). However in one single site study that collected detailed epidemiologic risk factors, persons with CA-MRSA infection were more likely to have had skin breaks and contact with infected persons when compared with those without CA-MRSA infections.[75] Additionally, high-risk sexual behavior, recent incarceration, homelessness, and visiting bars and raves were more common among patients with CA-MRSA infection.[75] MRSA risk factors, both "classical" and nonclassical (eg, recent hospitalization or exposure to the health care setting, recent incarceration, illicit drug use, or participation in contact sports), are extremely unreliable at differentiating patients with CA-MRSA from those with CA-MSSA

Box 1
The five (sometimes referred to as the six) Cs of community-associated MRSA infection transmission (see text for details)

1. Contact (eg, skin to skin contact with infected or colonized persons)

2. Cleanliness (eg, suboptimal personal hygiene, bathing, soap or antisepsis use; inadequate covering of infected wounds, and so forth)

3. Compromised skin integrity (eg, broken skin from cuts, abrasions, or dermatitis that allow MRSA to invade the skin)

4. Contaminated objects and surfaces and items (eg, fomites, such as shared items, razors, benches, towels, clothes, etc., that can facilitate acquisition of MRSA)

5. Crowded living conditions (eg, a large number of persons in a small space, which facilitates the spread of MRSA from one person to another).

6. Antibiotic Capsules (or liquids, pills, and so forth) (eg, recent consumption of an antibiotics, particularly antibiotics that have activity against CA-MSSA strains but not CA-MRSA strains)

Data from Minnesota Department of Health. Community-associated methicillin-resistant *Staphylococcus aureus* in Minnesota. Minnesota Department of Health Disease Control Newsletter 2004;32:61–72; and Ragan P. Community-acquired MRSA infection: an update. JAAPA 2006;19:24–9.

infections.[4,50] Many patients with endemic CA-MRSA, particularly children, have no discernable risks.

Larger population-based database studies have often found that ethnic minorities comprise the majority of CA-MRSA patients with infection rates typically higher than that of Caucasians.[76–79] Lower socioeconomic status has also been linked to increased CA-MRSA risk,[77,78] as has drug use, typically injection drug use.[4,49,75,80,81] A large study conducted by the CDC in three major metropolitan centers in the United States found that whereas persons of all ages are affected by CA-MRSA infection, persons younger than 2 years of age had higher incidences of CA-MRSA infection compared with those who were 2 years of age or older.[79] Data of risk factors for MSSA are generally lacking; although a study of risk factors for skin infections in the United States found that men, Medicaid recipients, and residents in the South and West were at highest risk.[39]

The transmission of CA-MRSA strains and infections to close contacts, including household contacts, has frequently been reported.[4,78,82,83] A prospective study among patients with CA–S aureus infections showed that reports of new skin infection among household members in the 30 days after the initial infection was 13% for CA-MRSA patients but just 4% for those who had CA-MSSA infections (although this difference was not statistically significant, $P = .20$).[84]

CLINICAL MANIFESTATIONS OF *STAPHYLOCOCCUS AUREUS* AND COMMUNITY-ASSOCIATED METHICILLIN-RESISTANT *STAPHYLOCOCCUS AUREUS* INFECTIONS
Skin and Soft Tissue Infections

Skin and soft tissue infections are by far the most common clinical manifestations of CA–S aureus infections in children and adults and account for approximately 85% to 95% of infections caused by this organism.[4,6,47,79,85–89] Abscesses, furuncles, carbuncles, and folliculitis are the predominant skin infections. Cellulitis is also commonly caused by S aureus.[90,91] The skin infections, especially those caused by CA-MRSA isolates, can be quite severe and necrotic appearing and can be confused with spider or other insect bites.[50,85] In a 6-year surveillance study at Texas Children's Hospital (TCH) in Houston, TX, for children with skin and soft tissue infections, overall 61% and 53% of the children with CA-MRSA and CA-MSSA isolates, respectively, were admitted to the hospital ($P = .0002$).[92] This suggests that the skin and soft tissue infections caused by CA-MRSA are more severe than those caused by CA-MSSA isolates. Although controversial, the necrotic nature of the skin lesions may be related, in part, to the production of the cytotoxin Panton-Valentine leukocidin, which is characteristic of the CA-MRSA isolates in the United States.[93] Virtually any area of skin can be infected but the extremities, trunk, perineum, and buttocks are particularly common sites.[94,95]

CA-MRSA is an important cause of breast abscesses among pregnant or nonpregnant women.[96,97] Recurrent skin infections are encountered in about 10% of patients with S aureus skin and soft tissue infections,[84,95] although a study of pregnant women with recurrent MRSA infection found a recurrence rate of over 50%.[97]

Head and neck CA-MRSA infections such as cervical lymphadenitis, otitis externa, otitis media with otorrhea, or acute mastoiditis and retropharyngeal abscess are also being encountered with increasing frequency.[86,98–102] The retropharyngeal abscesses can extend down into the mediastinum and may be associated with jugular vein thrombosis, similar to the classic Lemierre syndrome[101] (**Fig. 1**). An increasing number of patients with periorbital and orbital infections as well as other infections related to eye structures caused by CA-MRSA are being encountered in children and

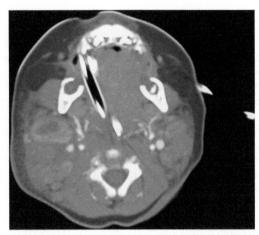

Fig. 1. Head CT scan of a 3-month old infant with a retropharyngeal abscess caused by CA-MRSA.

adults.[103,104] Although cases do occur, CA-MRSA is not a common etiology of acute otitis media or acute sinusitis.[105] However, S aureus is an important pathogen to consider in patients with intracranial complications of sinusitis such as epidural or subdural abscesses.[106]

Musculoskeletal Infections

Musculoskeletal infections are the most common invasive infections caused by CA–S aureus in children.[4,46–50] At TCH, acute hematogenous osteomyelitis is now most commonly caused by CA-MRSA isolates.[92] Over a 6-year surveillance study, 129 and 96 children had CA-MRSA and CA-MSSA osteomyelitis, respectively. This is also the case in a study from Memphis.[107] The most common sites of infection are the long bones such as the tibia and femur. The clinical manifestations of osteomyelitis caused by CA-MRSA versus CA-MSSA isolates differ somewhat in that multiple sites of infection are more common in patients with CA-MRSA.[108] Moreover, children with CA-MRSA osteomyelitis have a longer duration of fever and hospitalization than children with osteomyelitis caused by CA-MSSA isolates.[107,109]

The presence of the genes (pvl) encoding for the exotoxin Panton-Valentine leukocidin in CA–S aureus isolates was associated with both clinical and laboratory differences among our patients with acute osteomyelitis.[108] Children with isolates positive for pvl had greater measures of inflammation (white blood cell count, erythrocyte sedimentation rate, C–reactive protein) at admission as well as during the course of hospitalization, greater frequency of positive blood cultures, and greater frequency of subperiosteal or intraosseous abscesses than children whose isolates did not carry the pvl genes.[108] In addition, complications of osteomyelitis such as the development of chronic osteomyelitis or an associated deep venous thrombosis were more common in the children with pvl-positive isolates.[109] The increased inflammatory parameters occur in children with osteomyelitis caused by pvl-positive isolates regardless of the methicillin susceptibility of the isolate.[110] Arnold and colleagues[107] also reported a more complicated course including persistently positive blood cultures, subperiosteal abscesses and venous thrombosis among children with osteomyelitis caused by CA-MRSA compared with those caused by CA-MSSA. It should be noted that the role of pvl in the pathogenesis of S aureus infections is controversial. Animal studies of pneumonia and skin infection suggest that *pvl* simply may be a marker for other virulence factors rather than a critical gene for the pathogenesis of severe *S aureus* infection.[93,111–113]

Venous thrombophlebitis leading to septic pulmonary emboli and other sites of dissemination clearly occurs more commonly with the CA-MRSA isolates, especially the USA300 clone, for reasons that are yet to be determined.[107,114–116] In these patients the venous thrombosis typically occurs in a vein adjacent to the infected bone (**Fig. 2**). An erythematous, tender, and indurated streak may be apparent on physical examination, depending on the site of the osteomyelitis. In many cases, venous thrombosis is found with MRI studies. Typically bactericidal antibiotics are administered for endovascular infections and that is what we recommend for these patients for at least 6 weeks. In these circumstances, consultation should be sought with a hematologist with expertise in anticoagulation. Anticoagulation generally is provided until the thrombosis has resolved totally.

In adults, *S aureus* is also the most common cause of hematogenous osteomyelitis but the vertebrae are the most common sites of infection.[117] However, there are increasing reports of osteomyelitis in adults caused by the USA300 CA-MRSA strains.[79] Complications such as septic emboli or pathologic fractures are being reported as seen in children.[118,119]

S aureus isolates including CA-MRSA are less commonly isolated from children with septic arthritis than from children with acute osteomyelitis. Over the 6-year study, CA-MRSA and CA-MSSA isolates were recovered from 17 and 15 children, respectively, with septic arthritis. The clinical manifestations were no different for these two groups. In adults, *S aureus* is the most common cause of hematogenously acquired septic arthritis and is often associated with a catheter-related bacteremia or intravenous drug use.[120–122] In the CDC surveillance study of three communities, osteomyelitis and septic arthritis each accounted for 1% of the cases of CA-MRSA infections in 2001 to 2002.[79]

The CDC reported surveillance of invasive MRSA infections among all age groups from July 2004 through December 2005 for the ABC sites. Osteomyelitis accounted for 7.5% of all MRSA infections (community associated or health care associated).[123]

Myositis and pyomyositis are being recognized with increasing frequency in children with CA-MRSA infections, and multiple sites of muscle involvement and a concomitant osteomyelitis are common.[107,109,124] A preceding injury or vigorous use of muscles often precedes the onset of infection by several days. These patients typically complain of pain in the region with tenderness to palpation of the involved muscles. The muscles

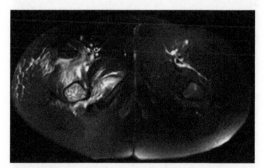

Fig. 2. Magnetic resonance imaging of the proximal right femur demonstrating osteomyelitis, surrounding myositis, and thrombosis of the superficial femoral vein in an adolescent with CA-MRSA osteomyelitis.

of the thigh or pelvis are most commonly involved. In large muscles of the extremities, swelling and warmth may be appreciated. As with most S aureus infections, pyomyositis and myositis are more common in the summer months.

Myositis or pyomyositis was associated with osteomyelitis in 28 or 45 children with pvl-positive isolates compared with 6 of 19 children with pvl-negative isolates (P = .05) in one study.[108] MRI shows inflammation or abscess formation of the muscle most readily of the imaging techniques and its greater use may, in part, explain the increasing recognition of this infection.[125,126] Multiple sites of myositis/pyomyositis and/or osteomyelitis can develop in the patient with disseminated S aureus infection (**Fig. 3**). Thus, physicians must carefully examine the patient daily to detect areas of infection that may not have been appreciated even the previous day. Repeat MRI, weekly in some cases, may be necessary to demonstrate these areas of inflammation and abscess formation as they develop. Pyomyositis caused by CA-MRSA isolates in particular also has been reported in adults, including postpartum women.[118,127,128] Previously these infections were seen mostly in tropical countries ("tropical pyomyositis"), but only rarely in temperate climates.[127]

Necrotizing fasciitis caused by CA-MRSA has been described in 14 adults, many of whom had a history of current or past injection-drug use or chronic underlying illnesses; CA-MRSA was the only pathogen in 10.[129] The buttocks, legs, arms, and shoulders were the most common areas affected. Symptoms were present an average of 6 days (range 3 to 21 days) before admission. Frequently the diagnosis was not expected at the time of surgery and more extensive debridement than anticipated preoperatively was required. USA300 was the only CA-MRSA clone identified. In another large series that included 29 adult patients with MRSA necrotizing fasciitis, 23 were CA-MRSA infections and only 2 overall were polymicrobial.[130] The mortality rate for MRSA necrotizing fasciitis in this study was 10%. This manifestation of CA-MRSA infection also has been described in a neonate.[131] Of note is that until recently necrotizing fasciitis was only rarely caused by monomicrobial S aureus infection and now several centers describe it as a major cause of necrotizing fasciitis at their center.[129,130]

Pneumonia with Empyema

Complicated pneumonias with empyema are more frequently encountered in children since CA-MRSA isolates have become so common. At TCH, CA-MRSA is now the most common pathogen isolated in children with pleural empyema.[132] Except for

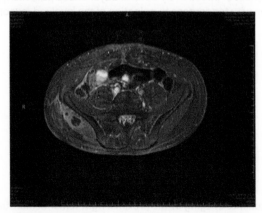

Fig. 3. Multiple sites of pyomyositis in the pelvic muscles in a 20-month old child with disseminated CA-MRSA infection.

the younger age of children with *S aureus* empyema, the clinical findings for pneumonia with empyema are similar for CA-MRSA infections compared with *Streptococcus pneumoniae*. The length of hospital stay for children with CA-MRSA empyema was longer (mean of 18.8 days) than seen in those with CA-MSSA empyema (mean 14.0 days). Among children with any invasive infection, CA–*S aureus* isolates carrying the genes encoding PVL are more likely to be associated with abnormal chest imaging (plain films, CT, MRI) than isolates negative for the *pvl* genes.[133]

Severe Sepsis

The number of children with severe invasive and disseminated CA-MRSA infections also has increased in many areas as CA-MRSA infections continue to increase. At TCH, over a 17-month period from September 2002 through January 2004, about 10% (16 of 150 children) of the children with invasive CA–*S aureus* infections were admitted to the intensive care.[134] Most were adolescents (14 of 16 patients were older than 10 years of age) with an average age of 12.9 years and mean weight of 63 kg. The USA300 CA-MRSA was the pathogen in 14 of 16 patients; USA300 CA-MSSA was found in the other 2 patients. Of the 14 children older than 10, most had skeletal infections, bacteremia, and pulmonary involvement; 11 required mechanical ventilation. Four had vascular thromboses. Evidence of disseminated disease such as multiple areas of pyomyositis or subcutaneous nodules may be noted (**Fig. 4**). The mean duration of bacteremia was 4 days (range 1 to 11 days); 8 patients were bacteremic for 4 days or longer. Three of the 14 older patients and 1 of the 2 younger patients died.

A purpura fulminans presentation in adults and children similar to severe meningococcemia has been associated with CA-MRSA isolates.[135,136] Clinical features in children included leukopenia, neutropenia, profound tachycardia, and lactic acidosis unresponsive to intensive care treatment.[135] Rapid onset of purpura may lead to amputation of extremities and a high likelihood of mortality. Adrenal hemorrhage may be noted at necropsy as observed in the Waterhouse-Friderichsen syndrome. The relationship of this clinical presentation to particular superantigens such as TSST-1, SEB, or SEC or the CA-MRSA clone (USA400 versus USA300) is unclear.

Endocarditis

S aureus is the leading cause of infective endocarditis in adults in many areas of the developed world, especially health care–related infective endocarditis.[137] In the

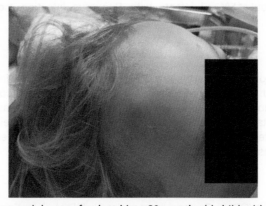

Fig. 4. Subcutaneous nodule over forehead in a 20-month old child with disseminated CA-MRSA infection.

United States, diabetes, hemodialysis and other chronic illnesses are noted in a high percentage of patients. S aureus is also a major cause of community-acquired infective endocarditis in individuals with or without a history of intravenous drug use. Stroke, other sites of systemic embolization, heart failure, and intracardiac abscess are common complications. Mortality exceeded 20% in patients in the United States in the international study of infective endocarditis conducted by Fowler and colleagues.[137]

Venous thrombosis is a common finding in patients with S aureus bacteremia associated with a central line. Clinical findings may be minimal and thus some experts recommend routine ultrasonography to detect thromboses even in the patient with an unremarkable physical examination.[138] Similarly, some experts suggest that adults with S aureus bacteremia of any nature undergo transthoracic echocardiography to help exclude the possibility of infective endocarditis.[139]

Despite the impressive increase in CA-MRSA infections overall and the invasive infections, in particular, an increase in the number of children with infective endocarditis caused by this organism has not been noted. Transthoracic echocardiograms are performed in virtually all patients with persistent bacteremia (> 4 days) at TCH; however, only very few children with vegetations have been identified.[133] In children with structurally normal hearts and S aureus bacteremia, abnormal echocardiograms are unusual.[140]

Neonates

CA-MRSA infections occur throughout the first year of life but are being recognized more commonly in the otherwise healthy neonate younger than 30 days of age.[141] Pustulosis either localized or diffuse is the most common manifestation in this age group. The buttocks and perineum are the most typical locations. Generally these babies with localized pustulosis are not ill, are afebrile, and have negative blood cultures.[142] Topical treatment with mupirocin appears to be adequate in most cases of localized pustulosis. For diffuse pustulosis, a blood culture is recommended but treatment could be an oral antibiotic such as clindamycin.

Abscesses, cellulitis including orbital cellulites, and other invasive infections occur less commonly but can be associated with bacteremia and more severe illness. Any infant with symptoms or with fever related to a potential S aureus infection should undergo a complete evaluation including blood and urine cultures and a cerebrospinal fluid (CSF) analysis and culture. Although not understood, a CSF pleocytosis may be noted in about 15% of infants with S aureus infection more severe than pustulosis.[142]

SUMMARY

CA-MRSA has rapidly become the predominant cause of S aureus infections in many parts of the world. This bacterium is notable for its predilection to cause infections in healthy persons and may disproportionately affect ethnic minorities and those of lower socioeconomic status. CA-MRSA isolates are also is notable for their ability to cause severe, life-threatening infections that include manifestations that were previously not or uncommonly associated with S aureus infection.

REFERENCES

1. Department WCDH. Community-associated MRSA infection surveillance in Washoe County final report for health care providers. Epi-News 2005;25:1–6.

2. Salgado CD, Farr BM, Calfee DP. Community-acquired methicillin-resistant *Staphylococcus aureus*: a meta-analysis of prevalence and risk factors. Clin Infect Dis 2003;36:131–9.
3. Minnesota Department of Health. Community-associated methicillin-resistant *Staphylococcus aureus* in Minnesota. Minnesota Department of Health Disease Control Newsletter 2004;32:61–72.
4. Miller LG, Perdreau-Remington F, Bayer AS, et al. Clinical and epidemiologic characteristics cannot distinguish community-associated methicillin-resistant *Staphylococcus aureus* infection from methicillin-susceptible *S. aureus* infection: a prospective investigation. Clin Infect Dis 2007;44:471–82.
5. Ito T, Katayama Y, Asada K, et al. Structural comparison of three types of staphylococcal cassette chromosome mec integrated in the chromosome in methicillin-resistant *Staphylococcus aureus*. Antimicrobial Agents Chemother 2001;45: 1323–36.
6. Naimi TS, LeDell KH, Como-Sabetti K, et al. Comparison of community- and health care-associated methicillin-resistant *Staphylococcus aureus* infection. JAMA 2003;290:2976–84.
7. Chien Y, Cheung AL. Molecular interactions between two global regulators, sar and agr, in *Staphylococcus aureus*. J Biolumin Chemilumin 1998;273:2645–52.
8. Sabersheikh S, Saunders NA. Quantification of virulence-associated gene transcripts in epidemic methicillin-resistant *Staphylococcus aureus* by real-time PCR. Mol Cell Probes 2004;18:23–31.
9. Daum RS, Ito T, Hiramatsu K, et al. A novel methicillin-resistance cassette in community-acquired methicillin-resistant *Staphylococcus aureus* isolates of diverse genetic backgrounds. J Infect Dis 2002;186:1344–7.
10. Aessopos A, Politou M, Farmakis D, et al. *Staphylococcus aureus* abscess of the spleen in a beta-thalassemia patient. Scand J Infect Dis 2002;34:466–8.
11. Weber JT. Community-associated methicillin-resistant *Staphylococcus aureus*. Clin Infect Dis 2005;41(Suppl 4):S269–72.
12. Eguia JM, Chambers HF. Community-acquired methicillin-resistant *Staphylococcus aureus*: epidemiology and potential virulence factors. Curr Infect Dis Rep 2003;5:459–66.
13. Deresinski S. Methicillin-resistant *Staphylococcus aureus*: an evolutionary, epidemiologic, and therapeutic odyssey. Clin Infect Dis 2005;40:562–73.
14. Kazakova SV, Hageman JC, Matava M, et al. A clone of methicillin-resistant *Staphylococcus aureus* among professional football players. N Engl J Med 2005;352:468–75.
15. Diep BA, Sensabaugh GF, Somboona NS, et al. Widespread skin and soft-tissue infections due to two methicillin-resistant *Staphylococcus aureus* strains harboring the genes for Panton-Valentine leucocidin. J Clin Microbiol 2004;42:2080–4.
16. Miller LG, Diep BA. Colonization, fomites, and virulence: rethinking the pathogenesis of community-associated methicillin-resistant *Staphylococcus aureus* infection. Clin Infect Dis 2008;46:742–50.
17. Larsen A, Stegger M, Goering R, et al. Emergence and dissemination of the methicillin resistant *Staphylococcus aureus* USA300 clone in Denmark (2000–2005). Euro Surveill 2007;12:22–4.
18. Gilbert M, MacDonald J, Gregson D, et al. Outbreak in Alberta of community-acquired (USA300) methicillin-resistant *Staphylococcus aureus* in people with a history of drug use, homelessness or incarceration. CMAJ 2006;175:149–54.
19. Tietz A, Frei R, Widmer AF. Transatlantic spread of the USA300 clone of MRSA. N Engl J Med 2005;353:532–3.

20. McDougal LK, Steward CD, Killgore GE, et al. Pulsed-field gel electrophoresis typing of oxacillin-resistant *Staphylococcus aureus* isolates from the United States: establishing a national database. J Clin Microbiol 2003;41:5113–20.

21. Four pediatric deaths from community-acquired methicillin-resistant *Staphylococcus aureus*—Minnesota and North Dakota, 1997–1999. MMWR Recomm Rep 1999;48:707–10.

22. Baba T, Takeuchi F, Kuroda M, et al. Genome and virulence determinants of high virulence community-acquired MRSA. Lancet 2002;359:1819–27.

23. Wang CC, Lo WT, Chu ML, et al. Epidemiological typing of community-acquired methicillin-resistant *Staphylococcus aureus* isolates from children in Taiwan. Clin Infect Dis 2004;39:481–7.

24. Wu KC, Chiu HH, Wang JH, et al. Characteristics of community-acquired methicillin-resistant *Staphylococcus aureus* in infants and children without known risk factors. J Microbiol Immunol Infect 2002;35:53–6.

25. Okuma K, Iwakawa K, Turnidge JD, et al. Dissemination of new methicillin-resistant *Staphylococcus aureus* clones in the community. J Clin Microbiol 2002;40: 4289–94.

26. Adhikari RP, Cook GM, Lamont I, et al. Phenotypic and molecular characterization of community occurring, Western Samoan phage pattern methicillin-resistant *Staphylococcus aureus*. J Antimicrob Chemother 2002;50:825–31.

27. Dufour P, Gillet Y, Bes M, et al. Community-acquired methicillin-resistant *Staphylococcus aureus* infections in France: emergence of a single clone that produces Panton-Valentine leukocidin. Clin Infect Dis 2002;35:819–24.

28. Witte W, Braulke C, Cuny C, et al. Emergence of methicillin-resistant *Staphylococcus aureus* with Panton-Valentine leukocidin genes in central Europe. Eur J Clin Microbiol Infect Dis 2005;24:1–5.

29. Witte W, Cuny C, Strommenger B, et al. Emergence of a new community acquired MRSA strain in Germany. Euro Surveill 2004;9:1–2.

30. Robinson DA, Kearns AM, Holmes A, et al. Re-emergence of early pandemic *Staphylococcus aureus* as a community-acquired methicillin-resistant clone. Lancet 2005;365:1256–8.

31. O'Brien FG, Pearman JW, Gracey M, et al. Community strain of methicillin-resistant *Staphylococcus aureus* involved in a hospital outbreak. J Clin Microbiol 1999;37:2858–62.

32. Seybold U, Kourbatova EV, Johnson JG, et al. Emergence of community-associated methicillin-resistant *Staphylococcus aureus* USA300 genotype as a major cause of health care-associated blood stream infections. Clin Infect Dis 2006;42: 647–56.

33. Healy CM, Hulten KG, Palazzi DL, et al. Emergence of new strains of methicillin-resistant *Staphylococcus aureus* in a neonatal intensive care unit. Clin Infect Dis 2004;39:1460–6.

34. Patel M, Kumar RA, Stamm AM, et al. USA300 genotype community-associated methicillin-resistant *Staphylococcus aureus* as a cause of surgical site infections. J Clin Microbiol 2007;45:3431–3.

35. Invasive methicillin-resistant *Staphylococcus aureus* infections among dialysis patients— United States, 2005. MMWR Morb Mortal Wkly Rep 2007;56:197–9.

36. Maree C, Daum RS, Boyle-Vavra S, et al. Community-associated methicillin-resistant *Staphylococcus aureus* strains causing healthcare-associated infections. Emerging Infect Dis 2007;13:236–42.

37. Folden DV, Machayya JA, Sahmoun AE, et al. Estimating the proportion of community-associated methicillin-resistant *Staphylococcus aureus*: two definitions

used in the USA yield dramatically different estimates. J Hosp Infect 2005;60: 329–32.

38. David MZ, Glikman D, Crawford SE, et al. What is community-associated methicillin-resistant *Staphylococcus aureus*? J Infect Dis 2008;197:1235–43.

39. McCaig LF, McDonald LC, Mandal S, et al. *Staphylococcus aureus*-associated skin and soft tissue infections in ambulatory care. Emerging Infect Dis 2006; 12:1715–23.

40. Chambers HF. The changing epidemiology of *Staphylococcus aureus*? Emerging Infect Dis 2001;7:178–82.

41. Udo EE, Pearman JW, Grubb WB. Genetic analysis of community isolates of methicillin-resistant *Staphylococcus aureus* in Western Australia. J Hosp Infect 1993;25:97–108.

42. Maguire GP, Arthur AD, Boustead PJ, et al. Emerging epidemic of community-acquired methicillin-resistant *Staphylococcus aureus* infection in the Northern Territory. Med J Aust 1996;164:721–3.

43. Herold BC, Immergluck LC, Maranan MC, et al. Community-acquired methicillin-resistant *Staphylococcus aureus* in children with no identified predisposing risk. JAMA 1998;279:593–8.

44. Groom AV, Wolsey DH, Naimi TS, et al. Community-acquired methicillin-resistant *Staphylococcus aureus* in a rural American Indian community. JAMA 2001;286: 1201–5.

45. Fergie JE, Purcell K. Community-acquired methicillin-resistant *Staphylococcus aureus* infections in south Texas children. Pediatr Infect Dis J 2001;20:860–3.

46. Moran GJ, Amii RN, Abrahamian FM, et al. Methicillin-resistant *Staphylococcus aureus* in community-acquired skin infections. Emerging Infect Dis 2005;11: 928–30.

47. Kaplan SL, Hulten KG, Gonzalez BE, et al. Three-year surveillance of community-acquired *Staphylococcus aureus* infections in children. Clin Infect Dis 2005;40:1785–91.

48. Frazee BW, Lynn J, Charlebois ED, et al. High prevalence of methicillin-resistant *Staphylococcus aureus* in emergency department skin and soft tissue infections. Ann Emerg Med 2005;45:311–20.

49. Young DM, Harris HW, Charlebois ED, et al. An epidemic of methicillin-resistant *Staphylococcus aureus* soft tissue infections among medically underserved patients. Arch Surg 2004;139:947–51.

50. Moran GJ, Krishnadasan A, Gorwitz RJ, et al. Methicillin-resistant *S. aureus* infections among patients in the emergency department. N Engl J Med 2006; 355:666–74.

51. Outbreaks of community-associated methicillin-resistant *Staphylococcus aureus* skin infections—Los Angeles County, California, 2002–2003. MMWR Morb Mortal Wkly Rep 2003;52:88.

52. Pan E, Moss N, Haller B, et al. Dramatic increase in methicillin-resistant Staphylococcus aureus (MRSA) due to a predominant clone in county jails between 1996 and 2001. Abstract P491, 12th European Congress of Clinical Microbiology and Infectious Diseases. Clin Microbiol Infect 2002;8 (Supp 1).

53. Methicillin-resistant *Staphylococcus aureus* infections in correctional facilities—Georgia, California, and Texas, 2001–2003. MMWR Morb Mortal Wkly Rep 2003; 52:992–6.

54. Zinderman CE, Conner B, Malakooti MA, et al. Community-acquired methicillin-resistant *Staphylococcus aureus* among military recruits. Emerging Infect Dis 2004;10:941–4.

55. LaMar JE, Carr RB, Zinderman C, et al. Sentinel cases of community-acquired methicillin-resistant *Staphylococcus aureus* onboard a naval ship. Mil Med 2003;168:135–8.
56. Lee NE, Taylor MM, Bancroft E, et al. Risk factors for community-associated methicillin-resistant *Staphylococcus aureus* skin infections among HIV-positive men who have sex with men. Clin Infect Dis 2005;40:1529–34.
57. Giordano S. CDC investigates CA-MRSA infections in gay men. Bay Windows. 2003. Available at: http://www.baywindows.com/news/2003/04/03/National News/Cdc-Investigates.CaMrsa.Infections.In.Gay.Men-407469.shtml. Accessed March 23, 2004.
58. Allen JE. Skin infection spreads among gay men in L.A. Los Angeles: Los Angeles Times; 2003.
59. Pan ES, Diep BA, Charlebois ED, et al. Population dynamics of nasal strains of methicillin-resistant *Staphylococcus aureus*—and their relation to community-associated disease activity. J Infect Dis 2005;192:811–8.
60. Saiman L, O'Keefe M, Graham PL 3rd, et al. Hospital transmission of community-acquired methicillin-resistant *Staphylococcus aureus* among postpartum women. Clin Infect Dis 2003;37:1313–9.
61. Begier EM, Frenette K, Barrett NL, et al. A high-morbidity outbreak of methicillin-resistant *Staphylococcus aureus* among players on a college football team, facilitated by cosmetic body shaving and turf burns. Clin Infect Dis 2004;39: 1446–53.
62. Murray RJ, Lim TT, Pearson JC, et al. Community-onset methicillin-resistant *Staphylococcus aureus* bacteremia in Northern Australia. Int J Infect Dis 2004; 8:275–83.
63. Kerttula AM, Lyytikainen O, Salmenlinna S, et al. Changing epidemiology of methicillin-resistant *Staphylococcus aureus* in Finland. J Hosp Infect 2004;58: 109–14.
64. Ho PL, Tse CW, Mak GC, et al. Community-acquired methicillin-resistant *Staphylococcus aureus* arrives in Hong Kong. J Antimicrob Chemother 2004;54:845–6.
65. Nagaraju U, Bhat G, Kuruvila M, et al. Methicillin-resistant *Staphylococcus aureus* in community-acquired pyoderma. Int J Dermatol 2004;43:412–4.
66. Fang YH, Hsueh PR, Hu JJ, et al. Community-acquired methicillin-resistant *Staphylococcus aureus* in children in northern Taiwan. J Microbiol Immunol Infect 2004;37:29–34.
67. Dong SL, Kelly KD, Oland RC, et al. ED management of cellulitis: a review of five urban centers. Am J Emerg Med 2001;19:535–40.
68. Swartz MN, Pasternack MS. Cellulitis and superficial infections. In: Mandell GL, Bennett JE, Dolin R, editors. Principles and practice of infectious disease. 6th edition. vol. 1. Philadelphia: Elsevier; 2005. p. 1172–94.
69. Nguyen DM, Mascola L, Brancoft E. Recurring methicillin-resistant Staphylococcus aureus infections in a football team. Emerging Infect Dis 2005;11:526–32.
70. Methicillin-resistant *Staphylococcus aureus* infections among competitive sports participants—Colorado, Indiana, Pennsylvania, and Los Angeles County, 2000–2003. MMWR Morb Mortal Wkly Rep 2003;52:793–5.
71. Baggett HC, Hennessy TW, Rudolph K, et al. Community-onset methicillin-resistant *Staphylococcus aureus* associated with antibiotic use and the cytotoxin Panton-Valentine leukocidin during a furunculosis outbreak in rural Alaska. J Infect Dis 2004;189:1565–73.
72. Ragan P. Community-acquired MRSA infection: an update. JAAPA 2006;19: 24–9.

73. Coronado F, Nicholas JA, Wallace BJ, et al. Community-associated methicillin-resistant *Staphylococcus aureus* skin infections in a religious community. Epidemiol Infect 2006;135:492–501.
74. Ellis MW, Hospenthal DR, Dooley DP, et al. Natural history of community-acquired methicillin-resistant *Staphylococcus aureus* colonization and infection in soldiers. Clin Infect Dis 2004;39:971–9.
75. Miller LG, Matayoshi K, Spellberg B, et al. A prospective investigation of community-acquired methicillin resistant Staphylococcus aureus (CA-MRSA) risk factors in infected and non-infected patients. Abstract 1058, 43rd Annual Meeting of the Infectious Disease Society of America, San Francisco, 2005.
76. Sattler CA, Mason EO Jr, Kaplan SL. Prospective comparison of risk factors and demographic and clinical characteristics of community-acquired, methicillin-resistant versus methicillin-susceptible *Staphylococcus aureus* infection in children. Pediatr Infect Dis J 2002;21:910–7.
77. Naimi TS, LeDell KH, Boxrud DJ, et al. Epidemiology and clonality of community-acquired methicillin-resistant *Staphylococcus aureus* in Minnesota, 1996–1998. Clin Infect Dis 2001;33:990–6.
78. Adcock PM, Pastor P, Medley F, et al. Methicillin-resistant *Staphylococcus aureus* in two child care centers. J Infect Dis 1998;178:577–80.
79. Fridkin SK, Hageman JC, Morrison M, et al. Methicillin-resistant *Staphylococcus aureus* disease in three communities. N Engl J Med 2005;352:1436–44.
80. Charlebois ED, Perdreau-Remington F, Kreiswirth B, et al. Origins of community strains of methicillin-resistant *Staphylococcus aureus*. Clin Infect Dis 2004;39:47–54.
81. Huang H C M, Flynn N, et al. Injection drug user (IDU) and community associated methicillin-resistant Staphylococcus aureus (CA-MRSA) Infection in Sacramento. Abstract, 43rd Annual Meeting of the Infectious Disease Society of America, San Francisco, 2005.
82. Zafar U, Johnson LB, Hanna M, et al. Prevalence of nasal colonization among patients with community-associated methicillin-resistant *Staphylococcus aureus* infection and their household contacts. Infect Control Hosp Epidemiol 2007;28:966–9.
83. Adam H, McGeer A, Simor A. Fatal case of post-influenza, community-associated MRSA pneumonia in an Ontario teenager with subsequent familial transmission. Can Commun Dis Rep 2007;33:45–8.
84. Miller LG, Quan C, Shay A, et al. A prospective investigation of outcomes after hospital discharge for endemic, community-acquired methicillin-resistant and susceptible *Staphylococcus aureus* skin infection. Clin Infect Dis 2007;44:483–92.
85. Daum RS. Clinical practice. Skin and soft-tissue infections caused by methicillin-resistant *Staphylococcus aureus*. N Engl J Med 2007;357:380–90.
86. Buckingham SC, McDougal LK, Cathey LD, et al. Emergence of community-associated methicillin-resistant *Staphylococcus aureus* at a Memphis, Tennessee Children's Hospital. Pediatr Infect Dis J 2004;23:619–24.
87. Purcell K, Fergie JE. Exponential increase in community-acquired methicillin-resistant *Staphylococcus aureus* infections in South Texas children. Pediatr Infect Dis J 2002;21:988–9.
88. Abi-Hanna P, Frank AL, Quinn JP, et al. Clonal features of community-acquired methicillin-resistant *Staphylococcus aureus* in children. Clin Infect Dis 2000;30:630–1.
89. Davis SL, Perri MB, Donabedian SM, et al. Epidemiology and outcomes of community-associated methicillin-resistant *Staphylococcus aureus* infection. J Clin Microbiol 2007;45:1705–11.

90. Weigelt J, Itani K, Stevens D, et al. Linezolid versus vancomycin in treatment of complicated skin and soft tissue infections. Antimicrobial Agents Chemother 2005;49:2260–6.
91. Jauregui LE, Babazadeh S, Seltzer E, et al. Randomized, double-blind comparison of once-weekly dalbavancin versus twice-daily linezolid therapy for the treatment of complicated skin and skin structure infections. Clin Infect Dis 2005;41:1407–15.
92. Kaplan SL, Hulten KG, Hammerman WA, et al. Six-year surveillance of community-acquired Staphylococcus aureus infections in children. 45th Annual Meeting of the Infectious Diseases Society of America. San Diego (CA), 2007.
93. Voyich JM, Otto M, Mathema B, et al. Is Panton-Valentine leukocidin the major virulence determinant in community-associated methicillin-resistant *Staphylococcus aureus* disease? J Infect Dis 2006;194:1761–70.
94. Lee MC, Rios AM, Aten MF, et al. Management and outcome of children with skin and soft tissue abscesses caused by community-acquired methicillin-resistant *Staphylococcus aureus*. Pediatr Infect Dis J 2004;23:123–7.
95. Jungk J, Como-Sabetti K, Stinchfield P, et al. Epidemiology of methicillin-resistant *Staphylococcus aureus* at a pediatric healthcare system, 1991–2003. Pediatr Infect Dis J 2007;26:339–44.
96. Moazzez A, Kelso RL, Towfigh S, et al. Breast abscess bacteriologic features in the era of community-acquired methicillin-resistant *Staphylococcus aureus* epidemics. Arch Surg 2007;142:881–4.
97. Laibl VR, Sheffield JS, Roberts S, et al. Clinical presentation of community-acquired methicillin-resistant *Staphylococcus aureus* in pregnancy. Obstet Gynecol 2005;106:461–5.
98. Santos F, Mankarious LA, Eavey RD. Methicillin-resistant *Staphylococcus aureus*: pediatric otitis. Arch Otolaryngol. Head Neck Surg 2000;126:1383–5.
99. Thomason TS, Brenski A, McClay J, et al. The rising incidence of methicillin-resistant *Staphylococcus aureus* in pediatric neck abscesses. Otolaryngol Head Neck Surg 2007;137:459–64.
100. Ossowski K, Chun RH, Suskind D, et al. Increased isolation of methicillin-resistant *Staphylococcus aureus* in pediatric head and neck abscesses. Arch Otolaryngol Head Neck Surg 2006;132:1176–81.
101. Fleisch AF, Nolan S, Gerber J, et al. Methicillin-resistant *Staphylococcus aureus* as a cause of extensive retropharyngeal abscess in two infants. Pediatr Infect Dis J 2007;26:1161–3.
102. Bothwell NE, Shvidler J, Cable BB. Acute rise in methicillin-resistant *Staphylococcus aureus* infections in a coastal community. Otolaryngol Head Neck Surg 2007;137:942–6.
103. McKinley SH, Yen MT, Miller AM, et al. Microbiology of pediatric orbital cellulitis. Am J Ophthalmol 2007;144:497–501.
104. Blomquist PH. Methicillin-resistant *Staphylococcus aureus* infections of the eye and orbit (an American Ophthalmological Society thesis). Trans Am Ophthalmol Soc 2006;104:322–45.
105. Huang WH, Hung PK. Methicillin-resistant *Staphylococcus aureus* infections in acute rhinosinusitis. Laryngoscope 2006;116:288–91.
106. Germiller JA, Monin DL, Sparano AM, et al. Intracranial complications of sinusitis in children and adolescents and their outcomes. Arch Otolaryngol Head Neck Surg 2006;132:969–76.

107. Arnold SR, Elias D, Buckingham SC, et al. Changing patterns of acute hematogenous osteomyelitis and septic arthritis: emergence of community-associated methicillin-resistant *Staphylococcus aureus*. J Pediatr Orthop 2006;26:703–8.
108. Bocchini CE, Hulten KG, Mason EO Jr, et al. Panton-Valentine leukocidin genes are associated with enhanced inflammatory response and local disease in acute hematogenous *Staphylococcus aureus* osteomyelitis in children. Pediatrics 2006;117:433–40.
109. Martinez-Aguilar G, Avalos-Mishaan A, Hulten K, et al. Community-acquired, methicillin-resistant and methicillin-susceptible *Staphylococcus aureus* musculoskeletal infections in children. Pediatr Infect Dis J 2004;23:701–6.
110. McCaskill ML, Mason EO Jr, Kaplan SL, et al. Increase of the USA300 clone among community-acquired methicillin-susceptible *Staphylococcus aureus* causing invasive infections. Pediatr Infect Dis J 2007;26:1122–7.
111. Labandeira-Rey M, Couzon F, Boisset S, et al. *Staphylococcus aureus* Panton-Valentine leukocidin causes necrotizing pneumonia. Science 2007;315:1130–3.
112. Wardenburg JB, Patel RJ, Schneewind O. Surface proteins and exotoxins are required for the pathogenesis of *Staphylococcus aureus* pneumonia. Infect Immun 2007;75:1040–4.
113. Bubeck Wardenburg J, Schneewind O. Vaccine protection against *Staphylococcus aureus* pneumonia. J Exp Med 2008;205:287–94.
114. Gonzalez BE, Teruya J, Mahoney DH Jr, et al. Venous thrombosis associated with staphylococcal osteomyelitis in children. Pediatrics 2006;117:1673–9.
115. Crary SE, Buchanan GR, Drake CE, et al. Venous thrombosis and thromboembolism in children with osteomyelitis. J Pediatr 2006;149:537–41.
116. Nourse C, Starr M, Munckhof W. Community-acquired methicillin-resistant *Staphylococcus aureus* causes severe disseminated infection and deep venous thrombosis in children: literature review and recommendations for management. J Paediatr Child Health 2007;43:656–61.
117. Lew DP, Waldvogel FA. Osteomyelitis. Lancet 2004;364:369–79.
118. Lin MY, Rezai K, Schwartz DN. Septic Pulmonary emboli and bacteremia associated with deep tissue infections caused by community-acquired methicillin-resistant *Staphylococcus aureus*. J Clin Microbiol 2008;46:1553–5.
119. Gelfand MS, Cleveland KO. Hematogenous vertebral osteomyelitis due to *Staphylococcus aureus* in the adult. South Med J 2005;98:853.
120. Raad I, Narro J, Khan A, et al. Serious complications of vascular catheter-related *Staphylococcus aureus* bacteremia in cancer patients. Eur J Clin Microbiol Infect Dis 1992;11:675–82.
121. Ross JJ. Septic arthritis. Infect Dis Clin North Am 2005;19:799–817.
122. Ghanem GA, Boktour M, Warneke C, et al. Catheter-related *Staphylococcus aureus* bacteremia in cancer patients: high rate of complications with therapeutic implications. Medicine 2007;86:54–60 (Baltimore).
123. Klevens RM, Morrison MA, Nadle J, et al. Invasive methicillin-resistant *Staphylococcus aureus* infections in the United States. JAMA 2007;298:1763–71.
124. Pannaraj PS, Hulten KG, Gonzalez BE, et al. Infective pyomyositis and myositis in children in the era of community-acquired, methicillin-resistant *Staphylococcus aureus* infection. Clin Infect Dis 2006;43:953–60.
125. Trusen A, Beissert M, Schultz G, et al. Ultrasound and MRI features of pyomyositis in children. Eur Radiol 2003;13:1050–5.
126. Karmazyn B, Kleiman MB, Buckwalter K, et al. Acute pyomyositis of the pelvis: the spectrum of clinical presentations and MR findings. Pediatr Radiol 2006;36: 338–43.

127. Ruiz ME, Yohannes S, Wladyka CG. Pyomyositis caused by methicillin-resistant *Staphylococcus aureus*. N Engl J Med 2005;352:1488–9.
128. Sokolov KM, Kreye E, Miller LG, et al. Postpartum iliopsoas pyomyositis due to community-acquired methicillin-resistant *Staphylococcus aureus*. Obstet Gynecol 2007;110:535–8.
129. Miller LG, Perdreau-Remington F, Rieg G, et al. Necrotizing fasciitis caused by community-associated methicillin-resistant *Staphylococcus aureus* in Los Angeles. N Engl J Med 2005;352:1445–53.
130. Lee TC, Carrick MM, Scott BG, et al. Incidence and clinical characteristics of methicillin-resistant *Staphylococcus aureus* necrotizing fasciitis in a large urban hospital. Am J Surg 2007;194:809–12 [discussion 812–3].
131. Dehority W, Wang E, Vernon PS, et al. Community-associated methicillin-resistant *Staphylococcus aureus* necrotizing fasciitis in a neonate. Pediatr Infect Dis J 2006;25:1080–1.
132. Schultz KD, Fan LL, Pinsky J, et al. The changing face of pleural empyemas in children: epidemiology and management. Pediatrics 2004;113:1735–40.
133. Gonzalez BE, Hulten KG, Dishop MK, et al. Pulmonary manifestations in children with invasive community-acquired *Staphylococcus aureus* infection. Clin Infect Dis 2005;41:583–90.
134. Gonzalez BE, Martinez-Aguilar G, Hulten KG, et al. Severe staphylococcal sepsis in adolescents in the era of community-acquired methicillin-resistant *Staphylococcus aureus*. Pediatrics 2005;115:642–8.
135. Adem PV, Montgomery CP, Husain AN, et al. *Staphylococcus aureus* sepsis and the Waterhouse-Friderichsen syndrome in children. N Engl J Med 2005;353:1245–51.
136. Kravitz GR, Dries DJ, Peterson ML, et al. Purpura fulminans due to *Staphylococcus aureus*. Clin Infect Dis 2005;40:941–7.
137. Fowler VG Jr, Miro JM, Hoen B, et al. *Staphylococcus aureus* endocarditis: a consequence of medical progress. JAMA 2005;293:3012–21.
138. Crowley AL, Peterson GE, Benjamin DK Jr, et al. Venous thrombosis in patients with short- and long-term central venous catheter-associated *Staphylococcus aureus* bacteremia. Crit Care Med 2008;36:385–90.
139. Fowler VG Jr, Li J, Corey GR, et al. Role of echocardiography in evaluation of patients with *Staphylococcus aureus* bacteremia: experience in 103 patients. J Am Coll Cardiol 1997;30:1072–8.
140. Valente AM, Jain R, Scheurer M, et al. Frequency of infective endocarditis among infants and children with *Staphylococcus aureus* bacteremia. Pediatrics 2005;115:e15–9.
141. Fortunov RM, Hulten KG, Hammerman WA, et al. Community-acquired *Staphylococcus aureus* infections in term and near-term previously healthy neonates. Pediatrics 2006;118:874–81.
142. Fortunov RM, Hulten KG, Hammerman WA, et al. Evaluation and treatment of community-acquired *Staphylococcus aureus* infections in term and late-preterm previously healthy neonates. Pediatrics 2007;120:937–45.

Staphylococcal Surgical Site Infections

Deverick J. Anderson, MD, MPH[a],*, Keith S. Kaye, MD, MPH[b]

KEYWORDS

• Surgical site infection • Epidemiology
• Antimicrobial prophylaxis

Significant advances have been made in the field of surgery and infection control over the past 150 to 200 years. As medicine has advanced, however, new types of infection risks have developed. For example, over the past 50 years, the frequency of surgical procedures has increased, procedures have become more invasive, a greater proportion of operative procedures include insertion of foreign objects, and procedures are performed on an increasingly morbid patient population. As a result, surgical site infections (SSIs) and, in particular, SSIs caused by *Staphyloccus aureus* remain a leading cause of morbidity and mortality in modern health care.

EPIDEMIOLOGY AND OUTCOMES
Epidemiology

SSIs are a devastating and common complication of hospitalization, occurring in 2% to 5% of patients undergoing surgery in the United States.[1] As many as 15 million procedures are annually performed in the United States; thus, this translates into 300,000 to 500,000 SSIs each year.[2] SSI is the second most common type of health care–associated infection (HAI).[3]

S aureus is the most common cause of SSI. *S aureus* is the primary pathogen in 20% of SSIs among hospitals that report to the Centers for Disease control and Prevention (CDC) (**Table 1**)[4] and causes as many as 37% of SSIs that occur in community hospitals.[5] The prevalence of SSI caused by *S aureus* has been increasing over the past few decades. From 1992 to 2002, the proportion of SSIs caused by *S aureus* at hospitals reporting SSI data to the CDC increased from 16.6% to 30.9% among patients undergoing coronary artery bypass grafting (CABG), cholecystectomy, colectomy, and total hip replacement.[6] *S aureus* is also becoming increasingly resistant to antibiotics. According to CDC data, the proportion of SSIs caused by *S aureus* that were methicillin

[a] Division of Infectious Diseases, Duke University Medical Center, DUMC Box 3605, Durham, NC 27710, USA
[b] Division of Infectious Diseases, Duke University Medical Center, DUMC Box 3152, Durham, NC 27710, USA
* Corresponding author.
E-mail address: dja@duke.edu (D.J. Anderson).

Infect Dis Clin N Am 23 (2009) 53–72
doi:10.1016/j.idc.2008.10.004
0891-5520/08/$ – see front matter © 2009 Elsevier Inc. All rights reserved.

id.theclinics.com

Table 1 Ten most common pathogens in surgical site infections among hospitals that report to the Centers for Disease Control and Prevention[4,12]	
Pathogen	Percentage of Infections
Staphylococcus aureus	20
Coagulase-negative staphylococci	14
Enterococci	12
Pseudomonas aeruginosa	8
Escherichia coli	8
Enterobacter species	7
Proteus mirabilis	3
Streptococci	3
Klebsiella pneumoniae	3
Candida albicans	2

resistant (MRSA) increased from 9% to 49% from 1992 to 2002.[6] MRSA is not only a common pathogen in tertiary care and academic institutions; in fact, MRSA has emerged as the single most common SSI pathogen in community hospitals.[5]

Outcomes

SSIs lead to increased duration of hospitalization, financial cost, and mortality. Each SSI leads to 7 to 10 additional postoperative hospital days.[2,7] The published costs attributable to SSI have varied widely, ranging from $3000 to $29,000 per patient per SSI.[8] Overall, SSI is believed to account for $1 billion to $10 billion in health care expenditure annually.[9-11] SSI increases mortality risk 2 to 11 fold.[10] Moreover, 77% of deaths in patients with SSI are attributed directly to the SSI.[12]

SSIs caused by S aureus are associated with particularly severe patient outcomes. Patients with any type of postoperative S aureus infection are at risk for adverse outcomes including 2 weeks of additional hospitalization, more than $49,000 of attributable extra costs, and a 5% increase in mortality.[13] For example, one case-control study comparing elderly patients with SSI caused by S aureus against uninfected elderly surgical patients demonstrated that patients with SSI caused by S aureus were at five times increased risk of death, had 2 weeks of additional hospitalization, and had an excess of $41,000 of attributable charges per SSI.[14] In an another study comparing 121 patients with SSI caused by MRSA to 193 uninfected postoperative control patients, patients with SSI caused by MRSA had more than an 11-fold increase in mortality, $29,000 of additional attributable costs, and approximately 2 extra weeks of hospitalization.[9]

Patients with infections caused by MRSA have worse outcomes and accumulate more hospital costs than patients with infections caused by methicillin-susceptible S aureus (MSSA).[15,16] A study comparing 127 patients with SSI caused by MRSA to 173 patients with SSI caused by MSSA demonstrated that patients with SSI caused by MRSA had 3.4 times higher mortality rates and $13,900 per SSI higher costs than patients with SSI caused by MSSA.[9] A cohort study of 441 SSIs caused by gram-positive bacteria reported that patients with SSI caused by MRSA had almost 50 days of additional hospitalization than patients with SSI caused by MSSA (71.9 days versus 26.6 days; $P < .05$).[17] Finally, another study examining the attributable impact of methicillin-resistance in patients undergoing cardiothoracic surgery demonstrated that patients with mediastinitis caused by MRSA had approximately five times higher rates of mortality at 1 year compared with patients with mediastinitis caused by MSSA (74% versus 16%, $P = .04$).[18]

DIAGNOSIS

Most SSIs that do not involve implants are diagnosable within 21days of surgery.[19] The CDC's National Nosocomial Infection Surveillance System (NNIS) has developed standardized surveillance criteria for defining SSIs that are widely used.[20] SSIs are classified as either incisional or organ/space (**Fig. 1**). Incisional SSIs are further classified into superficial (involving only skin or subcutaneous tissue of the incision) or deep (involving fascia and/or muscular layers). Organ/space SSIs include infections in any other anatomic site that was opened or manipulated during surgery. Definitions used for diagnosis of SSI are described in **Box 1**. For all classifications, infection is defined as occurring within 30 days after the operation if no implant was placed or within 1 year if an implant was placed and the infection is related to the incision. NNIS defines "implant" as a nonhuman-derived implantable foreign body (eg, prosthetic heart valve, nonhuman vascular graft, mechanical heart, or joint prosthesis) that is permanently placed in a patient.

Serum laboratory tests can be suggestive but not confirmatory for SSI. For example, basic hematologic abnormalities including increasing white blood cell count and neutrophil concentration are suggestive of infection. Leukocytosis of greater than 15,000/mm³ in the setting of hyponatremia (sodium < 135 mEq/L) is predictive of necrotizing soft tissue infection.[21] It is important to note that many SSIs occur without any hematologic or serologic laboratory abnormalities. Cultures, ideally obtained in the operative setting, should be sent to microbiology, on all suspected cases of deep and organ/space infections to guide therapy and determine the susceptibility of the infecting

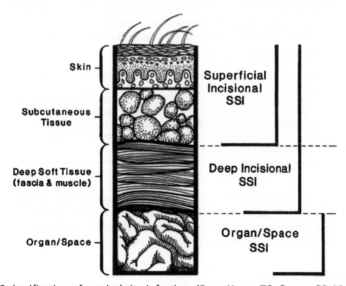

Fig. 1. CDC classification of surgical site infection. (*From* Horan TC, Gaynes RP, Martone WJ, et al. CDC definitions of nosocomial surgical site infections, 1992: a modification of CDC definitions of surgical wound infections. Infect Control Hosp Epidemiol 1992;13(10):606–8.)

Box 1
Criteria for defining a surgical site infection (SSI)

Incisional SSI

Superficial—infection involves skin or subcutaneous tissue of the incision *and* at least one of the following:

1. Purulent drainage, with or without laboratory confirmation, from the superficial incision.
2. Organisms isolated from an aseptically obtained culture from the superficial incision.
3. At least one of the following signs or symptoms: pain, localized swelling, erythema, or heat and superficial incision is deliberately opened by surgeon, unless incision is culture-negative.
4. Diagnosis of superficial incisional SSI by surgeon.

Deep—infection involves deep soft tissues (eg, fascial and muscle layers) of the incision *and* at least one of the following:

1. Purulent drainage from the deep incision, excluding organ/space.[a]
2. A deep incision that spontaneously dehisces or is deliberately opened by a surgeon when a patient has one or more of the following signs/symptoms: fever (>38°C), localized pain, unless site is culture-negative.
3. An abscess or other evidence of infection is found on direct examination, during repeat surgery, or by histopathologic or radiologic examination.
4. Diagnosis of a deep incisional SSI by surgeon.

Organ/Space SSI—infection involves any part of the anatomy (eg, organs or organ spaces) that was opened or manipulated during an operation and at least one of the following:

1. Purulent drainage from a drain that is placed through the stab wound into the organ/space.
2. Organisms isolated from an aseptically obtained culture from the organ/space.
3. An abscess or other evidence of infection involving organ/space that is found on examination (physical, histopathologic, or radiologic) or during repeat surgery.
4. Diagnosis of an organ/space SSI by surgeon.

[a] Report infection that involves both superficial and deep incision sites as a deep incisional SSI.
[b] Report an organ/space SSI that drains through the incision as a deep incisional SSI.
Adapted from Horan TC, Gaynes RP, Martone WJ, et al. CDC definitions of nosocomial surgical site infections, 1992: a modification of CDC definitions of surgical wound infections. Infect Control Hosp Epidemiol 1992;13(10):606–8. For all classifications, infection is defined as occurring within 30 days after the operation if no implant is placed or within 1 year if an implant is in place and the infection is related to the incision.

---

organism. *S aureus* cultured from a postoperative wound should not be considered to be a contaminant. Radiographic studies may be adjunctive for the diagnosis of SSI. Computed tomography (CT) is more reliable than plain radiographs for the detection of free air in soft tissue and the presence of deep abscess.

PATHOGENESIS OF INFECTION

The likelihood that an SSI will occur is a complex relationship between (1) microbial characteristics (eg, degree of contamination, virulence of pathogen), (2) patient characteristics (eg, immune status, diabetes), and (3) surgical characteristics (eg, introduction of foreign material, amount of damage to tissues).

Endogenous Contamination

The period of greatest risk for infection is from the time of incision to the time of wound closure.[11] Thus, gram-positive cocci from patients' endogenous flora at or near the site of surgery remain the leading cause of SSI.[22] Twenty percent of bacterial skin flora reside in skin appendages such as sebaceous glands, hair follicles, and sweat glands.[23] Thus, modern methods of pre- and perioperative antisepsis can reduce but not eliminate contamination of the surgical site by endogenous skin flora of the surgical patient. Inoculation of the surgical site by endogenous flora from remote sites of the patient may also occur infrequently. Experiments using albumin microspheres as tracer particles revealed that 100% of surgical wounds are contaminated with particles (skin squames) from sites from the surgical patient (eg, head, groin) that are distant in location to the surgical wound.[24] Finally, postsurgical inoculation of the surgical site secondary to a remote focus of infection (such as S aureus pneumonia) is an even less frequent cause of SSI.[25]

Exogenous Contamination

Exogenous sources of contamination, including colonized or infected surgical personnel, the operating room environment, and surgical instruments, are occasionally implicated in the pathogenesis of SSI. Infections caused by exogenous sources most commonly occur sporadically, but several exogenous point source outbreaks have been reported.[26–30]

Surgical personnel colonized with S aureus are occasionally identified as sources of S aureus causing SSI. One outbreak of SSIs caused by S aureus was described in pediatric patients. Three of four infection strains were identical by pulsed field gel electrophoresis (PFGE). None of the children were colonized with the epidemic strain, but approximately 25% of operating room personnel were colonized.[31] Another outbreak of SSIs caused by S aureus in patients admitted to a surgical intensive care unit involved a "cloud person" as an exogenous disseminator of S aureus.[32] One surgical resident who had a persistent upper respiratory tract infection during the epidemic was found to be colonized with the epidemic strain. Further experimentation revealed that large amounts of colony-forming units (CFUs) of S aureus were released into the air as a result of rhinoviral infection.[32] It is important to note, however, that the vast majority of SSIs caused by S aureus are not contracted from exogenous sources.

Burden of Inoculation

While many other factors contribute to the risk of SSI, the burden of pathogens inoculated into a surgical wound intraoperatively remains one of the most accepted risk factors. Simply, the greater the degree of surgical wound contamination, the higher the risk for infection. In the setting of appropriate antimicrobial prophylaxis, wound contamination with greater than 10^5 microorganisms is required to cause SSI.[33,34]

When foreign bodies are present, the bacterial inoculum required to cause SSI may be much lower.[35] For example, studies involving foreign bodies demonstrated that the presence of surgical sutures decreases the required inoculum for S aureus SSI by four logs (from 10^6 to 10^2 organisms).[36] Other models have demonstrated that the minimum inoculum for S aureus SSI is as few as 10 CFUs in the presence of polytetrafluoroethylene vascular grafts[37] and 1 CFU in the proximity of dextran beads.[38]

Virulence Factors of Staphylococcus aureus

S aureus has intrinsic virulence factors that enhance its ability to cause infection. For example, S aureus possesses microbial surface components recognizing adhesive matrix molecules (MSCRAMMs) that allow improved adhesion to extracellular matrix proteins such as collagen, fibrin, and fibronectin.[38,39] S aureus also has the ability to produce a biofilm rich in glycocalyx that shields the organism from most antimicrobial agents and the innate immune system.[40] S aureus is also shielded from the immune system by its polysaccharide capsule that inhibits opsonization and phagocytosis by host leukocytes.[41]

Once firmly entrenched in the wound, S aureus produces exotoxins that lead to host tissue damage,[42] interfere with leukocyte phagocytosis,[43] and alter cellular metabolism.[44] One notable S aureus exotoxin is coagulase, which creates a fibrin-rich environment in the wound by activating the coagulation protein cascade.[45] Another exotoxin that has gained recent notoriety in so-called "community-associated" strains is Panton-Valentine leukocidin (PVL), a potent inhibitor of human leukocytes. S aureus also possesses important endotoxins that stimulate host responses. The best example of an S aureus endotoxin is peptidoglycan, a major component of gram-positive bacterial cell walls. Peptidoglycan activates immune cells through Toll-like receptor and nucleotide-binding oligomerization domain[46,47] resulting in release of tumor necrosis factor-A, interleukin-1B, and interleukin-6.[48]

Antimicrobial resistance sometimes plays an important role in SSI pathogenesis. Some strains of S aureus harbor the type A variant of staphylococcal β-lactamase, which degrades less stable cephalosporins such as cefazolin, an agent commonly used for perioperative antimicrobial prophylaxis.[49] Animal models have demonstrated that the number of CFUs required to cause SSIs is significantly smaller in strains that harbor the type A β-lactamase compared with non-β-lactamase–producing strains of S aureus.[50]

The emergence of MRSA as the primary cause of SSI is concerning. Currently, standard recommended antimicrobial prophylaxis strategies do not include antimicrobial agents with activity against MRSA. This gap in MRSA coverage in standard prophylactic regimens is particularly concerning given the poor outcomes of patients with SSI caused by MRSA.[9]

RISK FACTORS

Most risk factors for SSI pertain to all pathogens and are not specific for S aureus. Risk factors for SSI typically are separated into patient-related (preoperative), procedure-related (perioperative), and postoperative categories (see **Table 2**).

In general patient-related risk factors for the development of SSI can be categorized as either unmodifiable or modifiable. One unmodifiable risk factor is age. In a recent cohort study of more than 144,000 patients, increasing age independently predicted an increased risk of SSI until age 65 years, but at ages 65 years and older, increasing age independently predicted a decreased risk of SSI.[51] The authors hypothesized that decreased risk of SSI in patients older than 65 years of age might represent a surgical patient selection bias or a "hardy survivor" effect. Modifiable risk factors include poorly controlled diabetes mellitus,[52] obesity,[53] tobacco use,[54,55] use of immunosuppressive medications,[56] and length of preoperative hospitalization.[11]

Procedure-related, perioperative risk factors include wound class (clean, clean-contaminated, contaminated, or dirty and infected),[57] length of surgery,[58] shaving of hair,[59,60] hypoxia,[61,62] and hypothermia.[63] In fact, the act of surgery itself leads to increased risk of infection. For example, the microbicidal activity of neutrophils harvested after surgery is 25% less than neutrophils harvested before surgery.[64] Additionally, neutrophils are affected by hypothermia induced by anesthetics. More specifically, neutrophils exhibit reduced chemotaxis and diminished superoxide production in the setting of perioperative hypothermia.[65] Finally, specific recommendations are available regarding personnel (traffic in the operating room) and operating room parameters (ventilation) to reduce the risk of exogenous seeding of the surgical wound as a result of personnel in and around the operating room.[12,66] In general, the degree of microbial contamination of the operating room air is directly proportional to the number of people in the room;[67] thus, traffic in and out of the room should be limited as much as possible.

Several risk factors that occur during the perioperative period (eg, glucose control, oxygenation, hypothermia) remain important during the immediate postoperative period. Diabetes mellitus and postoperative hyperglycemia are both clearly associated with increased risk of SSI.[52,68] Hyperglycemia leads to decreased host immune response by impairing the function of neutrophils and mononuclear phagocytes. In a retrospective study of 8910 patients undergoing cardiac surgery, rates of SSI decreased substantially after implementing an intensive intravenous insulin regimen to maintain postoperative glucose at less than 200 mg/dL for the first 48 hours after surgery.[52] As a result, aggressive postoperative glucose control is now standard of care for patients undergoing cardiac surgery. In contrast, strict glucose control in the intraoperative period has not been shown to decrease the risk of SSI and may actually lead to harm.[69]

Two additional risk variables that are present exclusively in the postoperative period are wound care and postoperative blood transfusions. Postoperative wound care is determined by the technique used for closure of the surgical site. Most wounds are closed primarily (ie, skin edges are approximated with sutures or staples) and these wounds should be kept clean by covering with a sterile dressing for 24 to 48 hours after surgery.[70] Finally, a meta-analysis of 20 studies of the associated risk of SSI following receipt of blood products demonstrated that patients who received even a single unit of blood in the immediate postoperative period were at increased risk for SSI (odds ratio [OR] = 3.45).[71]

Despite the increasing incidence of methicillin resistance among S aureus isolates and the emergence of MRSA as a leading cause of SSI, few studies have specifically examined risk factors for SSI caused by MRSA. In a prospective survey of 1757 surgical patients in Australia, patients with SSI caused by MRSA had longer lengths of preoperative hospitalization and higher rates of cancer compared with patients with SSI caused by MSSA and more often had wound drains and multiple operations compared with patients with SSI caused by other pathogens.[72] A recent case-control study comparing 77 patients with SSI caused by MRSA to 193 patients with SSI caused by other types of pathogens demonstrated that discharge to a long-term care facility and duration of postoperative antibiotic therapy of more than 1 day were significantly associated with SSI caused by MRSA.[73] Another case-control study that compared 64 patients with mediastinitis caused by MRSA to 80 uninfected cardiothoracic surgical patients identified diabetes (adjusted OR = 2.86), female sex (adjusted OR = 2.70), and age older than 70 years (adjusted OR = 3.43) as independent predictors of postoperative mediastinitis caused by MRSA.[74] Finally, a recent study of 150 patients with SSI caused by MRSA demonstrated that patients who required assistance with activities of daily living (ADLs) were at two- to fourfold higher risk of developing SSI caused by MRSA than were either uninfected patients or patients with SSI caused by MSSA.[75]

Table 2
Risk factors for and current recommendations to decrease the risk of surgical site infection

Risk Factor	Recommendation
Intrinsic, patient-related (Preoperative)	
Age	No formal recommendation: relationship to increased risk of SSI may be secondary to comorbidities or immunosenescence[51,58,116]
Glucose control, diabetes mellitus	Control serum blood glucose levels[117]
Obesity	Increase dosing of perioperative antimicrobial agent for morbidly obese patients[118]
Smoking cessation	Encourage smoking cessation within 30 days of procedure[117]
Immunosuppressive medications	No formal recommendation;[117] in general, avoid immunosuppressive medications in perioperative period if possible
Nutrition	Do not delay surgery to enhance nutritional support[117]
Remote sites of infection	Identify and treat all remote infections before elective procedures[117]
Preoperative hospitalization	Keep preoperative stay as short as possible[117]
Extrinsic, procedure-related (Perioperative)	
Preparation of patient	
Hair removal	Do not remove unless presence of hair will interfere with the operation;[117] if hair removal is necessary, remove by clipping and do not shave
Skin preparation	Wash and clean skin around incision site[117]
Chlorhexidine nasal and oropharyngeal rinse	No formal recommendation in most recent guidelines;[117] recent RCT of cardiac surgeries showed decreased incidence of postoperative nosocomial infections[98]
Surgical scrub (surgeon hands and forearms)	Use appropriate antiseptic agent to perform 2- to 5-minute preoperative surgical scrub[117]
Incision site	Use appropriate antiseptic agent[117]
Antimicrobial prophylaxis	Administer only when indicated[117]
Timing	Administer within 1 hour of incision to maximize tissue concentration[117]**
Choice	Select appropriate agents based on surgical procedure, most common pathogens causing SSI for a specific procedure, and published recommendations[117]
Duration of therapy	Stop agent within 24 hours after the procedure[87,117]
Surgeon skill/technique	Handle tissue carefully and eradicate dead space[117]
Incision time	No formal recommendation in most recent guidelines;[117] minimize as much as possible[119]
Maintain oxygenation with supplemental O_2	No formal recommendation in most recent guidelines;[117] RCTs have reported conflicting results in colorectal procedures[61,62,120]
Maintain normothermia	Avoid hypothermia in surgical patients whenever possible by actively warming the patient to > 36°C, particularly in colorectal surgery[121]

(continued on next page)

Table 2 (continued)	
Risk Factor	Recommendation
Operating room characteristic	
Ventilation	Follow American Institute of Architects' recommendations[66,117]
Traffic	Minimize operating room traffic[117]
Environmental surfaces	Use an Environmental Protection Agency–approved hospital disinfectant to clean visibly soiled or contaminated surfaces and equipment[117]

Abbreviations: RCT, randomized controlled trial; SSI, surgical site infection.

PREVENTION

An important component of improving outcomes of surgical patients is addressing all modifiable risk factors for SSI described previously during the perioperative period. Few interventions, however, are supported by data from randomized-controlled trials and even less data are available regarding risk factor modifications that specifically prevent SSI caused by *S aureus*. **Table 2** summarizes important risk factors and current guidelines for addressing each risk factor to decrease the risk of SSI. In particular, emphasis has recently been placed on the importance of perioperative antimicrobial prophylaxis and process measures.

Perioperative Antimicrobial Prophylaxis

The goal of surgical antimicrobial prophylaxis is to reduce the concentration of potential pathogens at or in close proximity to the surgical incision. The appropriate use of perioperative antimicrobial prophylaxis is a well-proven intervention to reduce the risk of SSI in elective procedures.[12,34,76] Four main principles override prophylactic antimicrobial use: (1) use antimicrobial prophylaxis for all elective operations that require entry into a hollow viscus (ie, clean-contaminated and contaminated procedures), operations that involve insertion of an intravascular prosthetic device or prosthetic joint, or operations in which an SSI would pose catastrophic risk;[77–80] (2) use antimicrobial agents that are safe, cost-effective, and bactericidal against expected pathogens for specific surgical procedures;[12] (3) time the infusion so that a bactericidal concentration of the agent is present in tissue and serum at the time of incision;[76] and (4) maintain therapeutic levels of the agent in tissue and serum throughout the entire operation (ie, until wound closure).[78,81,82] Thus, two important components of appropriate perioperative antimicrobial prophylaxis are using the correct agent at the correct dose and giving the agent at the correct time.

Administering antimicrobial prophylaxis shortly before incision reduces the rate of SSI.[76] The chosen agent should be given at a time that allows for maximum tissue concentration at the time of incision. The optimal administration time typically occurs within 1 to 2 hours before surgery, although some agents (eg, cefazolin) may be given within 30 minutes before incision.[83] In a retrospective study of approximately 3000 patients undergoing inpatient elective procedures, the lowest rates of infection occurred in the group of patients who received antimicrobial prophylaxis within 1 hour before incision.[76] If a procedure is expected to last several hours, prophylactic agents should be re-dosed intraoperatively.[12] For example, cefazolin should be re-infused if a procedure lasts longer than 3 to 4 hours.

Although not directly related to prevention of SSI, an additional measure related to perioperative surgical prophylaxis is the number of doses administered. Single-dose antimicrobial prophylaxis is equivalent to multiple perioperative doses for the prevention of SSI. A meta-analysis of over 40 studies comparing single doses of parenteral antimicrobials to placebo or multiple doses in hysterectomies; cesarean sections; colorectal procedures; gastric, biliary, and transurethral operations; and cardiothoracic procedures demonstrated that administering multiple doses of antibiotics provided no benefit over a single dose.[84] A more recent systematic review of 28 prospective, randomized studies comparing single versus multiple doses of perioperative antimicrobials also concluded that there was no additional benefit of more than a single prophylactic dose.[81] As a result, current recommendations state that prophylactic antibiotics should not be given for longer than 24 hours after surgery. Finally, prolongation of antimicrobial therapy beyond 24 hours may be harmful. Prolonged prophylaxis increases the risk of infections unrelated to the surgical site, increases the emergence of multidrug-resistant organisms, and may lead to *Clostridium difficile*–associated disease.[85]

Quality Improvement Programs and Process Measures to Decrease the Risk of Surgical Site Infections

The Centers for Medicare and Medicaid Services created the Surgical Infection Prevention Project (SIP) in 2002. After review of published guidelines, an expert panel identified three performance measures related to antimicrobial prophylaxis for quality improvement: delivery of intravenous antimicrobial prophylaxis within 1 hour before incision (2 hours are allowed for the administration of vancomycin and fluoroquinolones), use of an antimicrobial prophylactic agent consistent with published guidelines, and discontinuation of the prophylactic antimicrobial agent within 24 hours after surgery (discontinuation at 48 hours is allowable for cardiothoracic procedures).[86,87] SIP focuses on seven procedures: abdominal hysterectomy, vaginal hysterectomy, hip arthroplasty, knee arthroplasty, cardiothoracic surgery, vascular surgery, and colorectal surgery. SIP allows for the use of vancomycin for prophylaxis in cardiac, vascular, and orthopedic surgery if there is a documented reason (such as history of colonization with MRSA) in the medical record or a documented beta-lactam allergy. Many hospitals that implemented and improved compliance with SIP performance measures decreased their rates of SSI.[88]

The Surgical Care Improvement Project (SCIP) is a multiagency collaboration created in 2003 that essentially has become an extension of SIP. In addition to the three performance measures of SIP, SCIP also places focus on three additional evidence-supported process measures to prevent SSI: proper hair removal, controlling blood glucose during the immediate postoperative period for cardiac patients, and maintenance of perioperative normothermia in colorectal surgical patients (see preceding sections).[86]

The Institute for Healthcare Improvement (IHI) has created a nationwide quality improvement project to improve outcomes in hospitalized patients.[89] The IHI recommends the same six preventive measures recommended by the SCIP and has assembled the measures into a cohesive educational "bundle" that has been implemented across the United States.[89] In addition, the IHI has created an educational bundle to prevent the spread of MRSA in hospitals.

CONTROVERSIES IN PREVENTION OF SURGICAL SITE INFECTION CAUSED BY *STAPHYLOCOCCUS AUREUS*

Preoperative colonization with *S aureus* is strongly associated with an increased risk of SSI.[90,91] As a result, many studies have examined methods to decrease the burden of *S aureus* and, in some instances, MRSA, before surgery. Unfortunately, little data support preoperative bathing, the routine use of intranasal mupirocin for decolonization, or the routine use of vancomycin for surgical antimicrobial prophylaxis. Thus, these topics remain controversial and unresolved.

Preoperative Bathing

Showering or bathing with an antiseptic agent such as chlorhexidine, povidone-iodine, or triclorcarban-medicated soap decreases the amount of endogenous microbial flora on the skin.[92,93] Chlorhexidine, however, requires several applications for maximum microbial-reducing benefit.[94] Despite the proven reduction in preoperative microbial burden, this intervention has not yet been clearly demonstrated to lower rates of SSI in clinical trials.[95–97] In fact, a prospective, randomized-controlled, double-blinded trial comparing preoperative showers with soap containing chlorhexidine to preoperative showers with nonmedicated soap in 1400 patients found no significant difference in infection rates between the two groups.[95]

Decolonization of Staphylococcus aureus Carriage

Studies examining the utility of preoperative *S aureus* nasal decolonization with antimicrobial agents have produced inconsistent results. A recent randomized-controlled trial examined the utility of oral and nasal rinses with chlorhexidine gluconate (0.12%) before cardiothoracic surgery for the prevention of postoperative nosocomial infections.[98] Although the overall number of SSIs was not different in the two groups, the number of deep SSIs was significantly decreased in the chlorhexidine group (1.9% versus 5.2%, $P = .002$). Given the proven benefit, low toxicity, and lack of emerging resistance in long-term clinical studies of chlorhexidine,[99] preoperative treatment with chlorhexidine represents a promising intervention for the prevention of SSIs, particularly among cardiothoracic surgery patients. Unfortunately, this specific formulation is not available in the United States.

Studies examining the efficacy of decolonization of *S aureus* with mupirocin have generally shown that mupirocin is effective at decolonization, but the impact on SSI remains unclear. Studies have generally been underpowered to determine if *S aureus* infection is prevented by preoperative decolonization with mupirocin. One study reported that, regardless of *S aureus* carrier status, the preoperative application of mupirocin to the nares of operative patients led to a 67% decrease in the rate of SSI compared with historical controls following cardiothoracic surgery (from 7.3% to 2.8%).[100] A separate analysis of 854 consecutive cardiothoracic patients who received intranasal mupirocin compared with 992 consecutive cardiothoracic patients who did not receive intranasal mupirocin showed that the overall rate of SSI was lower in the mupirocin group (2.7% versus 0.9%, $P = .005$).[99] These findings, however, were not fully corroborated in a recent double-blinded randomized-controlled trial in which 1933 surgical patients randomized to receive preoperative mupirocin were compared with 1931 randomized to placebo.[101] Treatment with mupirocin led to lower rates of *S aureus* colonization and lower rates of overall postoperative nosocomial infections caused by *S aureus* (3.8% versus 7.6%, $P = .02$), but did not lead to a significant decrease in the rate of SSI caused by *S aureus* (3.6% versus 5.8%, OR = 2.9 [95% confidence interval, 0.8–3.4]).[101]

Unfortunately, *S aureus* resistance to mupirocin has rapidly emerged in some institutions.[102] For example, extensive use of mupirocin correlated with an increase in resistance to mupirocin among *S aureus* strains from 2.7% to 65.0% over a 4-year period in one European institution.[103] The emergence of mupirocin resistance is concerning and can negate the efficacy of preoperative decolonization.

Antimicrobial Prophylaxis with Vancomycin

Even though MRSA has emerged as the leading cause of SSI, the routine use of vancomycin for antimicrobial prophylaxis is not widely recommended.[104] A recent meta-analysis of seven studies comparing glycopeptides to beta-lactam antimicrobial prophylaxis before cardiothoracic surgery showed that there was no difference in rates of SSI between the two classes of antibiotics, supporting the view that beta-lactam antibiotics should remain the agents of choice.[105] Instead, the use of vancomycin should be reserved for specific clinical circumstances, such as during a proven outbreak of SSI caused by MRSA, if there is a "high" prevalence of MRSA in the hospital (note: there is no specific incidence of MRSA defined as "high"), or for patients who are identified to be at increased risk for SSI caused by MRSA (eg, prior history of MRSA infection or colonization).[74]

TREATMENT

Surgical opening of the incision with removal of necrotic tissue is the primary and most important aspect of therapy for many SSIs.[106] Deep incisional and organ/space infections almost universally require operative drainage of accumulated pus. Type of debridement and duration of postoperative antimicrobial therapy depend on the anatomic site of infection and invasiveness of the SSI. Antimicrobial therapy is an important adjunct to surgical debridement. A key consideration for both surgical and antimicrobial therapy is whether prosthetic material is infected.

According to expert opinion, postoperative patients with a temperature higher than 38.5°C or a heart rate greater than 110 beats/min generally require antibiotics in addition to opening of the suture line.[106] Few published data exist to support the use of specific agents or specific therapeutic durations for treatment of SSI caused by S aureus in the absence of infected prosthetic material. Decisions regarding the antimicrobial agent and length of therapy for SSI caused by S aureus are influenced by the location of the infection (eg, mediastinum, abdominal cavity, joint), the depth of infection, the adequacy or completeness of surgical debridement, and whether or not the S aureus pathogen is methicillin-resistant. As a rule of thumb, effective systemic antimicrobial therapy should be started as soon as a deep incisional or organ/space SSI is suspected. For example, in one study, patients with mediastinitis who received antimicrobial therapy active against the infecting pathogen within 7 days of debridement had a 60% reduction in mortality rates compared with patients who did not receive effective antimicrobial therapy.[107] First-generation cephalosporins and antistaphylococcal penicillins are frequently used for antimicrobial treatment of SSI caused by MSSA.[108] Patients with SSI caused by MRSA have traditionally been treated with vancomycin.[106]

Other agents with activity against MRSA, including linezolid, daptomycin, and tigecycline, have received Food and Drug Administration (FDA) indications for treatment of complicated skin and skin structure infections and, thus, represent alternatives to vancomycin for the treatment of SSI caused by MRSA. A recent subset analysis of a prospective, randomized controlled trial comparing linezolid to vancomycin for the treatment of skin and soft tissue infections focused exclusively on patients with SSI.[109] Linezolid and vancomycin were equivalent with respect to clinical resolution of symptoms of SSI. Patients receiving linezolid, however, had higher rates of microbial cure 7 days after initiation of therapy compared with vancomycin (84% versus 58%, $P = .007$); among patients with SSI caused by MRSA, the difference in microbial cure was even more pronounced (87% versus 48%, $P = .002$).[109] If linezolid therapy is administered for longer than 2 weeks, weekly hematological monitoring should be performed to screen for linezolid-associated thrombocytopenia.[110] Prolonged courses of linezolid can also cause neuropathy.

Both daptomycin and tigecycline have FDA indications for skin and soft tissue infections, but data on SSI are lacking. In a large randomized controlled study, daptomycin compared favorably to vancomycin for the treatment of complicated skin and skin structure infections. Data were not, however, specifically provided for the efficacy of daptomycin for SSI caused by S aureus.[111] Two randomized controlled trials compared tigecycline to the combination of vancomycin and aztreonam for the treatment of complicated skin and skin structure infections.[112] Overall, tigecycline was equivalent to the combination of vancomycin and aztreonam for the treatment of complicated skin and skin structure infections, but no data were presented on the efficacy of tigecycline specifically for the treatment of SSI.

Prosthetic joint infection caused by S aureus is a unique problem that usually requires surgical debridement and prolonged antimicrobial therapy. The choice of surgical modalities is a matter of clinical judgment that may be influenced by the operative findings, the skill or experience of individual surgeons, and/or the clinical stability of the patient. Surgical treatment for prosthetic joint infection includes the following different strategies: debridement with retention of the prosthesis, one- or two-stage exchange with reimplantation, resection arthroplasty, and amputation.[113] In all strategies, debridement is a critical component, as removal of foreign materials such as wires, bone wax, and devitalized tissues greatly improves the likelihood of cure.[114] Traditionally, a two-stage exchange has been the standard treatment modality used to cure an infected prosthesis. Two-stage exchange involves debridement and removal of the infected prosthesis, followed by prolonged antimicrobial therapy (often up to 6 to 8 weeks) and, finally, reimplantation of a new prosthesis. One-stage exchange involves debridement, removal of the prosthetic joint, and immediate reimplantation of a new prosthesis. In some cases of SSI caused by S aureus, the infected prosthesis can be salvaged through the combination of early surgical debridement in combination with effective antimicrobial therapy.[115] The likelihood of successful salvage of an infected prosthesis is improved if the following conditions are met: signs and symptoms of prosthetic joint infection with S aureus are detected within 3 weeks of implantation, the implant remains stable and functional, the surrounding soft tissue remains in good condition, and the patient is treated with appropriate systemic antimicrobials.[113] Antimicrobial therapy for SSIs caused by S aureus that involve prosthetic material is generally similar to therapy used for infections not involving prostheses. Patients with prosthetic joint infection caused by S aureus should undergo 6 to 8 weeks of intravenous antimicrobial therapy after explantation of the infected prosthesis before reimplantation.[113]

SUMMARY

SSI caused by S aureus is a major problem in the modern health care system and accounts for an increasing amount of health care resource expenditure, patient suffering, and death. In particular, SSI caused by MRSA has emerged as the leading cause of SSI in both tertiary and community hospitals. To prevent SSI caused by S aureus, improved adherence to evidence-based preventative measures and the development and implementation of novel approaches to SSI prevention are needed. In general, aggressive surgical debridement in combination with effective antimicrobial therapy are needed to optimize the treatment of SSI caused by S aureus.

REFERENCES

1. Graves HJ. National hospital discharge survey: annual summary 1987. Healthy People 2000 Stat Notes 1989;13:11.

2. Cruse P. Wound infection surveillance. Rev Infect Dis 1981;3(4):734–7.
3. Wenzel RP. Health care-associated infections: major issues in the early years of the 21st century. Clin Infect Dis 2007;45(Suppl 1):S85–8.
4. National Nosocomial Infections Surveillance (NNIS) report, data summary from October 1986–April 1996, issued May 1996. A report from the National Nosocomial Infections Surveillance (NNIS) System. Am J Infect Control 1996;24(5):380–8.
5. Anderson DJ, Sexton DJ, Kanafani ZA, et al. Severe surgical site infection in community hospitals: epidemiology, key procedures, and the changing prevalence of methicillin-resistant *Staphylococcus aureus*. Infect Control Hosp Epidemiol 2007;28(9):1047–53.
6. Jernigan JA. Is the burden of *Staphylococcus aureus* among patients with surgical-site infections growing? Infect Control Hosp Epidemiol 2004;25(6):457–60.
7. Cruse PJ, Foord R. The epidemiology of wound infection. A 10-year prospective study of 62,939 wounds. Surg Clin North Am 1980;60(1):27–40.
8. Anderson DJ, Kirkland KB, Kaye KS, et al. Underresourced hospital infection control and prevention programs: penny wise, pound foolish? Infect Control Hosp Epidemiol 2007;28(7):767–73.
9. Engemann JJ, Carmeli Y, Cosgrove SE, et al. Adverse clinical and economic outcomes attributable to methicillin resistance among patients with *Staphylococcus aureus* surgical site infection. Clin Infect Dis 2003;36(5):592–8.
10. Kirkland KB, Briggs JP, Trivette SL, et al. The impact of surgical-site infections in the 1990s: attributable mortality, excess length of hospitalization, and extra costs. Infect Control Hosp Epidemiol 1999;20(11):725–30.
11. Wong ES. Surgical site infections. In: Mayhall CG, editor. Hospital epidemiology and infection control. 3rd edition. Balitmore: Lippincott Williams and Wilkins; 2004.
12. Mangram AJ, Horan TC, Pearson ML, et al. Guideline for prevention of surgical site infection, 1999. Hospital Infection Control Practices Advisory Committee. Infect Control Hosp Epidemiol 1999;20(4):250–78, quiz 279–80.
13. Noskin GA, Rubin RJ, Schentag JJ, et al. The burden of *Staphylococcus aureus* infections on hospitals in the United States: an analysis of the 2000 and 2001 Nationwide Inpatient Sample Database. Arch Intern Med 2005;165(15):1756–61.
14. McGarry SA, Engemann JJ, Schmader K, et al. Surgical-site infection due to *Staphylococcus aureus* among elderly patients: mortality, duration of hospitalization, and cost. Infect Control Hosp Epidemiol 2004;25(6):461–7.
15. Cosgrove SE, Qi Y, Kaye KS, et al. The impact of methicillin resistance in *Staphylococcus aureus* bacteremia on patient outcomes: mortality, length of stay, and hospital charges. Infect Control Hosp Epidemiol 2005;26(2):166–74.
16. Cosgrove SE, Sakoulas G, Perencevich EN, et al. Comparison of mortality associated with methicillin-resistant and methicillin-susceptible *Staphylococcus aureus* bacteremia: a meta-analysis. Clin Infect Dis 2003;36(1):53–9.
17. Gleason TG, Crabtree TD, Pelletier SJ, et al. Prediction of poorer prognosis by infection with antibiotic-resistant gram-positive cocci than by infection with antibiotic-sensitive strains. Arch Surg 1999;134(10):1033–40.
18. Mekontso-Dessap A, Kirsch M, Brun-Buisson C, et al. Poststernotomy mediastinitis due to *Staphylococcus aureus*: comparison of methicillin-resistant and methicillin-susceptible cases. Clin Infect Dis 2001;32(6):877–83.
19. Sands K, Vineyard G, Platt R. Surgical site infections occurring after hospital discharge. J Infect Dis 1996;173(4):963–70.
20. Horan TC, Gaynes RP, Martone WJ, et al. CDC definitions of nosocomial surgical site infections, 1992: a modification of CDC definitions of surgical wound infections. Infect Control Hosp Epidemiol 1992;13(10):606–8.

21. Wall DB, Klein SR, Black S, et al. A simple model to help distinguish necrotizing fasciitis from nonnecrotizing soft tissue infection. J Am Coll Surg 2000;191(3):227–31.
22. Altemeier WA, Culbertson WR, Hummel RP. Surgical considerations of endogenous infections–sources, types, and methods of control. Surg Clin North Am 1968;48(1):227–40.
23. Tuazon CU. Skin and skin structure infections in the patient at risk: carrier state of Staphylococcus aureus. Am J Med 1984;76(5A):166–71.
24. Wiley AM, Ha'eri GB. Routes of infection. A study of using "tracer particles" in the orthopedic operating room. Clin Orthop Relat Res 1979;(139):150–5.
25. Edwards LD. The epidemiology of 2056 remote site infections and 1966 surgical wound infections occurring in 1865 patients: a four year study of 40,923 operations at Rush-Presbyterian-St. Luke's Hospital, Chicago. Ann Surg 1976;184(6):758–66.
26. Berkelman RL, Martin D, Graham DR, et al. Streptococcal wound infections caused by a vaginal carrier. JAMA 1982;247(19):2680–2.
27. Richet HM, Craven PC, Brown JM, et al. A cluster of Rhodococcus (Gordona) Bronchialis sternal-wound infections after coronary-artery bypass surgery. N Engl J Med 1991;324(2):104–9.
28. Lowry PW, Blankenship RJ, Gridley W, et al. A cluster of legionella sternal-wound infections due to postoperative topical exposure to contaminated tap water. N Engl J Med 1991;324(2):109–13.
29. Clegg HW, Foster MT, Sanders WE Jr, et al. Infection due to organisms of the Mycobacterium fortuitum complex after augmentation mammaplasty: clinical and epidemiologic features. J Infect Dis 1983;147(3):427–33.
30. Gartenberg G, Bottone EJ, Keusch GT, et al. Hospital-acquired mucormycosis (Rhizopus rhizopodiformis) of skin and subcutaneous tissue: epidemiology, mycology and treatment. N Engl J Med 1978;299(20):1115–8.
31. Weber S, Herwaldt LA, McNutt LA, et al. An outbreak of Staphylococcus aureus in a pediatric cardiothoracic surgery unit. Infect Control Hosp Epidemiol 2002; 23(2):77–81.
32. Sheretz RJ, Reagan DR, Hampton KD, et al. A cloud adult: the Staphylococcus aureus-virus interaction revisited. Ann Intern Med 1996;124(6):539–47.
33. Krizek TJ, Robson MC. Evolution of quantitative bacteriology in wound management. Am J Surg 1975;130(5):579–84.
34. Houang ET, Ahmet Z. Intraoperative wound contamination during abdominal hysterectomy. J Hosp Infect 1991;19(3):181–9.
35. James RC, Macleod CJ. Induction of staphylococcal infections in mice with small inocula introduced on sutures. Br J Exp Pathol 1961;42:266–77.
36. Elek SD, Conen PE. The virulence of Staphylococcus pyogenes for man: a study of the problems of wound infection. Br J Exp Pathol 1957;38(6):573–86.
37. Arbeit RD, Dunn RM. Expression of capsular polysaccharide during experimental focal infection with Staphylococcus aureus. J Infect Dis 1987; 156(6):947–52.
38. Froman G, Switalski LM, Speziale P, et al. Isolation and characterization of a fibronectin receptor from Staphylococcus aureus. J Biol Chem 1987; 262(14):6564–71.
39. Switalski LM, Patti JM, Butcher W, et al. A collagen receptor on Staphylococcus aureus strains isolated from patients with septic arthritis mediates adhesion to cartilage. Mol Microbiol 1993;7(1):99–107.
40. Mayberry-Carson KJ, Tober-Meyer B, Smith JK, et al. Bacterial adherence and glycocalyx formation in osteomyelitis experimentally induced with Staphylococcus aureus. Infect Immun 1984;43(3):825–33.

41. Kasper DL. Bacterial capsule—old dogmas and new tricks. J Infect Dis 1986; 153(3):407–15.
42. Rogolsky M. Nonenteric toxins of *Staphylococcus aureus.* Microbiol Rev 1979; 43(3):320–60.
43. Dossett JH, Kronvall G, Williams RC Jr, et al. Antiphagocytic effects of staphylococcal protein A. J Immunol 1969;103(6):1405–10.
44. Dellinger EP. Surgical infections and choice of antibiotics. In: Sabiston DC, editor. Textbook of surgery. 15th edition. Philadelphia: W.B. Saunders Co; 1997.
45. Kawabata S, Morita T, Iwanaga S, et al. Enzymatic properties of staphylothrombin, an active molecular complex formed between staphylocoagulase and human prothrombin. (Tokyo). J Biochem 1985;98(6):1603–14.
46. Aasen AO. The proenzyme functional inhibition index. A new parameter for evaluation of the severely injured and septic patient. Acta Chir Scand Suppl 1985; 522:211–31.
47. Aasen AO, Wang JE. Mediator responses in surgical infections. Surg Infect (Larchmt) 2006;7(Suppl 2):S3–4.
48. Wang JE, Dahle MK, Yndestad A, et al. Peptidoglycan of *Staphylococcus aureus* causes inflammation and organ injury in the rat. Crit Care Med 2004; 32(2):546–52.
49. Kernodle DS, Classen DC, Burke JP, et al. Failure of cephalosporins to prevent *Staphylococcus aureus* surgical wound infections. JAMA 1990;263(7): 961–6.
50. Kernodle DS, Voladri RK, Kaiser AB. Beta-lactamase production diminishes the prophylactic efficacy of ampicillin and cefazolin in a guinea pig model of *Staphylococcus aureus* wound infection. J Infect Dis 1998;177(3):701–6.
51. Kaye KS, Schmit K, Pieper C, et al. The effect of increasing age on the risk of surgical site infection. J Infect Dis 2005;191(7):1056–62.
52. Zerr KJ, Furnary AP, Grunkemeier GL, et al. Glucose control lowers the risk of wound infection in diabetics after open heart operations. Ann Thorac Surg 1997;63(2):356–61.
53. Lilienfeld DE, Vlahov D, Tenney JH, et al. Obesity and diabetes as risk factors for postoperative wound infections after cardiac surgery. Am J Infect Control 1988; 16(1):3–6.
54. Nagachinta T, Stephens M, Reitz B, et al. Risk factors for surgical-wound infection following cardiac surgery. J Infect Dis 1987;156(6):967–73.
55. Sorensen LT, Horby J, Friis E, et al. Smoking as a risk factor for wound healing and infection in breast cancer surgery. Eur J Surg Oncol 2002;28(8): 815–20.
56. Post S, Betzler M, von Ditfurth B, et al. Risks of intestinal anastomoses in Crohn's disease. Ann Surg 1991;213(1):37–42.
57. Berard F, Gandon J. Postoperative wound infections: the influence of ultraviolet irradiation of the operating room and of various other factors. Ann Surg 1964; 160(Suppl 1):1–192.
58. Pessaux P, Msika S, Atalla D, et al. Risk factors for postoperative infectious complications in noncolorectal abdominal surgery: a multivariate analysis based on a prospective multicenter study of 4718 patients. Arch Surg 2003;138(3):314–24.
59. Mishriki SF, Law DJ, Jeffery PJ. Factors affecting the incidence of postoperative wound infection. J Hosp Infect 1990;16(3):223–30.
60. Seropian R, Reynolds BM. Wound infections after preoperative depilatory versus razor preparation. Am J Surg 1971;121(3):251–4.

61. Belda FJ, Aguilera L, Garcia de la Asuncion J, et al. Supplemental perioperative oxygen and the risk of surgical wound infection: a randomized controlled trial. JAMA 2005;294(16):2035–42.

62. Greif R, Akca O, Horn EP, et al. Supplemental perioperative oxygen to reduce the incidence of surgical-wound infection. Outcomes Research Group. N Engl J Med 2000;342(3):161–7.

63. Melling AC, Ali B, Scott EM, et al. Effects of preoperative warming on the incidence of wound infection after clean surgery: a randomised controlled trial. Lancet 2001;358(9285):876–80.

64. El-Maallem H, Fletcher J. Effects of surgery on neutrophil granulocyte function. Infect Immun 1981;32(1):38–41.

65. Clardy CW, Edwards KM, Gay JC. Increased susceptibility to infection in hypothermic children: possible role of acquired neutrophil dysfunction. Pediatr Infect Dis 1985;4(4):379–82.

66. American Institute of Architects. Guidelines for design and construction of hospital and health care facilities. Washington, DC: American Institute of Architects Press; 1996.

67. Ayliffe GA. Role of the environment of the operating suite in surgical wound infection. Rev Infect Dis 1991;13(Suppl 10):S800–4.

68. Latham R, Lancaster AD, Covington JF, et al. The association of diabetes and glucose control with surgical-site infections among cardiothoracic surgery patients. Infect Control Hosp Epidemiol 2001;22(10):607–12.

69. Gandhi GY, Nuttall GA, Abel MD, et al. Intensive intraoperative insulin therapy versus conventional glucose management during cardiac surgery: a randomized trial. Ann Intern Med 2007;146(4):233–43.

70. Morain WD, Colen LB. Wound healing in diabetes mellitus. Clin Plast Surg 1990; 17(3):493–501.

71. Hill GE, Frawley WH, Griffith KE, et al. Allogeneic blood transfusion increases the risk of postoperative bacterial infection: a meta-analysis. J Trauma 2003;54(5):908–14.

72. Ross H. Postoperative wound infection with methicillin-resistant staphylococci in general surgical patients. Aust N Z J Surg 1985;55(1):13–7.

73. Manian FA, Meyer PL, Setzer J, et al. Surgical site infections associated with methicillin-resistant *Staphylococcus aureus*: do postoperative factors play a role? Clin Infect Dis 2003;36(7):863–8.

74. Dodds Ashley ES, Carroll DN, Engemann JJ, et al. Risk factors for postoperative mediastinitis due to methicillin-resistant *Staphylococcus aureus*. Clin Infect Dis 2004;38(11):1555–60.

75. Anderson DJ, Chen LF, Schmader KE, et al. Poor functional status predicts surgical site infection due to methicillin-resistant *Staphylococcus Aureus*. Infect Control Hosp Epidemiol 2008;29:832–9.

76. Classen DC, Evans RS, Pestotnik SL, et al. The timing of prophylactic administration of antibiotics and the risk of surgical-wound infection. N Engl J Med 1992; 326(5):281–6.

77. Kernodle DS, Kaiser AB. Surgical and trauma related infections. vol. 2. 5th edition. New York: Churchill Livingstone; 2000.

78. Antimicrobial prophylaxis in surgery. Med Lett Drugs Ther 1997;39(1012): 97–101.

79. Ehrenkranz NJ. Antimicrobial prophylaxis in surgery: mechanisms, misconceptions, and mischief. Infect Control Hosp Epidemiol 1993;14(2):99–106.

80. Nichols RL. Surgical antibiotic prophylaxis. Med Clin North Am 1995;79(3): 509–22.

81. McDonald M, Grabsch E, Marshall C, et al. Single- versus multiple-dose antimicrobial prophylaxis for major surgery: a systematic review. Aust N Z J Surg 1998; 68(6):388–96.
82. Nichols RL. Antibiotic prophylaxis in surgery. J Chemother 1989;1(3):170–8.
83. Page CP, Bohnen JM, Fletcher JR, et al. Antimicrobial prophylaxis for surgical wounds. Guidelines for clinical care. Arch Surg 1993;128(1):79–88.
84. DiPiro JT, Cheung RP, Bowden TA Jr, et al. Single dose systemic antibiotic prophylaxis of surgical wound infections. Am J Surg 1986;152(5):552–9.
85. Harbarth S, Samore MH, Lichtenberg D, et al. Prolonged antibiotic prophylaxis after cardiovascular surgery and its effect on surgical site infections and antimicrobial resistance. Circulation 2000;101(25):2916–21.
86. Bratzler DW, Hunt DR. The surgical infection prevention and surgical care improvement projects: national initiatives to improve outcomes for patients having surgery. Clin Infect Dis 2006;43(3):322–30.
87. Bratzler DW, Houck PM. Antimicrobial prophylaxis for surgery: an advisory statement from the National Surgical Infection Prevention Project. Clin Infect Dis 2004;38(12):1706–15.
88. Dellinger EP, Hausmann SM, Bratzler DW, et al. Hospitals collaborate to decrease surgical site infections. Am J Surg 2005;190(1):9–15.
89. Institute for Healthcare Improvement. A resource from the Institute of Healthcare Improvement. Available at: www.ihi.org. Accessed January 31, 2008.
90. Perl TM, Golub JE. New approaches to reduce *Staphylococcus aureus* nosocomial infection rates: treating *S aureus* nasal carriage. Ann Pharmacother 1998; 32(1):S7–16.
91. Kluytmans JA, Mouton JW, Ijzerman EP, et al. Nasal carriage of *Staphylococcus aureus* as a major risk factor for wound infections after cardiac surgery. J Infect Dis 1995;171(1):216–9.
92. Garibaldi RA. Prevention of intraoperative wound contamination with chlorhexidine shower and scrub. J Hosp Infect 1988;11(Suppl B):5–9.
93. Hayek LJ, Emerson JM, Gardner AM. A placebo-controlled trial of the effect of two preoperative baths or showers with chlorhexidine detergent on postoperative wound infection rates. J Hosp Infect 1987;10(2):165–72.
94. Kaiser AB, Kernodle DS, Barg NL, et al. Influence of preoperative showers on staphylococcal skin colonization: a comparative trial of antiseptic skin cleansers. Ann Thorac Surg 1988;45(1):35–8.
95. Rotter ML, Larsen SO, Cooke EM, et al. A comparison of the effects of preoperative whole-body bathing with detergent alone and with detergent containing chlorhexidine gluconate on the frequency of wound infections after clean surgery. The European Working Party on Control of Hospital Infections. J Hosp Infect 1988;11(4):310–20.
96. Leigh DA, Stronge JL, Marriner J, et al. Total body bathing with 'Hibiscrub' (chlorhexidine) in surgical patients: a controlled trial. J Hosp Infect 1983;4(3):229–35.
97. Lynch W, Davey PG, Malek M, et al. Cost-effectiveness analysis of the use of chlorhexidine detergent in preoperative whole-body disinfection in wound infection prophylaxis. J Hosp Infect 1992;21(3):179–91.
98. Segers P, Speekenbrink RG, Ubbink DT, et al. Prevention of nosocomial infection in cardiac surgery by decontamination of the nasopharynx and oropharynx with chlorhexidine gluconate: a randomized controlled trial. JAMA 2006;296(20):2460–6.
99. Cimochowski GE, Harostock MD, Brown R, et al. Intranasal mupirocin reduces sternal wound infection after open heart surgery in diabetics and nondiabetics. Ann Thorac Surg 2001;71(5):1572–8 [discussion 1578–9].

100. Kluytmans JA, Mouton JW, VandenBergh MF, et al. Reduction of surgical-site infections in cardiothoracic surgery by elimination of nasal carriage of *Staphylococcus aureus*. Infect Control Hosp Epidemiol 1996;17(12):780–5.

101. Perl TM, Cullen JJ, Wenzel RP, et al. Intranasal mupirocin to prevent postoperative *Staphylococcus aureus* infections. N Engl J Med 2002;346(24):1871–7.

102. Perl TM. Prevention of *Staphylococcus aureus* infections among surgical patients: beyond traditional perioperative prophylaxis. Surgery 2003;134 (5 Suppl):S10–7.

103. Miller MA, Dascal A, Portnoy J, et al. Development of mupirocin resistance among methicillin-resistant *Staphylococcus aureus* after widespread use of nasal mupirocin ointment. Infect Control Hosp Epidemiol 1996;17(12):811–3.

104. Recommendations for preventing the spread of vancomycin resistance. Recommendations of the Hospital Infection Control Practices Advisory Committee (HICPAC). MMWR Recomm Rep 1995;44(RR-12):1–13.

105. Bolon MK, Morlote M, Weber SG, et al. Glycopeptides are no more effective than beta-lactam agents for prevention of surgical site infection after cardiac surgery: a meta-analysis. Clin Infect Dis 2004;38(10):1357–63.

106. Stevens DL, Bisno AL, Chambers HF, et al. Practice guidelines for the diagnosis and management of skin and soft-tissue infections. Clin Infect Dis 2005;41(10):1373–406.

107. Karra R, McDermott L, Connelly S, et al. Risk factors for 1-year mortality after postoperative mediastinitis. J Thorac Cardiovasc Surg 2006;132(3):537–43.

108. Lewis RT. Soft tissue infections. World J Surg 1998;22(2):146–51.

109. Weigelt J, Kaafarani HM, Itani KM, et al. Linezolid eradicates MRSA better than vancomycin from surgical-site infections. Am J Surg 2004;188(6):760–6.

110. Gerson SL, Kaplan SL, Bruss JB, et al. Hematologic effects of linezolid: summary of clinical experience. Antimicrobial Agents Chemotheremother 2002;46(8):2723–6.

111. Arbeit RD, Maki D, Tally FP, et al. The safety and efficacy of daptomycin for the treatment of complicated skin and skin-structure infections. Clin Infect Dis 2004;38(12):1673–81.

112. Ellis-Grosse EJ, Babinchak T, Dartois N, et al. The efficacy and safety of tigecycline in the treatment of skin and skin-structure infections: results of 2 double-blind phase 3 comparison studies with vancomycin-aztreonam. Clin Infect Dis 2005;41(Suppl 5):S341–53.

113. Zimmerli W, Trampuz A, Ochsner PE. Prosthetic-joint infections. N Engl J Med 2004;351(16):1645–54.

114. El Oakley RM, Wright JE. Postoperative mediastinitis: classification and management. Ann Thorac Surg 1996;61(3):1030–6.

115. Brandt CM, Sistrunk WW, Duffy MC, et al. *Staphylococcus aureus* prosthetic joint infection treated with debridement and prosthesis retention. Clin Infect Dis 1997;24(5):914–9.

116. Raymond DP, Pelletier SJ, Crabtree TD, et al. Surgical infection and the aging population. Am Surg 2001;67(9):827–32 [discussion 832–23].

117. Mangram AJ, Horan TC, Pearson ML, et al. Guideline for prevention of surgical site infection, 1999. Centers for Disease Control and Prevention (CDC) Hospital Infection Control Practices Advisory Committee. Am J Infect Control 1999;27(2):97–132; quiz 133–4 [discussion 196].

118. Forse RA, Karam B, MacLean LD, et al. Antibiotic prophylaxis for surgery in morbidly obese patients. Surgery 1989;106(4):750–6 [discussion 756–7].

119. Haley RW, Culver DH, Morgan WM, et al. Identifying patients at high risk of surgical wound infection. A simple multivariate index of patient susceptibility and wound contamination. Am J Epidemiol 1985;121(2):206–15.
120. Pryor KO, Fahey TJ 3rd, Lien CA, et al. Surgical site infection and the routine use of perioperative hyperoxia in a general surgical population: a randomized controlled trial. JAMA 2004;291(1):79–87.
121. Kurz A, Sessler DI, Lenhardt R. Perioperative normothermia to reduce the incidence of surgical-wound infection and shorten hospitalization. Study of Wound Infection and Temperature Group. N Engl J Med 1996;334(19):1209–15.

Coagulase-Negative Staphylococcal Infections

Kathie L. Rogers, PhD[a], Paul D. Fey, PhD[a,b], Mark E. Rupp, MD[b,*]

KEYWORDS

- Coagulase-negative Staphylococci
- Staphylococcus epidermidis
- Intravascular catheter-associated bloodstream infection
- Biofilm • Prosthetic device infection
- *Staphylococcus haemolyticus*
- *Staphylococcus saprophyticus*

Coagulase-negative staphylococci (CNS) are differentiated from the closely related but more virulent *Staphylococcus aureus* by their inability to produce free coagulase. First identified in microbiological cultures in 1880 by Pasteur and Ogston when it was called *Staphylococcus albus*,[1] *Staphylococcus epidermidis* is the most commonly isolated CNS.[2] Currently, there are more than 40 recognized species of CNS. These organisms typically reside on healthy human skin and mucus membranes, rarely cause disease, and are most frequently encountered by clinicians as contaminants of microbiological cultures.[3,4] However, CNS have been increasingly recognized to cause clinically significant infections.[5–7] The conversion of the CNS from symbiont to human pathogen has been a direct reflection of the use of indwelling medical devices.[6,7] This review deals with the clinical syndromes, epidemiology, prevention, and management of infections caused by this unique group of organisms. Emphasis will be placed on *S. epidermidis*, with brief sections on *Staphylococcus lugdunensis*, *Staphylococcus saprophyticus*, and *Staphylococcus haemolyticus;* each an important member of the group capable of causing distinct infections.[8] The other members of the genus, most of which are only occasionally implicated in human disease, are generally indistinguishable from or less virulent than the infections caused by *S epidermidis*.[8]

[a] Department of Pathology and Microbiology, University of Nebraska Medical Center, 986280 Nebraska Medical Center, Omaha, NE 68198-6280, USA
[b] Department of Internal Medicine, University of Nebraska Medical Center, Nebraska Medical Center, Omaha, NE 68198-4031, USA
* Corresponding author.
E-mail address: merupp@unmc.edu (M.E. Rupp).

Infect Dis Clin N Am 23 (2009) 73–98
doi:10.1016/j.idc.2008.10.001
0891-5520/08/$ – see front matter © 2009 Elsevier Inc. All rights reserved.

CLINICAL SYNDROMES AND EPIDEMIOLOGY

The CNS, especially *S epidermidis*, are rarely implicated as the cause of infections of natural tissue.[9] They are found ubiquitously residing on human skin with healthy adults harboring 10 to 24 different strains of *S epidermidis*.[10] The number of CNS on human skin varies from 10 to 10^5 colony-forming units (CFU)/cm^2 on healthy adults in the community.[11] Their pathogenic potential lies in their ability to colonize and proliferate on biomaterials.[12] Every type of implanted biomaterial approved for use in humans has become prey to CNS infection.[13,14] These infections are often indolent and unresponsive to antimicrobials,[15,16] and frequently result in removal of the adulterated device.

INTRAVASCULAR CATHETER INFECTIONS

CNS are the most common cause of nosocomial bloodstream infection, responsible for 30% to 40% of these infections.[17] Most CNS bloodstream infections are the result of infections of intravascular catheters. Approximately 180 million peripheral intravascular catheters and 7 million central venous catheters (CVC) are used in the United States yearly.[18] Because of their transient nature (<72 hours usage) and placement sites (generally forearm or hand veins), peripheral intravascular catheters are not as commonly infected as CVCs. However, because of their ubiquitous usage, appreciable morbidity as a result of these infections does occur annually.[19]

A detailed description of the pathogenesis of these infections is beyond the scope of this monograph. Briefly, for peripheral intravenous catheters and short-term, nontunneled CVCs, infection most commonly results from CNS stemming from the patient's skin, migrating via the cutaneous surface of the catheter to gain access to the bloodstream.[20] However, for longer-term catheters and tunneled catheters, hub colonization (either from the patient's skin flora or from the health care environment) and migration of organisms via the luminal surface becomes increasingly important. Infrequently, catheter colonization occurs via hematogenous seeding or via infusate contamination.[19,21] As related later in this article, CNS have a number of adhesins that allow them to interact and adhere to the catheter surface and other factors that promote persistence.

It is estimated that approximately 250,000 cases of intravascular catheter-associated bloodstream infections occur yearly in the United States. The attributable mortality ranges widely in the literature from 1% to 2% to greater than 25% with an average additional cost per episode of $25,000 and excess hospital stay of 7 days or more.[19,22] It is estimated that many, if not most, of these infections are preventable, a topic addressed further in this article.[23,24]

Prompt and definitive diagnosis of these infections is necessary to decrease both morbidity and mortality, and to enable a decision to be made whether removal of the device is necessary or salvage is possible. Diagnosis of CNS intravascular device-related bloodstream infection is sometimes difficult because of the propensity for these organisms to cause blood culture contamination.[4,18,25,26] When diagnosing a bloodstream infection caused by CNS, it is imperative that at least two separate blood cultures be obtained, and if the patient has an indwelling CVC, that one of the blood cultures be collected through the catheter.[27] An incubation time to positivity of less than 25 hours has been considered consistent with true bacteremia.[28,29] In addition, the "differential time to positivity" test can be used to determine whether a vascular catheter is the source of bacteremia.[30] Blood drawn from the suspect catheter should have a higher inoculum, and turn positive more quickly, than blood obtained from the peripheral bloodstream. A 2-hour or more differential time has been demonstrated to be a sensitive and specific marker of catheter-associated bacteremia.[30,31]

In addition, the CNS isolates from the peripheral and catheter-drawn blood should have the same pulsed-field gel electrophoresis pattern and/or have the same antibiogram.[32] If quantitative blood cultures are used, a difference of three- to five-fold greater colony numbers in the catheter culture versus the peripheral bloodstream are indicative of a catheter-associated bloodstream infection.[33] The acridine orange leukocyte cytospin test is sometimes used to diagnose a catheter infection.[34] In this examination, a 50-μL aliquot of blood from the catheter is treated to lyse the red blood cells. The remaining microorganisms and white blood cells are centrifuged, placed on a slide, and examined under a UV microscope after staining with acridine orange. If the catheter is removed, the semiquantitative culture method described by Maki and colleagues,[35] in which a colony count of 15 CFU or higher is a positive result, may help determine the diagnosis of catheter infection. Other techniques used to culture the catheter include sonication or flushing the catheter segment.[36,37] Positive catheter-tip cultures in the absence of positive blood cultures or a clinical presentation of infection generally indicate colonization of the catheter and these patients should not be given antibiotics based on the culture results alone.[38] In general, catheters should not be cultured unless inflammation is present at the insertion site or the patient presents with clinical indications of bacteremia.[19] Generally, clinical signs of CNS bloodstream infection include classic signs of sepsis and include the presence of fever (greater than 38°C), leukocytosis, anemia, and hypotension.[39,40] Treatment consists of antimicrobial therapy appropriate for methicillin-resistant CNS usually combined with removal of the catheter[33] (see "Management of infections caused by coagulase-negative streptococci" later in this article).

VASCULAR GRAFT INFECTION

Prosthetic vascular graft infection incidence ranges from 1% to 6%, dependent on the graft location.[41] Infrainguinal grafts deriving from the groin have the highest rates of infection.[2] The CNS are the most common cause of these infections, which may occur within the first 30 days of surgery, but are more common months or years after implantation.[3] The type of material used in the graft does not appear to affect infection rates. Mortality rates of 17% and morbidity rates of 41% (usually amputation) with a 4-year survival rate of 70% are found with peripheral vascular graft infections.[3] Aortic graft infections have a mortality rate of about 50%, morbidity of 21%, and a 5-year survival rate of 50%.[3,41] Diagnosis is generally made by physical examination and radiographic imaging with the observation of a sinus tract or pseudoaneurysm at the vascular anastomosis site[41] (see "Management of infections caused by coagulase-negative streptococci" later in this article).

ENDOCARDITIS

Prosthetic valve endocarditis (PVE), although uncommon, is frequently caused by CNS. Those diagnosed with PVE caused by CNS (usually S epidermidis) comprise 15% to 40% of PVE cases.[3,42,43] Diagnosis is usually made by repeated positive blood cultures and echocardiograpy.[2,3] The infection is usually health care related (because of inoculation at the time of surgery) and manifests within 12 months of valve placement. These isolates are likely to be methicillin resistant because of their health care etiology.[2] The cases of PVE that present after this time period are less commonly caused by CNS, are usually associated with trauma to mucosal surfaces or incidental infection, and, if caused by CNS, are apt to be methicillin susceptible.[2] Heart failure occurs in 54% of cases and greater than 80% have complications including prosthetic valve dysfunction and intracardiac abscesses.[42,43] In addition to prolonged antibiotic therapy, valve replacement surgery is frequently required.[42] Despite aggressive therapy, the mortality caused by CNS PVE remains high at approximately 24% to 36%.[2,42–44]

Unlike PVE, native valve endocarditis caused by CNS is relatively rare, occurring in only 5% to 8% of endocarditis cases.[45–47] This infection is caused by hematogenous seeding of previously damaged or malformed heart valves and endocardium.[46] About half of these cases are health care associated (concomitant with the use of intravenous catheters or recent history of invasive procedure) and these isolates are usually methicillin resistant, whereas the organisms isolated in the other half of cases are considered to be community acquired and are most often methicillin susceptible.[45] Patients with native valve CNS endocarditis often have a very complicated clinical course because of embolic events, rhythm conduction abnormalities, and congestive heart failure.[44,48] Mortality may be as high as 36%.[44,45,48–50] More than half of these cases require valve replacement.[50]

CARDIAC DEVICES

Cardiac pacemaker infection occurs with an incidence of 0.13% to 19.9% and a mortality of 27% to 66%.[51] CNS (predominantly S epidermidis) account for at least 25% of these infections and may occur via inoculation at the time of device placement or by hematogenous seeding from another site.[2,3] One quarter of these infections occur within 1 to 2 months of insertion of the device. Clinically, patients present with inflammation at the pacer pocket site, bacteremia, or evidence of right-sided endocarditis. Diagnosis is generally made by culture of the generator pocket, culture of the device itself, or multiple positive sequential blood cultures with the same strain of CNS.[51] Radiologic and echocardiographic assessments may also aid in this diagnosis.[2,3] Successful treatment generally requires removal of the device and 4 to 6 weeks of intravenous antibiotics.[51] Relapse rates and mortality are increased if complete removal of the device is not accomplished.[52,53]

PROSTHETIC JOINT INFECTIONS

CNS are one of the most common causes of infection of prosthetic orthopedic devices.[54,55] These organisms are generally inoculated at the time of the arthroplasty and, owing to their relatively avirulent nature, may be quite indolent in their clinical presentation.[56] CNS prosthetic joint infections are usually caused by S epidermidis with a few cases caused by S lugdunensis or other CNS species.[3,57] Risk factors include previous joint surgery, duration of surgery, another infection at the time of surgery, and rheumatoid arthritis.[3] Infections are classified based on the length of the interval between surgery and diagnosis of the infection. Stage I infections occur within 3 months of surgery and are usually caused by S aureus. Stage II infections manifest between 3 months and 2 years after surgery and are often caused by CNS, whereas stage III infections occur after 2 years and are usually caused by hematogenous inoculation of organisms from some other source and are generally not caused by CNS.[3] CNS stage II infections are usually indolent and manifest as pain at the affected joint without fever or purulent drainage and must be treated with additional surgery and replacement of the infected joint. Diagnosis is made by the presence of an elevated erythrocyte sedimentation rate; radionuclide scans or other imaging techniques; and culture of the infected material obtained by needle aspiration, bone biopsy, or surgery.[57] The recovery of organisms can be optimized by sonication of the prosthesis at the time of removal.[58] CNS appear to be a prominent cause of "culture-negative" prosthetic joint infection that manifest as aseptic loosening of the joint.[59] It is thought that prior antibiotic therapy and induction of a metabolically quiescent population of CNS encased in biofilm may explain this condition.

CENTRAL NERVOUS SYSTEM SHUNT INFECTIONS

Although previously published infection rates were much higher, more recently examined series of patients indicate rates of infection of cerebrospinal fluid shunts of approximately 5%.[60] CNS are the predominant pathogen causing more than one half of these infections.[61,62] The risk of infection increases with the presence of abnormalities of the scalp at the time of shunt placement, a patient's age of younger than 6 months, reinsertion of shunt following previous infection, lack of experience of the surgeon, and the length of time of the operative procedure.[3] Clinically, the diagnosis should be suspected if the patient experiences unexplained fever within 2 months of shunt placement or shunt dysfunction. Definitive diagnosis is made by culturing cerebrospinal fluid obtained from the shunt or cerebral ventricles, or culture of the shunt itself upon removal.[3] Treatment always includes antimicrobial therapy and usually replacement of the shunt.[62]

SURGICAL SITE INFECTIONS

Further information regarding staphylococcal surgical site infections can be found in the section of this issue authored by Jhung and Jernigan. Surgical site infections caused by CNS occur frequently and are second only to *S aureus* as an etiologic agent.[3] The CNS are more often cultured from superficial incisional wounds than from deeper incisional wounds and they are more likely to cause infections in "clean" procedures rather than those performed in contaminated sites (bowel, genitourinary, and so forth).[3] These superficial incisional infections generally manifest within 1 to 10 days after surgery and are generally inoculated from the patient's endogenous flora or, less frequently, from the operating personnel or environment. Risk factors include length of surgical procedure, host factors (extremities of age, obesity, nutritional status, and so forth), experience of the surgical staff, and institution where the surgery is performed.[2,63] Diagnosis is made by culture of CNS either in pure culture or as the predominant isolate, or repeated isolation of the same organism in cultures of the site.[64] Occasionally, organ/space surgical site infections caused by the CNS occur and are a result of inoculation of the site at the time of surgery. Treatment is usually antimicrobial therapy and debridement and drainage of the wound if necessary.[65]

INFECTIONS INVOLVING OTHER PROSTHETIC DEVICES

Other implanted materials and devices that may become infected by the CNS include intraocular lenses, breast implants, and genitourinary prostheses, as well as virtually any other surgically inserted appliance.[5,66] As the list of such items in use in today's health care environment grows, it can be expected that infections caused by the CNS will also continue to increase in number.

COAGULASE-NEGATIVE STAPHYLOCOCCAL INFECTIONS IN NEONATES

Neonates are a particularly high-risk population for infections caused by CNS, as CNS are currently responsible for 31% of all nosocomial infections in neonatal intensive care units in the United States and 73% of all bacteremias in this setting.[67] In addition, the number of reported cases of infection caused by CNS in neonatal ICUs continues to increase each year.[68] This is in part because of the increase in the number of preterm infants requiring the use of umbilical and central venous catheters. This trend seems likely to continue as more women in modern society sustain high-risk pregnancies because of maternal age or multiple births as a result of in vitro fertilization.[69] However, unlike CNS infections in adults, in addition to vascular catheter-related infections, neonates may also develop wound abscesses, pneumonia, urinary tract infections, meningitis, enterocolitis, and omphalitis caused by CNS.[66] The microorganisms instigating these infections are acquired from the neonatal ICU environment resulting in rapid colonization of the skin, nares, umbilicus, and throat within several days of admission.[70] Risk factors for infection caused by CNS include very low birth weight (<1500 g), use of central venous catheters, mechanical ventilation, and total parenteral nutrition.[66] Although these infections are associated with a low mortality rate (0.3% to 1.6%), they often cause significant morbidity and result in longer hospital stays.[66,71] Therapy usually consists of antimicrobial treatment and often removal and replacement of indwelling catheters.[66,72]

OTHER SPECIES OF COAGULASE-NEGATIVE STAPHYLOCOCCI
Staphylococcus Saprophyticus

Besides *S epidermidis*, there are several other species of CNS that should be specifically discussed because of their documented pathogenic potential. The first of these, *S saprophyticus*, is a frequent cause of urinary tract infection (UTI) in young (18 to 35 years), sexually active women.[73–75] It is a member of the normal rectal or urogenital flora of 10% of females and is the second leading cause (behind *Escherichia coli*) of acute UTI in this population.[75–77] *S saprophyticus* possesses a unique adhesion protein, UafA, which allows it to adhere to human ureteral epithelial cells.[78] In addition, this bacterium also encodes several transport proteins enabling it to rapidly adjust to osmotic and pH changes. Finally, *S saprophyticus* produces abundant urease allowing it to proliferate in urine.[79] *S saprophyticus* is often distinguished in the clinical laboratory from other CNS by its resistance to novobiocin. UTIs caused by *S saprophyticus* are usually successfully treated with urinary tract antimicrobials with only rarely reported sequelae.[80]

Staphylococcus lugdunensis

S lugdunensis is unique among the CNS because the infections it causes are often similar in severity to those attributable to *S aureus*.[81] It is the second leading cause of CNS native valve endocarditis (responsible for up to 44% of cases),[82] and is an uncommon cause of myocarditis, brain abscess, sepsis, and chronic osteomyelitis.[81] Endocarditis caused by this organism is aggressive and frequently associated with valvular destruction and abscess formation resulting in a mortality rate of 50% to 70%.[81] *S lugdunensis* has also been implicated as a leading cause of skin and surgical wound infections, especially those occurring below the naval, as it is often found as part of the normal inguinal flora.[83] It is disposed to be more virulent than most other CNS because of the production of several virulence factors including a thermostable DNase, clumping factor, an extracellular glycocalyx, lipase, hemolysin, and a fatty acid enzyme-modifying enzyme. It also is capable of binding to human collagen, fibronectin, fibrinogen, human IgG, laminin, plasminogen, thrombospondin, and vitronectin.[84–88] Its prominent role in native valve endocarditis may be attributable to the production of a von Willebrand factor–binding protein, which allows it to bind to microscopic endothelial lesions.[87] Fortuitously, the organism is generally susceptible to most antistaphylococcal antibiotics, as beta-lactamase production is found in only about 25% of strains and methicillin resistance is uncommon.[81] Identification of this species by the clinical laboratory can be difficult. *S lugdunensis* can be easily confused with *S aureus* if identification is based only on the latex agglutination test, as the production of clumping factor by S lugdunensis will yield a positive test result.[81]

Staphylococcus haemolyticus

S haemolyticus is second to S epidermidis among the CNS in frequency of isolation from blood cultures especially in neonatal ICUs.[55,66,67] S haemolyticus expresses lipase, protease, and lyase and is often multiply antibiotic resistant.[89] This collection of putative virulence traits and antibiotic resistance determinants is believed to be a result of the large number of insertion sequences found in its genome, which may allow common gene rearrangement as the organism adapts to various environments.[89] This organism was the first of the CNS to exhibit decreased glycopeptide susceptibility, more commonly teicoplanin than vancomycin. Decreased susceptibility is attributable to alterations in the cell wall's peptidoglycan rather than acquisition of resistance genes via horizontal gene transfer.[90,91]

PATHOGENESIS AND VIRULENCE TRAITS

The virulence factors associated with the CNS are listed in **Table 1**. The single most important of these is the ability to produce a highly structured, tenacious biofilm on the surface of indwelling medical devices.[15] Biofilm formation is thought to occur in three distinct steps. First, the cells bind to the surface of the device in a reversible manner as a result of nonspecific forces such as polarity and hydrophobicity. Next, more specific adherence occurs as a result of the production of adhesins that specifically bind to human host proteins that quickly coat intravascular catheters or other devices. Once steadfastly bound, the cells then produce a thick biofilm consisting mainly of polysaccharide intercellular adhesion (PIA) (in S epidermidis),[92] thus creating an environment that results in antibiotic tolerance and evasion of host defense.[93,94] PIA is produced by the icaADBC operon in S epidermidis and the formation of biofilm in this species requires a functional ica locus.[95–97] The presence of this thick, sticky substance is at least partially responsible for the indolent, difficult-to-treat nature of these infections. It has been shown that the S epidermidis isolates found in the health care environment carry the ica locus more frequently than isolates found in the community.[96,98–100] Genetic regulation of the ica operon and biofilm production is complex.[101] Other virulence factors are noted in **Table 1**.

CLINICAL MICROBIOLOGY AND MOLECULAR TYPING

The CNS were originally divided on the basis of colony morphology and biochemical tests by Baird-Parker in the 1960s.[102] In the 1970s, Kloos and Schleifer,[103] developed a method for identifying CNS to the species level involving an array of morphologic descriptions, biochemical testing, physiologic testing, susceptibility testing results, and cell wall characterization. These have been adapted and modified to produce rapid identification kits and automated systems that differentiate the over 40 currently recognized species of CNS. In addition to biochemical tests, other typing analyses have historically included the use of the antibiogram, phage typing, multilocus enzyme electrophoresis, and plasmid profiling.[104–107] More recently, DNA-based techniques have been used to characterize CNS. These techniques include ribotyping, restriction fragment length polymorphism (RFLP) analysis, polymerase chain reaction (PCR)-based locus-specific RFLP analysis, random amplified polymorphic DNA (RAPD) assays, repetitive extragenic palindromic elements (REP)-PCR, amplified fragment length polymorphism (AFLP) testing, pulsed-field gel electrophoresis (PFGE), PCR amplification of ribosomal DNA spacer regions and transfer RNA intergenic regions, and finally,

Table 1
Staphylococcus epidermidis virulence factors

Virulence Factor	Mechanism	Gene(s)
Biofilm	Immune System Avoidance, Antimicrobialtolerance	
PIA	Polysaccharide component	*icaADBC*
Aap	Accumulation of biofilm cells	*aap*
Bhp	Accumulation	*bhp*
DNA	Structure of biofilm, nutrient, horizontal gene transfer	NA
Adhesin Molecules	Adherence to Host Proteins or Biomaterials	
Aae	Binds Fgn, Vn, Fn	*aae*
AtlE	Binds Vn	*atlE*
Bhp	Binds polystyrene	*bhp*
Ebp	Binds elastin	*ebp*
EmbP	Binds fibronectin	*empB*
Fbe(SdrG)	Binds fibrinogen	*sdrG*
GehD	Binds collagen	*gehD*
ScaA(Aae)	Binds Fgn, Vn, Fn	*scaA*
ScaB	Unknown ligand	*scaB*
SdrF	Binds collagen	*sdrF*
SdrG(Fbe)	Binds fibrinogen	*sdrG*
Ssp-1	Binds polystyrene	Unknown
Ssp-2	Binds polystyrene	Unknown
Teichoic acid	Binds fibronectin	*tagF* *yibD*
Other Virulence Traits	Various Mechanisms	
Peptidoglycan/ lipoteichoic acid	Stimulates cytokine production	*tagF, femA others*
Phenol-soluble modulins	Induction of cytokines, Immune system modulation	*psmα, psmβ*
	Biofilm dispersion	*psmδ, psmγ*
Poly-D-glutamic acid	Immune system avoidance Aid resistance of antimicrobial peptides	*cap* locus
Delta-toxin	Injury to host cells	*hld*
Exoenzymes		
Fatty-acid modifying enzyme	Inactivates fatty acids on skin	Unknown
Lipases	Skin and wound colonization	*gehC, gehD*
Proteases	Destruction of host tissue	*sspA, sspB* *sspC*

Abbreviations: Aap, accumulation-associated protein; Aae, autolysin/adhesion; AtlE, autolysin; Bhp, Bap homolog protein; Ebp, elastin-binding protein S; EmbP, extracellular matrix-binding protein; Fbe(SdrG), fibrinogen-binding protein; Fgn, fibrinogen; Fn, fibronectin; GehD, glycerol ester hydrolase; PIA, polysaccharide intercellular adhesion; ScaA(Aae), staphylococcal conserved antigen A; ScaB, staphylococcal conserved antigen B; SdrF, serine aspartate repeat protein F; SdrG(Fbe), serine aspartate repeat protein G; Ssp-1, staphylococcal surface protein 1; Ssp-2, staphylococcal surface protein 2; Vn, vitronectin.

genomic DNA sequencing.[108–110] A survey of the literature supports the notion that, of these methods, PFGE has been used most often and remains the most discriminatory method used in epidemiologic typing. Although PFGE is an excellent technique to explore local epidemiologic questions, it is not an appropriate tool to address questions of population structure. To define population biology, multilocus sequence typing

(MLST) has been recently developed for use in *S epidermidis*. MLST typically involves the partial sequencing and subsequent comparison of seven conserved housekeeping genes. Three MLST schemes have been proposed for *S epidermidis*, with the most recent scheme proposed by Thomas and colleagues[108] providing the highest level of discrimination. Monk and Archer[111] recently demonstrated that PCR and DNA sequence analysis of the repeat regions of both *sdrG* (fibrinogen-binding protein [Fbe]) and *aap* (accumulation-associated protein) in conjunction with MLST further enhances the discriminatory power of these methodologies.

PREVENTION OF COAGULASE-NEGATIVE STAPHYLOCOCCAL INFECTION

Because the infections presented by the CNS tend to be difficult to eradicate, an emphasis is placed on preventing both the exposure of the device to the pathogen as well as hindering colonization if exposure does occur. The first and foremost means for accomplishing these goals is strict adherence to good infection control practices. It has been estimated that 6% to 32% of all nosocomial infections could be prevented through improved application of infection control procedures.[24] More recently, studies suggest that most catheter-related bloodstream infections are preventable and that from 10% to 70% of all nosocomial infections can be prevented with implementation of institutionwide, well-organized infection control interventions.[24,112] This would save many lives and appreciably decrease health care costs.

A complete description of evidence-based practices to prevent a variety of health care–associated infections is available through the Centers for Disease Control and Prevention's Hospital Infection Control Practices Advisory Committee (http://www.cdc.gov/ncidod/dhqp/hicpac.html). A joint guideline from the Society for Healthcare Epidemiology of America (SHEA) and the Infectious Diseases Society of America (IDSA) regarding implementation of a variety of evidence-based practices to prevent healthcare-associated infections has recently been released. The interested reader is encouraged to review these guidelines at the official SHEA or IDSA websites (www.shea-online.org or www.idsociety.org). Some of these practices with particular impact on common CNS infections will be summarized in the following discussion.

PREVENTION OF INTRAVASCULAR CATHETER COAGULASE-NEGATIVE STAPHYLOCOCCAL INFECTIONS

The singular most critical factor in prevention of infections related to indwelling vascular devices is standardization of aseptic care. The first step involves careful site selection. The density of the skin flora at the insertion site plays a significant role in the risk of the catheter becoming infected[113] and it is recommended that the femoral site be avoided if possible.[114] Hand disinfection should be performed before placement or manipulation of vascular catheters.[115] Maximal sterile barrier precautions should be used when inserting a CVC and these consist of use of a mask, sterile gown, sterile gloves, cap, and a large sterile drape.[116] Site preparation is critical and disinfection of the skin should be performed with 2% aqueous chlorhexidine gluconate.[117,118] Prevention of hub contamination (often implicated in infections of long-term CVCs) begins with strict adherence to aseptic technique when manipulating the catheter. Catheter hubs, needleless connectors, and injection ports should be disinfected with a 70% alcohol saturated pad or alcoholic chlorhexidine before accessing the catheter. Limiting the number of catheter manipulations will assist in reducing infections as will use of a dedicated CVC care team.[119,120] "Bundling" these measures together, along with a daily checklist reminder to remove catheters as soon as they are not needed, has had a dramatic impact on catheter-related bacteremia in several settings.[112,121] This approach has been publicized and successfully promoted by the Institute for Health Care Improvement's 100,000 lives campaign (http://www.ihi.org/IHI/Programs/Campaign/).

A number of commercially available CVCs have been impregnated with antibiotics or antiseptics to prevent infection. CVCs coated with silver sulfadiazine and chlorhexidine have been demonstrated in well-designed, randomized, controlled clinical trials to reduce bacterial colonization and bloodstream infection in a cost-effective manner.[122–125] Similarly, catheters impregnated with rifampin and minocycline have been documented to prevent catheter infection.[126–128] Although concern has been expressed regarding the development of resistance to antibiotics used to coat catheters, this has not been observed in clinical studies.[129] Fewer clinical data are available for catheters coated with carbon, platinum, and silver.[130] A large variety of antibiotics has been used in experimental situations for coating catheters, including ampicillin, cefazolin, ciprofloxacin, clindamycin, dicloxacillin, flucloxacillin, fusidic acid, and teicoplanin, but none of these are commercially available. A variety of antiseptics, besides chlorhexidine or silver, have been incorporated into catheter coatings including benzalkonium chloride, a diphenyl ether derivative, gentian violet, and iodine. A silicone catheter that has electrically charged silver wires wrapped around its proximal end to generate low-amperage current and thus repulse microbial adherence is also in development.[131]

Because short-term catheters often become infected via the cutaneous surface, chlorhexidine-impregnated sponge dressings have been used to decrease the bacterial load on the skin and decrease the risk of infection.[132] More recently, a chlorhexidine-impregnated gel pad has been incorporated into a transparent dressing and been approved for marketing.[133] The use of a silver-impregnated subcutaneous collagen cuff left just below the skin insertion site has been used to intradict organisms migrating via the cutaneous surface.[134] Similarly, to decrease the burden of microbes at the cutaneous insertion site, povidone-iodine or polysporin ointments have been applied at hemodialysis catheter exit sites with documented benefit.[135,136] Although mupirocin ointment has been used for the same indication, many authorities recommend against such use because of the emergence of mupirocin resistance and potential damage to polyurethane dialysis catheters. To address the luminal route of inoculation, a catheter connector valve has recently been approved for marketing that is impregnated with silver nanoparticles.[137] Newer techniques using sutureless catheter securement devices may also confer an advantage in prevention of infections.[138]

Antimicrobial lock solutions have also been used to prevent CNS and other microbes from proliferating inside catheters. The lock solutions have included, alone or in combination, antiseptics such as alcohol or taurolidine, anticoagulants such as heparin or ethylenediaminetetraacetic acid (EDTA), as well as a variety of antibiotics such as vancomycin, teicoplanin, rifampin, ciprofloxacin, tigecycline, gentamicin, and minocycline.[139–141] Further studies are needed to define the optimum agents to use in these lock solutions that will result in maximal protection of the catheter with the least toxicity and propensity for emergence of resistance.

Many investigators have modified catheter biomaterials and surfaces in an attempt to develop a less infection-prone catheter. However, the search for the perfect intravascular biomaterial continues. Catheter material should be nonimmunogenic, nonthrombogenic, firm enough to allow insertion but soft and pliable enough to not damage tissues, totally smooth, and not prone to bacterial adherence. The use of Teflon or polyurethane catheters appears to be superior to polyvinyl chloride or polyethylene in terms of propensity for infection.[142] Polystyrene catheters modified with a copolymer of polyethylene oxide and polypropylene oxide exhibit reduced adherence of *S epidermidis* in in vitro studies.[143] Less adherence has also been demonstrated with the use of hydrophilic-coated polyurethane catheters.[66] Modified polymer surfaces can enable the covalent bonding of various chemicals that reduce in vitro adhesion of *S epidermidis* cells. Other bacterial adherence–reducing surface modifications of catheter polymers include using sulfonated polyethylene oxide as a surfactant in polyurethane or adding glycerophosphorylcholine as a chain extender on polyurethane.[144,145]

PREVENTION OF OTHER DEVICE-ASSOCIATED COAGULASE-NEGATIVE STAPHYLOCOCCAL INFECTIONS

Many surgically implanted prosthetic device infections can be prevented by strict adherence to recommendations for the prevention of surgical site infections. A complete description of these guidelines is beyond the scope of this monograph. Further information is available in the section of this issue on staphylococcal surgical site infections by Jhung and Jernigan and in the CDC Hospital Infection Control Practices Advisory Committee (HICPAC) guideline on prevention of surgical site infections.[146] In brief, some of the key points in prevention of surgical site infection include the appropriate delivery of prophylactic antibiotics (correct agent, administration within 1 hour of surgery, dosage correct for weight, redosing for prolonged procedures, and discontinuation of antibiotics within 24 hours), careful preparation of the surgical site (preoperative shower, correct hair removal, careful antiseptic scrub), maintenance of perioperative normothermia, maintenance of perioperative normoglycemia, meticulous attention to intraoperative aseptic procedures, careful surgical technique, appropriate postoperative wound management, and maintenance of the operative theater (eg, air handling, disinfection of the room and equipment, central sterile supply quality control).

The incorporation of antiseptics and antibiotics, similar to efforts described above for vascular catheters, has been accomplished for a variety of other devices. A limited synopsis of some of these efforts for some devices is noted later in this article. To prevent or treat orthopedic device infections, surgeons have for many years mixed vancomycin or gentamicin into bone cement. Similarly, polymethylmethacrylate beads can be impregnated with gentamicin, clindamycin, or fusidic acid and used to fill spaces in the treatment or prevention of bone and soft tissue infections.[147] Dacron vascular prostheses have been impregnated with amikacin or rifampin and in animal studies both proved effective at preventing infection with *S aureus*.[148] CNS shunts have been impregnated with various combinations of rifampin, clindamycin, trimethoprim, fusidic acid, mupirocin, and minocyline with excellent in vitro and in vivo success.[149]

A particularly novel approach to prevention of colonization and infection of implanted devices is the development of "intelligent polymers or devices"—devices that can sense the environment, discern when they are being colonized by microbes, and release their bound antimicrobial or antiseptic when necessary.[150] Truly exciting and promising research continues in the area of prevention of CNS device-associated infections, as a huge savings, both in terms of health care dollars and quality of life could be realized if more of these infections could be prevented. As the number of implanted medical devices continues to rise, prevention of infections becomes paramount.

MANAGEMENT OF INFECTIONS CAUSED BY COAGULASE-NEGATIVE STAPHYLOCOCCI

If prevention of these infections has been unsuccessful then it becomes imperative for the clinician to offer optimum therapy. A number of factors influence clinical decisions regarding the management of CNS device-associated infections including the need for the device, the clinical condition of the patient and anticipated course of any underlying disease, morbidity associated with device removal, antimicrobial susceptibility, and antimicrobial pharmacokinetic/dynamic considerations. Luckily, CNS are usually relatively avirulent and patients may be able to tolerate ongoing infection for a prolonged period without dire consequences.[151]

CNS prosthetic device–associated infections are one of the best examples of a biofilm-associated infection. Often underappreciated by clinicians is the recalcitrance of biofilm-associated CNS to antimicrobial agents. Although incompletely understood, there are a number of potential reasons why biofilm-associated CNS are tolerant of antibiotic levels that would normally suppress or kill them when existing in the planktonic state. These factors include the role of biofilms in the penetrance of antimicrobial agents, the rate of growth and metabolic state of biofilm-associated CNS, phenotypic plasticity, persister cells, and antibiotic depletion. The interested reader is referred to a number of recent works where these issues are more fully reviewed.[152,153] Briefly, biofilms are known to effect the diffusion of some antibiotics; however, most recent data indicate this is not the major reason for the lack of activity of antibiotics against biofilm-associated CNS. The CNS in biofilms experience various environmental conditions and some may be very slow growing or metabolically quiescent. As many antibiotics require rapidly growing cells to exert their influence, it stands to reason that the slowly growing cells would be relatively resistant to some antibiotics. Similarly, altered gene expression driven by quorum-sensing functions, stress response, or other environmental cues may radically change the ability of CNS to adapt or respond to antibiotics. Also, specialized survivor cells or persister cells may possess a significant temporary tolerance to antibiotics. Finally, the biofilm may promote neutralizing reactions between the antibiotic and biofilm constituents resulting in antibiotic depletion. In addition, the biofilm may interact and interfere with host defense cells and immunologic mechanisms. CNS biofilm-associated infections pose a formidable challenge to the clinician. In the following discussion a few salient issues will be pointed out regarding treatment of the most common types of infections due to CNS.

Intravascular Catheter Infections

As previously related, CNS are the most common cause of intravascular catheter infections. In general, infected short-term catheters should be promptly removed. In patients with tunneled catheters or totally implanted vascular access devices, removal of the device may not be immediately feasible and, in patients who are not septic, a careful trial of treatment with the catheter in situ may be reasonable. Combined systemic and lock antimicrobial therapy should be used with an antimicrobial agent to which the organism is susceptible. Most health care–associated CNS are methicillin-resistant strains and empiric therapy is usually initiated with vancomycin. A thorough evidence-based guideline for the treatment of intravascular catheter infections is available from the IDSA.[33] If the offending catheter is removed, most authorities feel a 7-day course of therapy is adequate.[22,33] If the catheter is retained, the clinician should be alert for relapse, as this occurs in a significant minority of patients.[154] Relapse of CNS bacteremia represents a strong indication for catheter removal. To more completely assist clinicians in choosing an antibiotic, some laboratories offer testing to determine the minimum biofilm eradication concentration.[155] A couple of interesting issues are the utility of lysostaphin and ultrasound. The use of lysostaphin, an endopeptidase specific for the cell wall peptidoglycan of staphylococci, has been studied in the management of CNS catheter infections.[156] The use of ultrasound is often used to disrupt bacteria from the surface of foreign bodies in the laboratory and the use of ultrasound, in combination with antibiotics, is being investigated as a means to treat *S epidermidis* biofilm-associated infection.[157]

Prosthetic Joint Infections

A more complete description of treatment of prosthetic joint infections can be found in the section of this issue by Karchmer. Briefly, CNS prosthetic joint infections are most successfully treated with a two-stage replacement procedure.[158] In the first stage, the involved prosthesis and infected tissues are resected. This is followed by approximately 6 weeks of antibiotics, usually vancomycin. Sterilization of tissues is documented by a period of time off antibiotics, which is followed by joint reimplantation. Success rates of over 90% are typical. The role of antibiotic-impregnated beads, spacers, or temporary prostheses is not completely defined, but they are frequently employed.[158]

Other treatment options include a one-stage replacement procedure, which has the advantage of a single operation but typically is less successful in eradication of the infection. Resection arthroplasty without replacement of the joint is almost always successful in eradicating infection, but has the obvious limitation of loss of mobility and is usually limited to nonambulatory patients. Debridement and retention of the involved prosthesis is occasionally attempted in patients with early and acute infection, a stable prosthesis, and no sinus tract. In patients in whom a potentially curative procedure is not possible, and who do not exhibit systemic symptoms of infection, chronic suppressive therapy can be administered.

Cerebrospinal Fluid Shunt Infections

Infections of cerebrospinal fluid shunts are optimally treated with antibiotic therapy and removal of the shunt with external ventricular drainage.[62] The shunt is best replaced after CSF sterility is achieved, for if the shunt is removed and immediately replaced, there is a greater chance for relapse. The least optimal treatment is antibiotic therapy alone. Antibiotic therapy is usually a combination of parenteral as well as intraventricular delivery of vancomycin, gentamicin, and rifampin. Vancomycin and gentamicin can be given both systemically as well as intraventricularly. Rifampin is usually administered orally, as it has excellent bioavailability and readily crosses the blood brain barrier to reach adequate concentration in the CSF.[2,62] If the causative bacteria are methicillin susceptible, a semisynthetic penicillinase-resistant penicillin should be given parenterally.

Treatment of Other Coagulase-Negative Staphylococcal Infected Prosthetic Devices

The treatment principles discussed previously are germane to infections involving other devices. In general, the greatest chance for cure is associated with removal of the device, debridement of infected tissues, administration of antibiotics until inflammatory markers (erythrocyte sedimentation rate, C-reactive protein) have normalized (typically 4 to 8 weeks), and then reimplantation of the device. However, this course is tempered by the underlying disease and the need for the device. Obviously, the luxury of antibiotic administration without the presence a foreign body is not possible in the case of prothetic valve endocarditis, vascular graft infection, or pacer infection in a patient with a pacer-dependent cardiac dysrhythmia. In these cases, the infected device is removed and replaced while the patient is receiving optimal antibiotic therapy. It is often remarkable how few of the replacement devices suffer recurrent infection.

Table 2
Anti-staphylococcal antibiotics, resistance rates and mechanisms of resistance

Antibiotic Class	Antibiotic	Site of Action	Mechanism of Resistance	Means of Acquisition	% CNS Susceptible	
					MRCNS	MSCNS
Cell-Wall Biosynthesis Inhibitors						
Beta-lactam	Penicillin	Cell wall	β-lactamase (blaZ)	Plasmid: Tn	0	<10
Beta-lactam	Oxacillin	Cell wall	Altered PBP (mecA)	SCCmec	0	100
Glycopeptide	Vancomycin	Cell wall	Mutations (VISA), vanA	Plasmid: Tn	>99	100
Transcription Inhibitors						
Rifamycin	Rifampin	RNA polymerase	rpoB mutation	Point mutations	80–85	95–99
DNA Inhibitors						
Flouroquinolone	Ciprofloxacin	DNA gyrase, topoisomerase IV	Mutations in: grlA, grlB, gyrA, and gyrB, Mutation in NorA MDR pump	Series of point mutations	40–45	90–95
Protein Synthesis Inhibitors						
Aminoglycoside	Gentamicin	Ribosome	Aminoglycoside-modifying enzymes (aac, aph)	Plasmid, Plasmid: Tn	40–45	90–95
Tetracycline	Tetracycline	Ribosome	Active efflux, ribosomal protection	Plasmid	75–80	80–85
Chloramphenicol	Chloramphenicol	Ribosome	Acetylation of antibiotic	Plasmid	72–77	90–95
Macrolide	Erythromycin	Ribosome	Ribosomal methylases (ermA, ermB, ermC), Efflux (msrA)	Plasmid	20–25	60–65

Lincosamide	Clindamycin	Ribosome	Ribosomal methylases,	Plasmid	40–50	88–92
Streptogramin	StreptograminB	Ribosome	Ribosomal methylases	Plasmid	Resistance rare	
Streptogramin	StreptograminA	Ribosome	Acetyltransferases, efflux	Plasmid	Resistance rare	
Oxazolidinone	Linezolid	Ribosome	23S rRNA mutation (rrn) Mutations in genes for 50S ribosomal subunit	Point mutations	Resistance rare	
Glycylcycline	Tigecycline	Ribosome	Unknown	Unknown	Resistance rare	
Small Molecule Biosynthesis Inhibitors						
Sulfonamide	Sulfamethoxazole	Dihydropterate synthetase	Overproduction of p-aminobenzoic acid (sulA)	Chromosome	Trimethoprim/sulfamethoxazole: 42–48	88–92
DHFR Inhibitor	Trimethoprim	Dihydrofolate reductase	Reduced affinity for DHFR	Chromosome		
Membrane Alteration						
Lipopeptide	Daptomycin	Cell membrane	Unknown	Stepwise mutations	Resistance rare	
New antibiotics						
Glycopeptide	Oritavancin	Cell wall	NA	NA	New	
Glycopeptide	Telavancin	Cell wall, lipid production, membrane	NA	NA	New	
Glycopeptide	Dalbavancin	Cell wall	NA	NA	New	
Cephalosporin	Ceftobiprole	Cell wall	NA	NA	New	
DHFR inhibitor	Iclaprim	Dihydrofolate reductase	DHFR	NA	New	

Abbreviations: CNS, coagulase-negative staphylococci; DHFR, dihydrofolate reductase; MRCNS, methicillin-resistant coagulase-negative staphylococci; MSCNS, methicillin-susceptible coagulase-negative staphylococci; MDR, multidrug-resistance pump; PBP, penicillin-binding protein; Tn, transposon; VISA, vancomycin intermediate-susceptible *Staphylococcus aureus*.

ANTIMICROBIAL RESISTANCE IN COAGULASE-NEGATIVE STAPHYLOCOCCI

Antistaphylococcal antibiotics are covered more fully in another article in this issue. **Table 2** summarizes information regarding antistaphylococcal antibiotics, resistance rates, and mechanisms of resistance. Briefly, when dealing with antimicrobial resistance in CNS, it is useful to distinguish hospital-acquired strains from community strains. Typically, those isolates causing disease in the community have lower rates of resistance than isolates acquired in the hospital environment.[159,160] Unfortunately, most infections caused by CNS result from the inoculation of organisms at the time of device implantation in the hospital or, in the case of many intravascular catheter infections, occur in seriously ill patients who have undergone alterations in their normal cutaneous flora to favor more resistant strains. Nosocomial isolates of CNS generally possess the *mecA* gene conferring resistance to methicillin and all of the β-lactam antibiotics. In addition, many of these strains are resistant to a variety of other antibiotic classes. The coagulase-negative staphylococci, similar to *S aureus*, may show heterotypic expression of resistance to methicillin (oxacillin) wherein only 1 in 10^4 to 10^8 cells of a genetically homogeneous population tested will be resistant.[161] Therefore, the Clinical and Laboratory Standards Institute (CLSI) has lowered the breakpoint for oxacillin to greater than or equal to 0.5 μg/mL to detect resistance in the CNS (except for *S lugdunensis,* which remains at greater than ore equal to 4 μg/mL).[162] This breakpoint detects oxacillin resistance in *S epidermidis*, *S haemolyticus,* and *S hominis* but may indicate false resistance to oxacillin in other strains of CNS.[163] For these isolates, instead of phenotypic susceptibility tests for the detection of methicillin resistance, tests that detect the *mecA* gene or PBP 2a should be used. During the 1990s, methicillin-resistance rates for CNS ranged globally from 75% to 90%.[164] The glycopeptides vancomycin (so named because of its use in "vanquishing" penicillin-resistant staphylococci) was developed in the 1950s and until the 1990s *S epidermidis* remained susceptible to this drug. Since the 1990s, there have been increasing reports of both vancomycin-intermediate as well as vancomycin-resistant strains, and overall minimum inhibitory concentration "creep."[165,166] Glycopeptides with greater potency against staphylococci that are in various stages of development include televancin, dalbovancin, and oritavancin.[167] As previously mentioned, many methicillin-resistant CNS are resistant to multiple other classes of antibiotics including aminoglycosides, tetracyclines, macrolides, and fluoroquinolones. Among the older classes of antibiotics, CNS often remain susceptible to trimethoprim-sulfamethoxazole (20% to 40% resistance) and rifampin. However, mutations conferring resistance to rifampin readily occur, and, therefore, if rifampin is used, it should be combined with another antimicrobials. CNS are generally susceptible to the streptogrammin combination quinipristin-dalfopristin, introduced in 1999; the oxazolidinone linezolid, introduced in 2001; daptomycin, a lipopeptide, approved by the Food and Drug Administration (FDA) in 2003; and tigecycline, a glycylcycline, FDA approved in 2005. Other antibiotics in development that appear to have excellent activity against methicillin-resistant CNS include a beta-lactam antibiotic, ceftobiprole, and a dihydrofolate inhibitor, iclaprim.

SUMMARY

The CNS, in particular *S epidermidis,* are uniquely qualified pathogens of modern medical care. They typically reside harmlessly on human skin and mucus membranes as a prominent part of the normal flora. However, this environmental niche gives them ready access to prosthetic devices that traverse the dermal tissues or are surgically implanted. Once these organisms gain access to the device, they are able to adhere and proliferate. *S epidermidis* is able to elaborate a thick, tenacious biofilm and establish a mature biomaterial-based infection. Recently, we have come to appreciate that the CNS biofilm-associated community is a complex ecosystem that allows the cells to shield themselves from host immunity and survive in a potentially hostile environment that includes high concentrations of antibiotic agents. Because of this stubbornness, these infections are difficult to treat and involved devices often have to be removed. However, many of these infections can be prevented or delayed by rigorous application of traditional infection control techniques. In the future, it is hoped that an increased understanding of the pathogenesis of these infections will lead to innovative prosthetic devices that are less prone to infection, novel means to prevent bacterial adherence and biofilm production, and antimicrobial agents that can eradicate CNS from biofilm-associated environments.

REFERENCES

1. Ogston A. Report upon micro-organisms in surgical diseases. Br Med J 1881;1: 369–75.
2. Archer GL, Climo MW. *Staphylococcus epidermidis* and other coagulase- negative staphylococci. In: Mandell GL, Bennett JE, Dolin R, editors. Principles and practice of infectious disease, vol. 2. Philadelphia: Elsevier Churchill Livingstone; 2005. p. 2352–9.
3. Boyce JM. Coagulase-negative staphylococci. In: Mayhall CG, editor. Hospital epidemiology and infection control, 3rd edition, vol. 1. Philadelphia: Lippincott, Williams and Wilkins, 2004. p. 495–516.
4. Weinstein MP, Towns ML, Quartey SM, et al. The clinical significance of positive blood cultures in the 1990s: a prospective comprehensive evaluation of the microbiology, epidemiology, and outcome of bacteremia and fungemia in adults. Clin Infect Dis 1997;24(4):584–602.
5. Rupp ME, Archer GL. Coagulase-negative staphylococci: pathogens associated with medical progress. Clin Infect Dis 1994;19(2):231–43 [quiz: 244–5].
6. Rupp ME. Infections of intravascular catheters and vascular devices. In: Crossley K, Archer G, editors. The staphylococci in human disease, vol. 1. New York: Churchill Livingstone Inc.; 1997. p. 379–99.
7. Banerjee SN, Emori TG, Culver DH, et al. Secular trends in nosocomial primary bloodstream infections in the United States, 1980–1989. National Nosocomial Infections Surveillance System. Am J Med 1991;91(3B):86S–9S.
8. Tristan A, Lina G, Ettienne J, et al. Biology and pathogenicity of staphylococci other than *Staphylococcus aureus* and *Staphylococcus epidermidis*. In: Fischetti VA, Novick RP, Ferretti JJ, editors. 2nd Edition, Gram-positive pathogens, vol. 1. Washington (DC): ASM Press American Society for Microbiology; 2006.
9. Refsahl K, Andersen BM. Clinically significant coagulase-negative staphylococci: identification and resistance patterns. J Hosp Infect 1992;22(1):19–31.
10. Kloos WE, Musselwhite MS. Distribution and persistence of *Staphylococcus* and *Micrococcus* species and other aerobic bacteria on human skin. Appl Microbiol 1975;30(3):381–5.
11. Kloos WE. Natural populations of the genus *Staphylococcus*. Annu Rev Microbiol 1980;34:559–92.
12. Gotz F. *Staphylococcus* and biofilms. Mol Microbiol 2002;43(6):1367–78.
13. Fleer A, Verhoef J. New aspects of staphylococcal infections: emergence of coagulase-negative staphylococci as pathogens. Antonie Van Leeuwenhoek 1984;50(5–6):729–44.

14. Huebner J, Goldmann DA. Coagulase-negative staphylococci: role as pathogens. Annu Rev Med 1999;50:223–36.
15. Mack D, Rohde H, Harris LG, et al. Biofilm formation in medical device-related infection. Int J Artif Organs 2006;29(4):343–59.
16. von Eiff C, Peters G, Heilmann C. Pathogenesis of infections due to coagulase-negative staphylococci. Lancet Infect Dis 2002;2(11):677–85.
17. Rupp ME. Nosocomial bloodstream infections. In: Mayhall CG, editor. Hospital epidemiology and infection control, 3rd Edition, vol. 1. Philadelphia: Lippincott Williams and Wilkins; 2004. p. 253–66.
18. Hanna R, Raad II. Diagnosis of catheter-related bloodstream infection. Curr Infect Dis Rep 2005;7(6):413–9.
19. O'Grady NP, Alexander M, Dellinger EP, et al. Guidelines for the prevention of intravascular catheter-related infections. Centers for disease control and prevention. MMWR Recomm Rep 2002;51(RR-10):1–29.
20. Rupp ME. Infections associated with intravascular catheters. In: Baddour LM, Gorbach SL, editors. Therapy of infectious disease, vol. 1. Philadelphia: Elsevier Science; 2003. p. 141–52.
21. Eggimann P, Sax H, Pittet D. Catheter-related infections. Microbes Infect 2004; 6(11):1033–42.
22. Raad I, Hanna H, Maki D. Intravascular catheter-related infections: advances in diagnosis, prevention, and management. Lancet Infect Dis 2007;7(10):645–57.
23. Halton K, Graves N. Economic evaluation and catheter-related bloodstream infections. Emerg Infect Dis 2007;13(6):815–23.
24. Harbarth S, Sax H, Gastmeier P. The preventable proportion of nosocomial infections: an overview of published reports. J Hosp Infect 2003;54(4):258–66 [quiz: 321].
25. Rupp ME. Coagulase-negative staphylococcal infections; an update regarding recognition and management. In: Remington JS, Swartz MN, editors. Current clinical topics in infectious disease, vol. 1. Maldon (MA): Blackwell Science; 1997. p. 51–87.
26. Herwaldt LA, Geiss M, Kao C, et al. The positive predictive value of isolating coagulase-negative staphylococci from blood cultures. Clin Infect Dis 1996; 22(1):14–20.
27. Richter SS, Beekmann SE, Croco JL, et al. Minimizing the workup of blood culture contaminants: implementation and evaluation of a laboratory-based algorithm. J Clin Microbiol 2002;40(7):2437–44.
28. Martinez JA, Pozo L, Almela M, et al. Microbial and clinical determinants of time-to-positivity in patients with bacteraemia. Clin Microbiol Infect 2007;13(7): 709–16.
29. Yebenes JC, Serra-Prat M, Miro G, et al. Differences in time to positivity can affect the negative predictive value of blood cultures drawn through a central venous catheter. Intensive Care Med 2006;32(9):1442–3.
30. Gaur AH, Flynn PM, Giannini MA, et al. Difference in time to detection: a simple method to differentiate catheter-related from non-catheter-related bloodstream infection in immunocompromised pediatric patients. Clin Infect Dis 2003;37(4): 469–75.
31. Raad I, Hanna HA, Alakech B, et al. Differential time to positivity: a useful method for diagnosing catheter-related bloodstream infections. Ann Intern Med 2004; 140(1):18–25.
32. Garcia P, Benitez R, Lam M, et al. Coagulase-negative staphylococci: clinical, microbiological and molecular features to predict true bacteraemia. J Med Microbiol 2004;53(Pt 1):67–72.

33. Mermel LA, Farr BM, Sherertz RJ, et al. Guidelines for the management of intra-vascular catheter-related infections. Clin Infect Dis 2001;32(9):1249–72.
34. Kite P, Dobbins BM, Wilcox MH, et al. Rapid diagnosis of central-venous-cathe-ter-related bloodstream infection without catheter removal. Lancet 1999; 354(9189):1504–7.
35. Maki DG, Weise CE, Sarafin HW. A semiquantitative culture method for identify-ing intravenous-catheter-related infection. N Engl J Med 1977;296(23):1305–9.
36. Bouza E, Alvarado N, Alcala L, et al. A prospective, randomized, and compar-ative study of 3 different methods for the diagnosis of intravascular catheter colonization. Clin Infect Dis 2005;40(8):1096–100.
37. Sherertz RJ, Heard SO, Raad II. Diagnosis of triple-lumen catheter infection: comparison of roll plate, sonication, and flushing methodologies. J Clin Microbiol 1997;35(3):641–6.
38. Safdar N, Fine JP, Maki DG. Meta-analysis: methods for diagnosing intravascu-lar device-related bloodstream infection. Ann Intern Med 2005;142(6):451–66.
39. Bates DW, Lee TH. Rapid classification of positive blood cultures. Prospective validation of a multivariate algorithm. JAMA 1992;267(14):1962–6.
40. Bates DW, Cook EF, Goldman L, et al. Predicting bacteremia in hospitalized patients. A prospectively validated model. Ann Intern Med 1990;113(7): 495–500.
41. O'Brien T, Collin J. Prosthetic vascular graft infection. Br J Surg 1992;79(12): 1262–7.
42. Lalani T, Kanafani ZA, Chu VH, et al. Prosthetic valve endocarditis due to coag-ulase-negative staphylococci: findings from the International Collaboration on Endocarditis Merged Database. Eur J Clin Microbiol Infect Dis 2006;25(6): 365–8.
43. Wang A, Athan E, Pappas PA, et al. Contemporary clinical profile and outcome of prosthetic valve endocarditis. JAMA 2007;297(12):1354–61.
44. Whitener C, Caputo GM, Weitekamp MR, et al. Endocarditis due to coagulase-negative staphylococci. Microbiologic, epidemiologic, and clinical consider-ations. Infect Dis Clin North Am 1993;7(1):81–96.
45. Chu VH, Woods CW, Miro JM, et al. Emergence of coagulase-negative staphy-lococci as a cause of native valve endocarditis. Clin Infect Dis 2008;46(2): 232–42.
46. Demitrovicova A, Hricak V, Karvay M, et al. Endocarditis due to coagulase-neg-ative staphylococci: data from a 22-year national survey. Scand J Infect Dis 2007;39(6–7):655–6.
47. Hricak V, Kovacik J, Marks P, et al. Aetiology and outcome in 53 cases of native valve staphylococcal endocarditis. Postgrad Med J 1999;75(887):540–3.
48. Caputo GM, Archer GL, Calderwood SB, et al. Native valve endocarditis due to coagulase-negative staphylococci. Clinical and microbiologic features. Am J Med 1987;83(4):619–25.
49. Chu VH, Cabell CH, Abrutyn E, et al. Native valve endocarditis due to coagulase-negative staphylococci: report of 99 episodes from the International Collaboration on Endocarditis Merged Database. Clin Infect Dis 2004;39(10): 1527–30.
50. Etienne J, Eykyn SJ. Increase in native valve endocarditis caused by coagulase negative staphylococci: an Anglo-French clinical and microbiological study. Br Heart J 1990;64(6):381–4.
51. Gandelman G, Frishman WH, Wiese C, et al. Intravascular device infections: epidemiology, diagnosis, and management. Cardiol Rev 2007;15(1):13–23.

52. Chua JD, Wilkoff BL, Lee I, et al. Diagnosis and management of infections involving implantable electrophysiologic cardiac devices. Ann Intern Med 2000; 133(8):604–8.
53. del Rio A, Anguera I, Miro JM, et al. Surgical treatment of pacemaker and defibrillator lead endocarditis: the impact of electrode lead extraction on outcome. Chest 2003;124(4):1451–9.
54. Rupp ME. Pathogenesis of Staphylococcus epidermidis prosthetic joint infection: adherence and biofilm formation. Semin Arthroplasty 1998;9(4):274–80.
55. Gentry LO. Osteomyelitis and other infections of bones and joints. In: Crossley KB, Archer GL, editors. The Staphylococci in Human Disease, 1st editon. New York: Churchill Livingstone; 1997. p. 455–73.
56. Brause BD. Infections with prostheses in bones and joints. In: Mandell GL, Bennett E, Dolin R, editors. Principles and practices of infectious diseases, 6th edition, vol. 1. Philadelphia: Elsevier; 2005. p. 1332–7.
57. Lentino JR. Infections associated with prosthetic knee and prosthetic hip. Curr Infect Dis Rep 2004;6(5):388–92.
58. Trampuz A, Piper KE, Jacobson MJ, et al. Sonication of removed hip and knee prostheses for diagnosis of infection. N Engl J Med 2007;357(7):654–63.
59. Berbari EF, Marculescu C, Sia I, et al. Culture-negative prosthetic joint infection. Clin Infect Dis 2007;45(9):1113–9.
60. Tunkel AR, Kaufman BA. Cerebrospinal fluid shunt infections. In: Mandell GL, Bennett JE, Dolin R, editors. Principles and Practice of Infectious Diseases, 6th editon. Philadelphia: Elsevier; 2005. p. 1126–32.
61. Kestle JR, Garton HJ, Whitehead WE, et al. Management of shunt infections: a multicenter pilot study. J Neurosurg 2006;105(Suppl 3):177–81.
62. Schreffler RT, Schreffler AJ, Wittler RR. Treatment of cerebrospinal fluid shunt infections: a decision analysis. Pediatr Infect Dis J 2002;21(7):632–6.
63. Wong ES. Surgical site infections. In: Mayhall CG, editor. Hospital epidemiology and infection control, vol. 1. Philadelphia: Lippincott, Williams and Wilkins; 2004. p. 287–306.
64. Horan TC, Gaynes RP, Martone WJ, et al. CDC definitions of nosocomial surgical site infections, 1992: a modification of CDC definitions of surgical wound infections. Infect Control Hosp Epidemiol 1992;13(10):606–8.
65. Homer-Vanniasinkam S. Surgical site and vascular infections: treatment and prophylaxis. Int J Infect Dis 2007;11(Suppl 1):S17–22.
66. von Eiff C, Jansen B, Kohnen W, et al. Infections associated with medical devices: pathogenesis, management and prophylaxis. Drugs 2005;65(2): 179–214.
67. Anday EK, Talbot GH. Coagulase-negative Staphylococcus bacteremia—a rising threat in the newborn infant. Ann Clin Lab Sci 1985;15(3):246–51.
68. Gaynes RP, Martone WJ, Culver DH, et al. Comparison of rates of nosocomial infections in neonatal intensive care units in the United States. National Nosocomial Infections Surveillance System. Am J Med 1991;91(3B):192S–6S.
69. Benzies KM. Advanced maternal age: are decisions about the timing of childbearing a failure to understand the risks? CMAJ 2008;178(2):183–4.
70. Klingenberg C, Ronnestad A, Anderson AS, et al. Persistent strains of coagulase-negative staphylococci in a neonatal intensive care unit: virulence factors and invasiveness. Clin Microbiol Infect 2007;13(11):1100–11.
71. Khadilkar V, Tudehope D, Fraser S. A prospective study of nosocomial infection in a neonatal intensive care unit. J Paediatr Child Health 1995;31(5):387–91.

72. Venkatesh MP, Placencia F, Weisman LE. Coagulase-negative staphylococcal infections in the neonate and child: an update. Semin Pediatr Infect Dis 2006; 17(3):120–7.
73. Latham RH, Running K, Stamm WE. Urinary tract infections in young adult women caused by *Staphylococcus saprophyticus*. JAMA 1983;250(22):3063–6.
74. Hovelius B, Mardh PA. *Staphylococcus saprophyticus* as a common cause of urinary tract infections. Rev Infect Dis 1984;6(3):328–37.
75. Rupp ME, Soper DE, Archer GL. Colonization of the female genital tract with *Staphylococcus saprophyticus*. J Clin Microbiol 1992;30(11):2975–9.
76. Wallmark G, Arremark I, Telander B. *Staphylococcus saprophyticus*: a frequent cause of acute urinary tract infection among female outpatients. J Infect Dis 1978;138(6):791–7.
77. Jordan PA, Iravani A, Richard GA, et al. Urinary tract infection caused by *Staphylococcus saprophyticus*. J Infect Dis 1980;142(4):510–5.
78. Kuroda M, Yamashita A, Hirakawa H, et al. Whole genome sequence of *Staphylococcus saprophyticus* reveals the pathogenesis of uncomplicated urinary tract infection. Proc Natl Acad Sci U S A 2005;102(37):13272–7.
79. Gatermann S, John J, Marre R. *Staphylococcus saprophyticus* urease: characterization and contribution to uropathogenicity in unobstructed urinary tract infection of rats. Infect Immun 1989;57(1):110–6.
80. Gillespie WA, Sellin MA, Gill P, et al. Urinary tract infection in young women, with special reference to *Staphylococcus saprophyticus*. J Clin Pathol 1978;31(4):348–50.
81. Frank KL, Del Pozo JL, Patel R. From clinical microbiology to infection pathogenesis: how daring to be different works for *Staphylococcus lugdunensis*. Clin Microbiol Rev 2008;21(1):111–33.
82. Jones RM, Jackson MA, Ong C, et al. Endocarditis caused by *Staphylococcus lugdunensis*. Pediatr Infect Dis J 2002;21(3):265–8.
83. van der Mee-Marquet N, Achard A, Mereghetti L, et al. *Staphylococcus lugdunensis* infections: high frequency of inguinal area carriage. J Clin Microbiol 2003;41(4):1404–9.
84. Hebert GA. Hemolysins and other characteristics that help differentiate and biotype *Staphylococcus lugdunensis* and *Staphylococcus schleiferi*. J Clin Microbiol 1990;28(11):2425–31.
85. Mitchell J, Tristan A, Foster TJ. Characterization of the fibrinogen-binding surface protein Fbl of *Staphylococcus lugdunensis*. Microbiology 2004;150 (Pt 11):3831–41.
86. Lambe DW Jr, Ferguson KP, Keplinger JL, et al. Pathogenicity of *Staphylococcus lugdunensis*, *Staphylococcus schleiferi*, and three other coagulase-negative staphylococci in a mouse model and possible virulence factors. Can J Microbiol 1990;36(7):455–63.
87. Nilsson M, Bjerketorp J, Wiebensjo A, et al. A von Willebrand factor-binding protein from *Staphylococcus lugdunensis*. FEMS Microbiol Lett 2004;234(1): 155–61.
88. Donvito B, Etienne J, Denoroy L, et al. Synergistic hemolytic activity of *Staphylococcus lugdunensis* is mediated by three peptides encoded by a non-agr genetic locus. Infect Immun 1997;65(1):95–100.
89. Takeuchi F, Watanabe S, Baba T, et al. Whole-genome sequencing of *Staphylococcus haemolyticus* uncovers the extreme plasticity of its genome and the evolution of human-colonizing staphylococcal species. J Bacteriol 2005;187(21): 7292–308.

90. Nunes AP, Teixeira LM, Iorio NL, et al. Heterogeneous resistance to vancomycin in *Staphylococcus epidermidis, Staphylococcus haemolyticus* and *Staphylococcus warneri* clinical strains: characterisation of glycopeptide susceptibility profiles and cell wall thickening. Int J Antimicrob Agents 2006; 27(4):307–15.

91. Billot-Klein D, Gutmann L, Bryant D, et al. Peptidoglycan synthesis and structure in *Staphylococcus haemolyticus* expressing increasing levels of resistance to glycopeptide antibiotics. J Bacteriol 1996;178(15):4696–703.

92. O'Gara JP, Humphreys H. *Staphylococcus epidermidis* biofilms: importance and implications. J Med Microbiol 2001;50(7):582–7.

93. Vuong C, Otto M. *Staphylococcus epidermidis* infections. Microbes Infect 2002; 4(4):481–9.

94. Vuong C, Durr M, Carmody AB, et al. Regulated expression of pathogen-associated molecular pattern molecules in *Staphylococcus epidermidis*: quorum-sensing determines pro-inflammatory capacity and production of phenol-soluble modulins. Cell Microbiol 2004;6(8):753–9.

95. Heilmann C, Schweitzer O, Gerke C, et al. Molecular basis of intercellular adhesion in the biofilm-forming *Staphylococcus epidermidis*. Mol Microbiol 1996; 20(5):1083–91.

96. Arciola CR, Baldassarri L, Montanaro L. Presence of icaA and icaD genes and slime production in a collection of staphylococcal strains from catheter-associated infections. J Clin Microbiol 2001;39(6):2151–6.

97. Rupp ME, Ulphani JS, Fey PD, et al. Characterization of *Staphylococcus epidermidis* polysaccharide intercellular adhesin/hemagglutinin in the pathogenesis of intravascular catheter-associated infection in a rat model. Infect Immun 1999; 67(5):2656–9.

98. Rupp ME, Archer GL. Hemagglutination and adherence to plastic by *Staphylococcus epidermidis*. Infect Immun 1992;60(10):4322–7.

99. Arciola CR, Baldassarri L, Montanaro L. In catheter infections by *Staphylococcus epidermidis* the intercellular adhesion (ica) locus is a molecular marker of the virulent slime-producing strains. J Biomed Mater Res 2002;59(3):557–62.

100. Galdbart JO, Allignet J, Tung HS, et al. Screening for *Staphylococcus epidermidis* markers discriminating between skin-flora strains and those responsible for infections of joint prostheses. J Infect Dis 2000;182(1):351–5.

101. Handke LD, Slater SR, Conlon KM, et al. SigmaB and SarA independently regulate polysaccharide intercellular adhesin production in *Staphylococcus epidermidis*. Can J Microbiol 2007;53(1):82–91.

102. Baird-Parker AC. Staphylococci and their classification. Ann N Y Acad Sci 1965; 128(1):4–25.

103. Kloos WE, Schleifer KH. Simplified scheme for routine identification of human *Staphylococcus* species. J Clin Microbiol 1975;1(1):82–8.

104. Casey AL, Worthington T, Lambert PA, et al. Evaluation of routine microbiological techniques for establishing the diagnosis of catheter-related bloodstream infection caused by coagulase-negative staphylococci. J Med Microbiol 2007; 56(Pt 2):172–6.

105. Combe M, Lemeland J, Pestel-Caron M, et al. Multilocus enzyme analysis in aerobic and anaerobic bacteria using gel electrophoresis-nitrocellulose blotting. FEMS Microbiol Lett 2000;185(2):169–74.

106. Parisi JT, Lampson BC, Hoover DL, et al. Comparison of epidemiologic markers for *Staphylococcus epidermidis*. J Clin Microbiol 1986;24(1):56–60.

107. Schlichting C, Branger C, Fournier JM, et al. Typing of *Staphylococcus aureus* by pulsed-field gel electrophoresis, zymotyping, capsular typing, and phage typing: resolution of clonal relationships. J Clin Microbiol 1993;31(2):227–32.

108. Thomas JC, Vargas MR, Miragaia M, et al. Improved multilocus sequence typing scheme for *Staphylococcus epidermidis*. J Clin Microbiol 2007;45(2):616–9.

109. Turner KM, Feil EJ. The secret life of the multilocus sequence type. Int J Antimicrob Agents 2007;29(2):129–35.

110. Wang XM, Noble L, Kreiswirth BN, et al. Evaluation of a multilocus sequence typing system for *Staphylococcus epidermidis*. J Med Microbiol 2003;52 (Pt 11):989–98.

111. Monk AB, Archer GL. Use of outer surface protein repeat regions for improved genotyping of *Staphylococcus epidermidis*. J Clin Microbiol 2007;45(3):730–5.

112. Pronovost P, Needham D, Berenholtz S, et al. An intervention to decrease catheter-related bloodstream infections in the ICU. N Engl J Med 2006;355(26): 2725–32.

113. Goetz AM, Wagener MM, Miller JM, et al. Risk of infection due to central venous catheters: effect of site of placement and catheter type. Infect Control Hosp Epidemiol 1998;19(11):842–5.

114. Merrer J, De Jonghe B, Golliot F, et al. Complications of femoral and subclavian venous catheterization in critically ill patients: a randomized controlled trial. JAMA 2001;286(6):700–7.

115. Larson EL. APIC guideline for handwashing and hand antisepsis in health care settings. Am J Infect Control 1995;23(4):251–69.

116. Raad II, Hohn DC, Gilbreath BJ, et al. Prevention of central venous catheter-related infections by using maximal sterile barrier precautions during insertion. Infect Control Hosp Epidemiol 1994;15(4 Pt 1):231–8.

117. Chaiyakunapruk N, Veenstra DL, Lipsky BA, et al. Chlorhexidine compared with povidone-iodine solution for vascular catheter-site care: a meta-analysis. Ann Intern Med 2002;136(11):792–801.

118. Maki DG, Ringer M, Alvarado CJ. Prospective randomised trial of povidone-iodine, alcohol, and chlorhexidine for prevention of infection associated with central venous and arterial catheters. Lancet 1991;338(8763):339–43.

119. Tomford JW, Hershey CO, McLaren CE, et al. Intravenous therapy team and peripheral venous catheter-associated complications. A prospective controlled study. Arch Intern Med 1984;144(6):1191–4.

120. Mermel LA. Prevention of central venous catheter-related infections: what works other than impregnated or coated catheters? J Hosp Infect 2007;65(Suppl 2): 30–3.

121. Berenholtz SM, Pronovost PJ, Lipsett PA, et al. Eliminating catheter-related bloodstream infections in the intensive care unit. Crit Care Med 2004;32(10): 2014–20.

122. Veenstra DL, Saint S, Saha S, et al. Efficacy of antiseptic-impregnated central venous catheters in preventing catheter-related bloodstream infection: a meta-analysis. JAMA 1999;281(3):261–7.

123. Veenstra DL, Saint S, Sullivan SD. Cost-effectiveness of antiseptic-impregnated central venous catheters for the prevention of catheter-related bloodstream infection. JAMA 1999;282(6):554–60.

124. Maki DG, Stolz SM, Wheeler S, et al. Prevention of central venous catheter-related bloodstream infection by use of an antiseptic-impregnated catheter. A randomized, controlled trial. Ann Intern Med 1997;127(4):257–66.

125. Rupp ME, Lisco SJ, Lipsett PA, et al. Effect of a second-generation venous catheter impregnated with chlorhexidine and silver sulfadiazine on central catheter-related infections: a randomized, controlled trial. Ann Intern Med 2005;143(8): 570–80.

126. Darouiche RO, Raad II, Heard SO, et al. A comparison of two antimicrobial-impregnated central venous catheters. Catheter Study Group. N Engl J Med 1999;340(1):1–8.

127. Falagas ME, Fragoulis K, Bliziotis IA, et al. Rifampicin-impregnated central venous catheters: a meta-analysis of randomized controlled trials. J Antimicrob Chemother 2007;59(3):359–69.

128. Raad I, Darouiche R, Dupuis J, et al. Central venous catheters coated with minocycline and rifampin for the prevention of catheter-related colonization and bloodstream infections. A randomized, double-blind trial. The Texas Medical Center Catheter Study Group. Ann Intern Med 1997;127(4):267–74.

129. Sampath LA, Tambe SM, Modak SM. In vitro and in vivo efficacy of catheters impregnated with antiseptics or antibiotics: evaluation of the risk of bacterial resistance to the antimicrobials in the catheters. Infect Control Hosp Epidemiol 2001;22(10):640–6.

130. Ranucci M, Isgro G, Giomarelli PP, et al. Impact of oligon central venous catheters on catheter colonization and catheter-related bloodstream infection. Crit Care Med 2003;31(1):52–9.

131. Liu WK, Tebbs SE, Byrne PO, et al. The effects of electric current on bacteria colonising intravenous catheters. J Infect 1993;27(3):261–9.

132. Ho KM, Litton E. Use of chlorhexidine-impregnated dressing to prevent vascular and epidural catheter colonization and infection: a meta-analysis. J Antimicrob Chemother 2006;58(2):281–7.

133. Maki DG, Stahl J, Jacobson C, et al. A novel integrated chlorhexidine transparent dressing for prevention of vascular catheter-related bloodstream infections: Three comparative studies. 18th Annual Meeting of the Society for Healthcare Epidemiology of America. Orlando, FL, April 5–8, 2008. Abstract 159.

134. Maki DG, Cobb L, Garman JK, et al. An attachable silver-impregnated cuff for prevention of infection with central venous catheters: a prospective randomized multicenter trial. Am J Med 1988;85(3):307–14.

135. Levin A, Mason AJ, Jindal KK, et al. Prevention of hemodialysis subclavian vein catheter infections by topical povidone-iodine. Kidney Int 1991;40(5):934–8.

136. Lok CE, Stanley KE, Hux JE, et al. Hemodialysis infection prevention with polysporin ointment. J Am Soc Nephrol 2003;14(1):169–79.

137. Rupp ME, Struve PS, Burleson GR, et al. Effect of a silver-coated, luer-activated, intravenous catheter connector valve in a rat model of MRSA central venous catheter associated bloodstream infection. 48th Annual Interscience Conference on Antimicrobial Agents and Chemotherapy and the 46th Annual Meeting of the Infectious Diseases Society of America, Washington DC, October 25–28, 2008. Abstract K3400a.

138. Yamamoto AJ, Solomon JA, Soulen MC, et al. Sutureless securement device reduces complications of peripherally inserted central venous catheters. J Vasc Interv Radiol 2002;13(1):77–81.

139. Bleyer AJ, Mason L, Russell G, et al. A randomized, controlled trial of a new vascular catheter flush solution (minocycline-EDTA) in temporary hemodialysis access. Infect Control Hosp Epidemiol 2005;26(6):520–4.

140. Safdar N, Maki DG. Use of vancomycin-containing lock or flush solutions for prevention of bloodstream infection associated with central venous access

devices: a meta-analysis of prospective, randomized trials. Clin Infect Dis 2006; 43(4):474–84.

141. Henrickson KJ, Axtell RA, Hoover SM, et al. Prevention of central venous catheter-related infections and thrombotic events in immunocompromised children by the use of vancomycin/ciprofloxacin/heparin flush solution: a randomized, multicenter, double-blind trial. J Clin Oncol 2000;18(6):1269–78.

142. Sheth NK, Franson TR, Rose HD, et al. Colonization of bacteria on polyvinyl chloride and Teflon intravascular catheters in hospitalized patients. J Clin Microbiol 1983;18(5):1061–3.

143. Bridgett MJ, Davies MC, Denyer SP. Control of staphylococcal adhesion to polystyrene surfaces by polymer surface modification with surfactants. Biomaterials 1992;13(7):411–6.

144. Baumgartner JN, Yang CZ, Cooper SL. Physical property analysis and bacterial adhesion on a series of phosphonated polyurethanes. Biomaterials 1997;18(12):831–7.

145. Han DK, Park KD, Kim YH. Sulfonated poly(ethylene oxide)-grafted polyurethane copolymer for biomedical applications. J Biomater Sci Polym Ed 1998;9(2):163–74.

146. Mangram AJ, Horan TC, Pearson ML, et al. Guideline for prevention of surgical site infection, 1999. Hospital Infection Control Practices Advisory Committee. Infect Control Hosp Epidemiol 1999;20(4):250–78 [quiz: 279–80].

147. Neut D, Hendriks JG, van Horn JR, et al. Antimicrobial efficacy of gentamicin-loaded acrylic bone cements with fusidic acid or clindamycin added. J Orthop Res 2006;24(2):291–9.

148. Ginalska G, Kowalczuk D, Osinska M. Amikacin-loaded vascular prosthesis as an effective drug carrier. Int J Pharm 2007;339(1–2):39–46.

149. Hampl J, Schierholz J, Jansen B, et al. In vitro and in vivo efficacy of a rifampin-loaded silicone catheter for the prevention of CSF shunt infections. Acta Neurochir (Wien) 1995;133(3–4):147–52.

150. Ehrlich Garth D, Hu FZ, Lin Qiao, et al. Intelligent implants to battle biofilms. ASM News 2004;70(3):127–33.

151. Raad I, Costerton W, Sabharwal U, et al. Ultrastructural analysis of indwelling vascular catheters: a quantitative relationship between luminal colonization and duration of placement. J Infect Dis 1993;168(2):400–7.

152. Ghannoum M, O'Toole GA, editors. Microbial biofilms, 1st Edition. vol. 1. Washington (DC): ASM Press; 2004.

153. Pace JL, Rupp ME, Finch RG, editors. Biofilms, infection and antimicrobial therapy, 1st Edition. vol. 1. New York: Taylor and Francis; 2006.

154. Raad I, Davis S, Khan A, et al. Impact of central venous catheter removal on the recurrence of catheter-related coagulase-negative staphylococcal bacteremia. Infect Control Hosp Epidemiol 1992;13(4):215–21.

155. Ceri H, Olson ME, Morck DW, et al. Minimal biofilm eradication concentration (MBEC) assay; susceptibility testing for biofilms. In: Pace JL, Rupp ME, Finch RG, editors. Biofilms, Infection and Antimicrobial Therapy. New York: Taylor and Francis; 2006. p. 257–70.

156. Walencka E, Sadowska B, Rozalska S, et al. Lysostaphin as a potential therapeutic agent for staphylococcal biofilm eradication. Pol J Microbiol 2005;54(3):191–200.

157. Carmen JC, Roeder BL, Nelson JL, et al. Ultrasonically enhanced vancomycin activity against Staphylococcus epidermidis biofilms in vivo. J Biomater Appl 2004;18(4):237–45.

158. Antonios V, Berbari E, Osmon D. Treatment protocol of infection of orthopedic devices. In: Pace JL, Rupp ME, Finch RG, editors. Biofilms, Infection and Antimicrobial Therapy. New York: Taylor and Francis; 2006. p. 449–76.

159. Archer GL, Armstrong BC. Alteration of staphylococcal flora in cardiac surgery patients receiving antibiotic prophylaxis. J Infect Dis 1983;147(4):642–9.

160. Cove JH, Eady EA, Cunliffe WJ. Skin carriage of antibiotic-resistant coagulase-negative staphylococci in untreated subjects. J Antimicrob Chemother 1990; 25(3):459–69.

161. Tomasz A, Nachman S, Leaf H. Stable classes of phenotypic expression in methicillin-resistant clinical isolates of staphylococci. Antimicrob Agents Chemother 1991;35(1):124–9.

162. Clinical and Laboratory Standards Institute. Performance Standards for Antimicrobial Susceptibility Testing; Eighth Informational Supplement, CLSI document M100-S18. Wayne, PA: Clinical and Laboratory Standards Institute; 2008.

163. Hussain Z, Stoakes L, Massey V, et al. Correlation of oxacillin MIC with mecA gene carriage in coagulase-negative staphylococci. J Clin Microbiol 2000; 38(2):752–4.

164. Diekema DJ, Pfaller MA, Schmitz FJ, et al. Survey of infections due to *Staphylococcus* species: frequency of occurrence and antimicrobial susceptibility of isolates collected in the United States, Canada, Latin America, Europe, and the Western Pacific region for the SENTRY Antimicrobial Surveillance Program, 1997–1999. Clin Infect Dis 2001;32(Suppl 2):S114–32.

165. Jones RN. Microbiological features of vancomycin in the 21st century: minimum inhibitory concentration creep, bactericidal/static activity, and applied breakpoints to predict clinical outcomes or detect resistant strains. Clin Infect Dis 2006;42(Suppl 1):S13–24.

166. Deresinski S. Counterpoint: vancomycin and *Staphylococcus aureus*—an antibiotic enters obsolescence. Clin Infect Dis 2007;44(12):1543–8.

167. Aksoy DY, Unal S. New antimicrobial agents for the treatment of Gram-positive bacterial infections. Clin Microbiol Infect 2008;14:411–20.

Antistaphylococcal Agents

Howard S. Gold, MD*, Satish K. Pillai, MD

KEYWORDS

- *Staphylococcus* aureus • β-Lactam drugs
- Methicillin-resistant *S aureus*
- Vancomycin-intermediate *S aureus*

These are interesting times in the treatment of infections caused by *Staphylococcus aureus*, with shifting epidemiology of antibiotic resistance; changing prevalence of clinical syndromes (probably reflecting changes in virulence of circulating strains); and the recent availability of a variety of new agents with activity against multidrug-resistant gram-positive cocci. In the wake of the well-documented explosion in methicillin resistance in *S aureus*, one can confidently predict more limited use for currently approved β-lactam drugs for the treatment of *S aureus* infections, although several investigational β-lactams have clinically useful activity against methicillin-resistant *S aureus* (MRSA). Despite initial reports showing general susceptibility to non–β-lactam drugs (with the exception of erythromycin), it has become increasingly apparent that at least some community-associated MRSA (CA-MRSA) have become multidrug resistant and this trend is almost certain to continue as these clones cause more infections and are exposed to more courses of various non–β-lactam drugs.[1] After 40 years of vancomycin use for treatment of MRSA infections and for methicillin-susceptible *S aureus* (MSSA) in β-lactam–allergic patients, there is gathering evidence hinting at reduced efficacy of that drug. Clearly, there are isolated reports of vancomycin-resistant *S aureus* (VRSA) and vancomycin-intermediate *S aureus* (VISA), but some experts have begun to debate the efficacy of vancomycin even against isolates that test susceptible to vancomycin using the updated Clinical and Laboratory Standards Institute (CLSI) breakpoint for susceptibility of 2 μg/mL.[2–4] The magnitude of this evidence has perhaps been amplified by the efforts of pharmaceutical companies to position newer Food and Drug Administration (FDA)–approved and premarket branded agents. However, it is impossible to ignore reports of rising vancomycin minimum inhibitory concentrations (MICs), despite the fact that this has not been a universal finding,[5,6] and the effect that higher vancomycin MICs within the susceptible range seem to have on treatment outcomes in some retrospective

Silverman Institute for Health Care Quality and Safety, Division of Infectious Diseases, Beth Israel Deaconess Medical Center, 330 Brookline Avenue, LMOB-6A, Boston, MA 02215, USA
* Corresponding author.
E-mail address: hogold@caregroup.harvard.edu (H.S. Gold).

Infect Dis Clin N Am 23 (2009) 99–131
doi:10.1016/j.idc.2008.10.008
0891-5520/08/$ – see front matter © 2009 Elsevier Inc. All rights reserved.

series[7] and one prospective observational study,[8] not to mention the observations of increased vancomycin toxicity at currently used higher trough concentrations.[9] The abundance of riches in new drugs for the multidrug-resistant gram-positive space is timely, and these agents show great potential, but as yet have incompletely tested durability and comparative efficacy. This article reviews the advantages and disadvantages of the variety of antistaphylococcal agents by providing basic information including mechanism of action; mechanisms of resistance; clinical use (including dosing for and data supporting common indications); drug toxicities; and major drug interactions.

β-LACTAMS

The family of β-lactam antibiotics is a large and diverse group of drugs that have variable degrees of activity against S aureus. A detailed review of these agents is encyclopedic and beyond the scope of this article, but can be found in various standard texts.[10–13] Thus, we will limit our consideration to agents that are currently available in the United States, focusing on common themes, common usage of these drugs for staphylococcal infection, and notable exceptions. β-lactams act by binding to so-called "penicillin-binding proteins," which are proteins involved in cell-wall synthesis. These drugs are typically bactericidal against susceptible staphylococci in a time-dependent manner.[14] Resistance to β-lactam drugs in S aureus is mediated by two major mechanisms. The first is a highly prevalent narrow-spectrum β-lactamase that confers resistance to penicillins exclusive of the penicillinase-resistant penicillins dicloxacillin, oxacillin, and nafcillin. Most cephalosporins and the carbapenems are not greatly hydrolyzed by this enzyme, and β-lactamase inhibitors can protect otherwise vulnerable penicillins. The other major mechanism of resistance is the presence of the penicillin-binding protein PBP2a, mediated by the mecA gene that confers resistance to all currently FDA-approved β-lactams creating the MRSA phenotype.[11]

The adverse drug reactions caused by β-lactams include a number of class effects that occur to varying degrees after exposure to these agents and several effects that are particularly prominent with specific agents. The former can include various hypersensitivity reactions ranging from urticaria to allergic interstitial nephritis to anaphylaxis; rash; drug fever; serum sickness; gastrointestinal toxicity (particularly, although not exclusively, with oral formulations); hematologic toxicity; and seizures (relatively rare). Most β-lactams have relatively limited drug interactions, eg, most increase the anticoagulant effects of warfarin; whereas others (antistaphylococcal penicillins) actually reduce this effect and so interactions should always be reviewed for specific agents.[15,16]

Penicillins

Most S aureus isolates produce a narrow-spectrum β-lactamase that inactivates penicillins (other than nafcillin, oxacillin, and dicloxacillin). The current prevalence of β-lactamase–producing S aureus is difficult to assess because the substrate drugs are not typically tested in large surveys; however, 72.5% of 690 community-acquired lower respiratory tract isolates of S aureus from Europe and the United States from 1992 to 1993 produced β-lactamase.[17] This is much greater susceptibility than is seen in the authors' center currently, where 99% of all S aureus isolates tested were resistant to penicillin. Against the relatively rare penicillin-susceptible S aureus, penicillin (or ampicillin or amoxicillin) may be used for treatment of infections. Because most MSSA isolates are resistant to penicillin (and ampicillin, amoxicillin, piperacillin, and ticarcillin), the penicillinase-resistant penicillins, nafcillin, oxacillin, and dicloxacillin are typically used and are the mainstay of treatment. The MICs of these drugs for penicil-linase-positive and -negative MSSA are typically 0.25 to 0.4 µg/mL.[11] Oxacillin and nafcillin are the most frequently used parenteral drugs in this group, and dicloxacillin is the major oral formulation. Nafcillin and oxacillin are typically dosed at 1 to 2 g every 4–6 hours depending on the severity of the infection. Dicloxacillin is given at 250 or 500 mg four times a day.[11,13] These drugs are primarily metabolized by the liver, so dose adjustments are not made for reduced renal function. Because of their hepatic metab-olism, these drugs may interact with other medications metabolized by the liver (eg, the known interaction between warfarin and nafcillin or dicloxacillin that may result in larger warfarin doses to maintain a desirable international normalized ratio).[16,18] In addition to the standard penicillin class adverse drug reactions, these drugs may cause elevations of liver enzymes, perhaps oxacillin to a greater extent than nafcillin,[19] and it is prudent to follow liver enzymes in patients on high doses of these agents. Also, these drugs may cause other significant reactions including neutropenia, allergic interstitial nephritis, hypokalemia, and tissue necrosis from extravasation.[11,13,20] These drugs are the drugs of choice for treating serious infections caused by MSSA, and as such are recommended in guidelines for treatment for endocarditis, community-acquired pneumonia, and meningitis caused by MSSA,[21–23] in addition to their standard use in the treatment of skin and soft tissue infections (SSTI) and os-teomyelitis. Because of their status as standard-of-care treatment, these agents are often used as the control arm in clinical trials of newer drugs; their relative efficacy against those agents is discussed further in later sections.[24–30]

β-Lactam–β-Lactamase Inhibitor Combinations

The β-lactam–β-lactamase inhibitor combinations (amoxicillin-clavulanate, only avail-able in oral formulation in the United States; ticarcillin-clavulanate [IV]; ampicillin-sul-bactam [IV]; and piperacillin-tazobactam [IV]) all have good activity against MSSA, but not MRSA, and are active against anaerobes and gram-negative bacilli to varying de-grees, making them appropriate choices for the treatment of polymicrobial infections including MSSA, such as complicated SSTI.[12] For example, in a randomized, double-blinded trial, outcomes of treatment of limb-threatening diabetic foot infections were similar with ampicillin-sulbactam and imipenem-cilastatin.[31]

Cephalosporins

Cephalosporins are among the most frequently prescribed antibiotic medications and have a long record of efficacy and relative safety. They possess the typical β-lactam class adverse drug reactions. Cephalosporins are generally grouped into so-called "generations" based on antimicrobial spectrum of activity.[10] The first-generation drugs include the parenteral agent cefazolin (typically dosed at 1 g every 8 hours, but as much as 1.5 g every 6 hours can be used) and the oral drug cephalexin (typically dosed at 500 mg four times a day).[10,13] These drugs have good activity against MSSA (MIC that inhibits 90% of isolates tested [MIC_{90}] of 2–4 µg/mL) and Streptococcus pyogenes, but only limited activity against gram-negative bacilli. Some second-gener-ation drugs, such as cefuroxime, maintain good antistaphylococcal activity (MIC_{90} of 2 µg/mL) with somewhat greater gram-negative activity. The MICs of the cephamy-cins, however, such as cefotetan and cefoxitin (also grouped in the second genera-tion), versus MSSA are higher (MIC_{90} of 8–16 µg/mL). The third-generation drugs have even broader gram-negative spectrum and several are active against MSSA. The notable exceptions (ie, drugs lacking clinically useful activity against MSSA) in-clude the antipseudomonal cephalosporin ceftazidime and the oral third-generation drugs cefixime and ceftibuten. The more recently developed fourth-generation drug cefepime has very broad gram-negative activity and maintains clinically useful activity against MSSA with MIC_{90} of 4.[10]

The first-generation cephalosporins are drugs of choice for the treatment of MSSA infections in patient who are unable to tolerate antistaphylococcal penicillins. In the absence of a severe penicillin allergy, such as anaphylaxis (because of concerns for cross-reactivity), they are favored over use of vancomycin in this setting.

Carbapenems

Carbapenems are broad-spectrum β-lactam antibiotics with activity against anaerobes, gram-negative bacteria, and gram-positive bacteria, including MSSA. As a class, currently approved carbapenems lack clinically useful activity against MRSA. In the United States, carbapenems available for clinical use include imipenem, meropenem, ertapenem, and doripenem. Side effects associated with this class are essentially similar between these agents and are similar to those seen among other β-lactams, with the exception that seizures seem to be more associated with imipenem than the other carbapenems.[12] In vitro data reveal that imipenem and doripenem have slightly greater activity against MSSA than either meropenem or ertapenem, as assessed by the MIC_{90}.[32] As a class they have been shown to be effective against *S aureus* in numerous clinical studies.[33–39]

Imipenem has the broadest spectrum of FDA approval for the treatment of *S aureus* infections, including lower respiratory tract, urinary tract, intra-abdominal, gynecologic, orthopedic, and SSTI, in addition to endocarditis, bacterial septicemia caused by penicillinase-producing MSSA, and polymicrobial infections that include non–penicillinase-producing *S aureus* (ie, penicillin-susceptible).[40] Meropenem is approved by the FDA for the treatment of complicated SSTI caused by *S aureus* (MSSA).[41] Ertapenem has been approved for the treatment of MSSA-related complicated SSTI, including diabetic foot infections (excluding osteomyelitis).[42] Although doripenem demonstrates in vitro against MSSA and has been approved by the FDA for the treatment of complicated intra-abdominal infections and complicated urinary tract infections, it has not been specifically approved for the treatment of *S aureus* infections.[43]

Given their broad-spectrum of activity, the carbapenems may be most appropriate in settings that require broad, empiric therapy that includes MSSA coverage or when treating a polymicrobial infection that includes MSSA. If culture data subsequently reveal a monomicrobial MSSA infection, narrowing the antibiotic spectrum may be prudent to prevent the selection of antibiotic-resistant bacteria.

Monobactams

The monobactam drug aztreonam is a parenteral agent with activity against aerobic gram-negative bacilli, but lacks clinically relevant activity against *S aureus*.[12]

VANCOMYCIN

Vancomycin is a glycopeptide antibiotic derived from the actinomycete *Streptomyces orientalis* and was first approved by the FDA for clinical use in 1958.[44] It is not absorbed from the gastrointestinal tract in clinically relevant concentrations, and so it must be used as a parenteral agent for systemic infections. For adult patients with normal renal function, vancomycin is typically dosed at 30 mg/kg in divides doses, typically 1 g every 12 hours or 500 mg every 6 hours, but must be adjusted for reduced renal function. Although the pharmacokinetics of the drug are fairly predictable for many patients and despite the evidence that serum concentrations are not well-correlated to clinical outcomes, the testing of trough levels is advisable for patients receiving concurrent treatment with a nephrotoxic drug; those with rapidly changing renal function; patients undergoing hemodialysis or continuous venovenous hemofiltration; and patients who are morbidly obese, have severe burns, or have an infection where maintaining adequate therapeutic levels might be particularly critical, such as endocarditis, osteomyelitis, pneumonia, or meningitis. There is also some evidence from in vitro studies that exposure to subtherapeutic concentrations may tend to select for reduced susceptibility to vancomycin.[45,46] Testing of peak serum vancomycin concentrations is rarely required, but may be reasonable for patients receiving unusually high doses (>2–3 g/d) or being maintained with high trough concentrations (>25 μg/mL) of vancomycin. It is generally viewed as a slowly bactericidal drug against S aureus with time-dependent killing and acts by binding to the terminus of the peptidoglycan precursor, the building block for the bacterial cell wall.[47,48] In most large series, most S aureus isolates are inhibited by 1 μg/mL of vancomycin (roughly 94% in almost 30,000 S aureus isolates from the SENTRY database).[5] In vitro resistance to vancomycin in clinical isolates of staphylococci was unknown until 1996 when the first of what is currently referred to as VISA (MIC of vancomycin 4–8 μg/mL) was reported from a pediatric patient in Japan.[49] The mechanism of this resistance seems to be the development of a thickened abnormal cell wall that essentially traps vancomycin by providing an excess of target molecules.[50,51] Isolates with this mechanism remain uncommon,[5,52] but because of the limitations in current antimicrobial susceptibility testing methods and perhaps geographic differences, the prevalence of isolates with heterogeneous reduced susceptibility to vancomycin (hVISA) is much less certain and possibly significantly higher.[53,54] This is concerning because the current understanding is that under selective pressure from vancomycin, a series of sequential mutations are selected for as an organism transitions from full susceptibility to hVISA to VISA.[51] More recently, there have been isolated reports of fully VRSA (MIC of vancomycin ≥16 μg/mL) from the United States, but these remain quite rare.[55] The mechanism in these cases seems to be the transfer of the vancomycin resistance gene cluster from vancomycin-resistant enterococci into S aureus.[56]

The toxicities associated with vancomycin are well known, but may have been overestimated historically because of impurities of early preparations of the drug.[44] Phlebitis is a relatively common adverse reaction, and a variety of hypersensitivity reactions including rash may occur in a small number of patients. These must be distinguished from the "red-man syndrome" and hypotension, which have typically been associated with rapid infusion of the drug and do not represent true drug allergies.[57] These infusion-related events can often be avoided by using a slower vancomycin infusion. The frequency of these events may be higher in uninfected patients receiving vancomycin (eg, receiving vancomycin for surgical prophylaxis) than in infected patients.[58,59] Nephrotoxicity is often attributed to vancomycin, but is relatively uncommon in clinical use unless the drug is used at high trough levels (eg, >15 μg/mL) or combined with other nephrotoxic agents, such as aminoglycosides.[9,60] This synergistic nephrotoxicity is also vancomycin's most significant drug interaction.[9,60] Ototoxicity, historically associated with vancomycin, is actually uncommon.[44]

Vancomycin remains the standard treatment for serious MRSA infections and serious MSSA infections in patients with β-lactam allergies. Its label notes the effectiveness of vancomycin in the treatment of staphylococcal endocarditis and other indications including septicemia, bone infections, lower respiratory tract infections, and skin and skin structure infections.[61] For treatment of S aureus endocarditis, vancomycin has been noted to produce a relatively slow clinical response. In a study of vancomycin (with and without rifampin) treatment of S aureus endocarditis predominated by right-sided endocarditis cases, the median duration of fever and bacteremia were 7 and 9 days, respectively.[62] The efficacy of vancomycin (when combined with an aminoglycoside) was not statistically inferior to daptomycin in a recent clinical trial of *S aureus* bacteremia and endocarditis.[28] In the current version of the American Heart Association endocarditis treatment guidelines (endorsed by the Infectious Diseases Society of America), vancomycin remains the recommended treatment for native (6 weeks) and prosthetic valve endocarditis (PVE; at least 6 weeks) caused by MRSA and for MSSA infections in patients with anaphylactic reactions to β-lactams.[21] For the native-valve endocarditis, the potential benefit (likely nominal) of 3 to 5 days of an aminoglycoside must be balanced with the risk of synergistic nephrotoxicity, whereas for PVE vancomycin is typically combined with 2 weeks of treatment with an aminoglycoside and a full 6 weeks or more of rifampin.[21] Whereas the American Heart Association guideline suggests trough vancomycin concentration of 10 to 15 μg/mL and a peak concentration of 30 to 40 μg/mL, some expert opinion suggests higher trough concentrations (15–20 μg/mL) and less attention to peak concentrations unless the daily dose of vancomycin exceeds 2 g. A nonrandomized study of patients with MSSA bacteremia requiring hemodialysis found that the group treated with vancomycin (typically using a loading dose of vancomycin of 15 mg/kg followed by 500 mg after each dialysis session with a resulting median serum concentration of 14 μg/mL) failed treatment more often (31% versus 13%) than those treated with cefazolin (dosed at 2–3 g after each session of hemodialysis).[63] In vitro, it has been reported that β-lactams kill more rapidly than vancomycin.[47] The study by Stryjewski and colleagues[63] adds further support to a bit of staphylococcal treatment dogma: the concept that because of superior efficacy MSSA infections should be treated with β-lactams, not vancomycin, whenever possible. Additional clinical evidence in this regard was found in a retrospective study of *S aureus* bacteremias compiled by Chang and colleagues[64] that found that receipt of vancomycin (versus nafcillin) was associated with a higher rate of persistent bacteremia and relapse. The preference for β-lactams is also favored from a microbial ecology standpoint to reduce selective pressure for vancomycin-resistant gram-positive flora.[65] For the treatment of staphylococcal pneumonia, often hospital-acquired MRSA and often ventilator-associated, vancomycin remains one of the drugs of choice, as noted in the American Thoracic Society and the Infectious Diseases Society of America guidelines for the management of adults with hospital-acquired, ventilator-associated, and health care–associated pneumonia.[66] Those guidelines suggest a trough concentration of vancomycin of 15 to 20 μg/mL for the treatment of hospital-acquired pneumonia and ventilator-associated pneumonia based on poor outcomes of treatment of *S aureus* pneumonias and pharmacokinetic modeling.[66,67] Vancomycin achieves lower epithelial-lining fluid concentrations than linezolid and there has been considerable discussion of the results of a post hoc subset analysis of patients with MRSA from two clinical trials that suggested linezolid was superior to vancomycin for the treatment of hospital-acquired pneumonia.[68–70] Although biologically plausible, this purported superiority has yet to be demonstrated in a prospective fashion (see the section on linezolid for additional details). Vancomycin remains the standard of care for treatment of SSTI (caused by MSSA in patients with severe hypersensitivity to β-lactams and for MRSA) requiring parenteral therapy and has often been used as the standard treatment arm for many clinical trials testing new drugs for the treatment of complicated SSTI.[71] Cure rates in clinical trials including more than 5000 patients with MRSA infections ranged from 69% to 90%, as summarized by Stryjewski and Chambers,[72] and in no blinded study did the new agent show statistically superior efficacy to vancomycin. Vancomycin is often recommended as a standard treatment for osteomyelitis caused by MRSA or MSSA in β-lactam–intolerant patients, but there are only limited clinical data to support this common practice.[13,73] Vancomycin is recommended for treatment of cases of S aureus meningitis (MRSA or in the presence of β-lactam allergy), but achieves relatively low concentrations in the central nervous system (better for inflamed than noninflamed meninges) prompting some recommendations for using higher than standard dosing (30–45 mg/kg) and consideration of the addition of rifampin for methicillin-resistant staphylococcal meningitis, particularly in the setting of a cerebrospinal fluid shunt infection.[23,74]

Vancomycin remains a drug of choice for the treatment of serious MRSA infections or MSSA infections in patients with severe β-lactam allergy. It is a slowly bactericidal drug and has been shown to produce a similarly slow response in the treatment of some staphylococcal infections. Because of poor penetration into epithelial lining fluid, vancomycin may ultimately be supplanted by successor drugs for the treatment of MRSA pneumonia, but conclusive clinical trials are still pending. Concerns have arisen regarding possible deterioration in efficacy in recent years, but most clinical trials have not demonstrated superiority of newer agents.

DAPTOMYCIN

Daptomycin is a cyclic lipopeptide antibiotic derived from Streptomyces reseosporus.[75] It achieves bactericidal activity against gram-positive bacteria by inserting into cell membranes and causing membrane depolarization.[76] It has an MIC_{90} of 0.5 µg/mL for both MSSA and MRSA.[77] Daptomycin has been approved in the United States for use in the treatment of adults with complicated SSTI caused by gram-positive pathogens including S aureus (methicillin susceptible and resistant) at a dose of 4 mg/kg intravenously once daily by and S aureus bacteremia and right-sided endocarditis at a dose of 6 mg/kg once daily by the intravenous route. Dosing should be adjusted for renal function. In addition, there are no currently established dosing regimens for populations under the age of 18.[78]

Daptomycin has been compared with β-lactam and vancomycin in several clinical studies. For the treatment of complicated SSTI, pooled data from two prospective, randomized, controlled trials comparing daptomycin with either vancomycin or a penicillinase-resistant penicillin revealed that among 761 microbiologically evaluable patients cure rates for daptomycin were equivalent to the comparator drugs for both MSSA (85.9% and 87%, respectively) and MRSA infections (75% and 69.4%, respectively).[27]

Another prospective, randomized, controlled study evaluated the treatment of S aureus bacteremia (including right-sided endocarditis) with daptomycin versus the combination of low-dose gentamicin plus either vancomycin or an antistaphylococcal penicillin. The modified intention-to-treat analysis consisted of 120 patients in the daptomycin-treated arm and 115 patients in the comparator arm. In this analysis, daptomycin was noninferior to the comparator regimen at the 6-week posttreatment test-of-cure assessment, with a successful outcome achieved in 44.2% of patients in the daptomycin versus 41.7% in the comparator group. Success in the MITT group was defined as those patients with documented clinical improvement who did not suffer treatment-limiting adverse events; did not receive additional, potentially active non-study antibiotics; did not prematurely discontinue the study medication; and had documented negative posttreatment blood cultures. When considering only those patients that failed therapy because of lack of clinical efficacy of the treatment, success rates were 70% (daptomycin recipients) and 68.7% (comparator recipients). MRSA accounted for about 38% of isolates in both arms of the study, and whereas time to clearance of bacteremia was greater for MRSA infections (8–9 days) versus MSSA infections (3–4 days), the times to clearance did not differ between daptomycin and the comparator agents. Adverse events that occurred significantly more often in the daptomycin-treated patients included creatinine kinase elevation and bacteremia, whereas peripheral neuropathy, arthralgias, nausea, bronchospasms, and renal insufficiency were significantly less common in the daptomycin-treated patients when compared with patients receiving either vancomycin or an antistaphylococcal penicillin plus gentamicin.[28]

A post-hoc analysis of the bacteremia study was conducted to assess the efficacy of daptomycin for the treatment of osteoarticular infections (septic arthritis or osteomyelitis) Thirty-two cases of osteoarticular infections were identified among the enrolled patients with complicated S aureus bacteremia (21 receiving daptomycin, 7 receiving antistaphylococcal penicillin, 4 receiving vancomycin). At the posttreatment follow-up visit, a clinically successful outcome was achieved in 67% and 55% of patients in the daptomycin and comparator groups, respectively. The authors acknowledged, however, that the small numbers of patients with osteoarticular infections limited their ability to assess for significant differences between the two treatment groups.[29]

Following the exclusion of patients who received any other effective antibiotic therapy before study enrollment, pooled data from two clinical trials comparing daptomycin (dosed at 4 mg/kg/d) with ceftriaxone (given 2 g/d) for the treatment of community-acquired pneumonia revealed that daptomycin was associated with significantly worse overall clinical outcome compared with ceftriaxone.[79] Furthermore, eradication rates of S aureus were lower for patients receiving daptomycin (69.2%) compared with ceftriaxone (90.5%) and this difference approached statistical significance. The lack of efficacy of daptomycin for the treatment of bronchoalveolar pneumonia has been attributed to surfactant-mediated inhibition of daptomycin.[80]

Of note, early studies investigating the emergence of daptomycin resistance indicated a spontaneous mutation frequency of less than 10^{-10} for S aureus.[81] Subsequently, there have been reports of clinical failures of daptomycin therapy for the treatment of S aureus infections with the associated emergence of daptomycin nonsusceptible S aureus.[82,83] In the previously mentioned study evaluating the efficacy of daptomycin for the treatment of S aureus bacteremia, daptomycin nonsusceptible S aureus isolates emerged in 6 of the 19 patients who had microbiologic failure while receiving daptomycin therapy.[28] The authors noted that most cases of microbiologic failure occurred in settings of inadequate surgical debridement of deep-seated infections. In addition to these findings, other investigators have shown a positive in vitro correlation between reduced daptomycin susceptibility and vancomycin-intermediate susceptibility among S aureus that is independent of prior daptomycin exposure.[84,85]

Pharmacy acquisition costs should never be the sole determinant of antibiotic selection and must be balanced by considerations of efficacy, toxicity, drug interactions, drug allergies, and so forth. It is notable, however, that the average weighted price of a 500-mg vial of daptomycin, the daily dose at the 6 mg/kg dose for a 83-kg patient, is $232.09 versus the daily cost of $34.24 for 2 g (about 24 mg/kg) of vancomycin.[86]

Daptomycin is a bactericidal agent with potent in vitro activity against S aureus (MSSA and MRSA) and has been shown to be noninferior to β-lactams and vancomycin in clinical trials of SSTI and bacteremia. Clinicians should be aware of the lack of efficacy in treating bronchoalveolar pneumonia. Development of daptomycin nonsusceptible S aureus during treatment, although rare, has been documented, particularly in the setting of deep-seated S aureus infections that require surgical debridement in addition to antibiotic therapy. Finally, given that cross-resistance to daptomycin has been noted in VISA, clinicians should confirm daptomycin susceptibility before switching to this agent in patients failing vancomycin therapy for *S aureus* infections.

LINEZOLID

Approved in 2000, linezolid was the second of the newer generation of agents (following quinupristin-dalfopristin in 1998) with antimicrobial activity against resistant gram-positive pathogens, and the first new drug in 50 years with an FDA-approved indication for treatment of infections caused by MRSA. Linezolid is an oxazolidinone and the only approved agent in this class. Although there are and have been a number of oxazolidinones in development, to date none have progressed to late-stage clinical trials. These drugs act by binding to the bacterial ribosome, inhibiting protein synthesis. They are generally considered bacteriostatic against staphylococci using the standing definition of a 3-log kill in 24 hours.[87] Initially, it was thought that cross-resistance to linezolid was not conferred by mechanisms of resistance against agents acting on the ribosome; however, the more recently described typically plasmid-mediated ribosomal methyltransferase encoded by *cfr* does confer cross-resistance to linezolid, chloramphenicol, lincosamides, streptogramin A, and pleuromutilins.[88,89] Despite 8 years of rapidly escalating use of linezolid, resistance to this drug among staphylococci remains distinctly uncommon, with a recent survey of United States isolates showing nonsusceptibility (MIC >4) in fewer than 0.1% of *S aureus* isolates and 1.6% of coagulase-negative staphylococci, and only 0.5% of coagulase-negative staphylococci and no *S aureus* isolates in a recent survey of non–United States isolates.[90,91] There have been a number of reports of linezolid resistance in *S aureus* and coagulase-negative staphylococci at individual centers, and some evidence of clonal clusters of linezolid-resistant coagulase-negative staphylococci isolates,[90] so susceptibility should never be assumed.

A major advantage of linezolid is that it has excellent, nearly 100% absorption from the gastrointestinal tract. It also has an IV formulation. It can be dosed twice daily because of a half-life of approximately 5 hours without regard for renal function, but because it is a dializable drug (about one third of the drug is removed by a standard high-flux hemodialysis session), it should be dosed after hemodialysis.[92,93] Standard dosing is 600 mg every 12 hours (IV and by mouth). A 400-mg dose was approved for uncomplicated skin infections, but it has not been manufactured in the United States. Pediatric dosing is 10 mg/kg every 8 hours for children up to 11 years of age, and adult dosing for children 12 years of age and older. Its major drug interaction liabilities relate the linezolid's activity as a monoamine oxidase inhibitor, and the propensity to potentiate serotonergic and adrenergic drugs (rarely resulting in the serotonin syndrome and a pressor response, respectively).[94–96] Because of the potential for a pressor response, foods containing large quantities of tyramine (>100 mg during a meal) should be avoided, although this is probably only rarely clinically relevant.[97,98] The most common side effects of linezolid in clinical trials were diarrhea, headache, and nausea in descending frequency. A prominent toxicity of this drug is on the bone marrow, primarily but not exclusively manifested by thrombocytopenia occurring after 2 weeks of treatment, prompting the recommendation to check complete blood counts weekly in patients receiving linezolid.[92,98] Other serious but uncommon toxicities, mostly occurring after prolonged use, include optic neuritis, peripheral neuropathy, and lactic acidosis.[99–101]

Current FDA-approved indications for linezolid include complicated skin and skin structure infections caused by S aureus including MRSA, but only including MSSA for uncomplicated skin infections, and hospital-acquired pneumonia caused by S au-reus including MRSA, but only including MSSA for community-acquired pneumonia.

The only published randomized double-blind trial of linezolid for complicated SSTI excluded MRSA infections.[24] In that study, wherein patients could receive aztreonam for gram-negative activity if necessary, linezolid intravenous or oral showed statistically equivalent efficacy to intravenous oxacillin and oral dicloxacillin with clinical cure rates in the intent-to-treat population of 69.8% versus 64.9%, respectively (P = .141; 95% confidence interval [CI], 1.58–85.8). A company-sponsored open-label study comparing the efficacy of linezolid intravenous or oral with vancomycin intravenous for the treatment of suspected or proved MRSA-complicated SSTI did show superior efficacy for the linezolid arm, but only in the subset of patients found to have MRSA.[102]

Linezolid plus aztreonam was equivalent to vancomycin plus aztreonam in two double-blind studies of hospital-acquired pneumonia (the second study being a continuation of the first), including cases caused by MRSA.[103,104] A post hoc subset analysis of patients from the two trials suggested superior efficacy for linezolid versus vancomycin for MRSA hospital-acquired pneumonia.[69] Because of the distinct advantage of attainment of excellent epithelial-lining fluid concentrations achieved by linezolid (essentially 100% of serum levels),[70] it is plausible that linezolid is the more active drug for this indication versus vancomycin (which achieves only about a 1:6 ratio of epithelial-lining fluid/serum),[68] but this has yet to be demonstrated in a prospective, double-blinded fashion. A Letter to the Editor written by authors at the FDA in response to the report by Wunderink and colleagues[104] raised substantial questions about the conclusions drawn by authors of the aforementioned study.[105] A company-sponsored phase IV clinical trial is currently enrolling to test this hypothesis in a more definitive fashion and has an estimated completion date of March 2012.[106]

Current FDA-approved indications for linezolid do not explicitly include S aureus or co-agulase-negative staphylococcal bacteremia; however, pooled data from randomized clinical trials suggest linezolid is noninferior to vancomycin for patients with secondary S aureus bacteremia.[107] Somewhat perplexing results came from a large study of catheter-related bloodstream infections treated with linezolid versus vancomycin with potential switch to oxacillin-dicloxacillin and use of aztreonam or an aminoglycoside antibiotic for known or suspected gram-negative infection at the discretion of the investigators. Linezolid was reported to be noninferior, but there was excess mortality in linezolid-treated patients with blood cultures that grew gram-negative organisms or were sterile, prompting a warning to be issued by FDA regarding lack of FDA approval for use of linezolid to treat catheter-related bloodstream infections and a reminder to providers that the drug lacks gram-negative activity.[25,108] Case reports have described the use of linezolid to treat infective endocarditis, as summarized by Falagas and colleagues,[109] but this indication has not been studied in a clinical trial. Because of its activity as an inhibitor of protein synthesis, an effect that is shared by clindamycin, linezolid may be a useful agent in staphylococcal toxin-mediated diseases, including toxic shock syndrome and necrotizing pneumonia.[110–112]

Pediatric use of linezolid has been studied directly in pharmacokinetic studies,[113] and in a few randomized clinical trials. The largest pediatric clinical study was a randomized, open label, multicenter study of hospitalized subjects from birth to 12 years of age comparing linezolid with vancomycin in the treatment of nosocomial pneumonia, complicated skin and skin structure infections, catheter-associated bacteremia, bacteremia of unknown source or other systemic infections caused predominantly by S aureus and coagulase-negative staphylococci. The two drugs showed comparable efficacy and linezolid had fewer adverse drug reactions (19% versus 34%; P<.001).[114] There was a randomized, blinded, multicenter study of hospitalized subjects from 5 to 17 years of age that demonstrated equivalence of linezolid to cefadroxil in the treatment of uncomplicated skin and skin structure infections.[115] The package insert includes pediatric use for nosocomial pneumonia, community-acquired pneumonia, and complicated skin and skin structure infections for pediatric patients from birth to 11 years of age, and uncomplicated skin and skin structure infections in patients from 5 to 17 years of age.[92]

No discussion of the clinical use of linezolid is complete without consideration of the cost of the drug. At the current (September 2008) average wholesale price per day of $173.80 for the oral form and $222.70 for the IV formulation, linezolid is approximately 5.1- and 6.5-fold more expensive than vancomycin (respectively) by pharmacy cost.[86] Despite the substantially higher pharmacy costs, a number of studies have concluded that use of linezolid could be cost-effective. For example, one analysis showed a shorter hospital length of stay in clinically evaluable patients with SSTI treated with linezolid median 8 days (95% CI, 6–13; P = .0025), mean of 15.4 days (SE 1.9; P = .0025) versus vancomycin (median 16 days [95% CI, 13–19]; mean of 20.3 days [SE 1.7]).[116]

Linezolid is a very useful but expensive antistaphylococcal agent. It remains active against most S aureus isolates. Because of its excellent bioavailability, the option of oral treatment is very appealing and can reduce hospital length of stay. In clinical trials published to date and in a meta-analysis, when only blinded clinical trials are considered, linezolid has not been demonstrated to be superior to comparators.[117]

TRIMETHROPRIM-SULFAMETHAXAZOLE

Both trimethoprim and sulfonamides inhibit enzymes in the bacterial folate biosynthesis pathway. Combining the trimethoprim with a sulfonamide achieves bactericidal activity and reduces the emergence of bacterial resistance.[118] Trimethoprim-sulfamethaxazole (TMP-SMX) is available in oral and IV formulations. Because of its renal elimination dosing must be adjusted for renal function. Among the side effects associated with TMP-SMX are gastrointestinal upset; dermatologic reactions (ranging from rash to Stevens-Johnson syndrome); cytopenias; and hepatic and renal dysfunction.[119] In a recent study, sulfonamides (along with clindamycin and moxifloxacin) was one of the drugs associated with the highest frequency of estimated emergency department visits (per prescription visit) for antibiotic-associated adverse drug reactions, and had the highest frequency of moderate-to-severe allergic reactions.[120] Folate antagonists, such as TMP-SMX, are not recommended for use during pregnancy.[121] Although antibacterial drugs in general may affect the anticoagulant effects of warfarin, TMP-SMX seems to be a particularly problematic agent in this regard and relatively frequently causes supratherapeutic international normalized ratios.[15]

In terms of antistaphylococcal activity, in vitro studies have shown that the combination of TMP-SMX is synergistic and bactericidal against MSSA and MRSA,[122–125] and demonstrates significantly greater activity than either of the drugs alone in an MRSA mouse intraperitoneal infection model.[123]

Despite these in vitro data, a review summarizing the existing literature on the use of TMP-SMX for the treatment of S aureus infections reported a cumulative failure rate of 50% among 221 patients treated between 1972 and 2005.[118] It is important to note, however, that the studies included in this review varied greatly in their designs (prospective versus retrospective, different routes of drug administration, and whether the efficacy of TMP-SMX was being compared with that of another antibiotic). In addition, the studies included multiple types of infection (bacteremia, right-sided endocarditis, SSTI, bone and joint infections, meningitis, bronchiectasis, and perito-neal dialysis catheter infection). Because of these differences, it is difficult accurately to assess the efficacy of TMP-SMX for the treatment of S aureus from these aggregate data. Some of the individual studies included in this review, however, provide some insights into the potential role of TMP-SMX in the treatment of S aureus infections.

A small prospective, randomized clinical trial compared TMP-SMX (160 mg/800 mg orally twice a day) with doxycyline (100 mg orally twice a day) for 7 days for the treat-ment of SSTI following incision and drainage of the wound.[126] Most infections were caused by CA-MRSA (68%) and intention-to-treat analysis failed to demonstrate a sig-nificant difference between the two treatment arms at the 10- to 14-day follow-up (11 of 14 patients cured in TMP-SMX arm versus 19 of 20 cured in doxycycline arm). Szumowski and colleagues[127] conducted a retrospective analysis of 200 cases of SSTI caused by MRSA presenting to a community health clinic. The authors found that improved clinical outcomes coincided with the increased use of TMP-SMX as the empiric antibiotic of choice for these patients. This statistically significant difference persisted even after controlling for the use of wound incision and drainage. Taken to-gether, these data suggest TMP-SMX is a viable oral option for the treatment of SSTI caused by S aureus infections, especially when resistance rates to other antistaphyl-coccal agents in the community are high. This is reflected in the Infectious Diseases Society of America's treatment guidelines for SSTI, in which TMP-SMX is one of the options for disease caused by either MSSA or MRSA for both adult and pediatric pa-tients. For adults the recommended dosing is one to two double-strength TMP-SMX tablets (160 mg of trimethoprim in each double-strength tablet) twice daily and in pe-diatric patients the dose is 8 to 12 mg/kg (based on trimethoprim component) in two to four daily divided doses depending on route of administration.[71]

In a randomized, controlled trial comparing the efficacy of intravenous TMP-SMX (320 mg/1600 mg IV every 12 hours) with vancomycin (1 g IV every 12 hours) for the treatment of S aureus infections among parenteral drug users (including SSTI, bone and joint infections, right-sided endocarditis, and suppurative thrombophlebitis), Markowitz and colleagues[128] evaluated 101 (43 in the TMP-SMX arm, 58 in the vanco-mycin arm). Among the study population, nearly two thirds were bacteremic and nearly half of the infections were caused by MRSA. Overall, there were no statistically significant differences between the two arms in terms of duration of positive S aureus cultures, duration of fever, or hospital stay. The cure rate in the TMP-SMX arm (86%) was significantly lower, however, compared with the vancomycin arm (98% cure rate). Interestingly, in subgroup analysis, the difference in cure rates between the two arms of the study occurred because of reduced efficacy of TMP-SMX against MSSA infec-tions (cure rates of 73% versus 97% for vancomycin). All patients with MRSA infection were cured in both arms.

Other investigators have looked at the use of TMP-SMX in the treatment of MRSA osteomyelitis.[124] In this noncomparative study, four (67%) of six patients treated with oral TMP-SMX for a minimum of 8 weeks had a positive clinical response.

In an era of increasing community-associated MRSA SSTI, TMP-SMX may be an attrac-tive therapeutic option, contingent on local susceptibility patterns. Susceptibility to this drug seems to be largely preserved, even in otherwise multidrug-resistant CA-MRSA.[1] The studies by Markowitz and colleagues[128] and Yeldandi and colleagues[124] suggest that in more complicated or invasive staphylococcal infections, TMP-SMX could be con-sidered a treatment alternative if other first-line antistaphylcoccal antibiotics fail, are not tolerated, or are otherwise contraindicated. Also, TMP-SMX may be an oral "step-down" treatment option for certain complicated S aureus infections (eg, osteomyelitis) following initial clinical improvement with a course of appropriate IV antibiotic therapy.

TETRACYCLINES AND GLYCYLCYCLINES

The tetracyclines are bacteriostatic agents that act by binding to the bacterial ribosome to inhibit protein synthesis. Doxycycline and minocycline have greater staphylococcal activity than tetracycline, and tigecycline is the most active agent of this group against MRSA. The tetracyclines (tetracycline, doxycycline, and minocycline) are highly bioavailable and can be administered either orally or parenterally; however, the IV formulation of minocycline is not currently available in the United States. Tigecycline is only available as a parenteral drug. Side effects are varied and include photosensitivity; lupus-like reactions (seen with minocycline); gastrointestinal symptoms (notably tigecycline); hepatotoxicity; vestibular toxicity (seen with minocycline); and pseudotumor cerebrii. They are also contraindicated in children less than 8 years old and pregnant women because of the accumulation in developing bone and teeth.[129–131]

Doxycycline and Minocycline

In a review of the literature regarding the use of long-acting tetracyclines (doxycycline and minocycline) for the treatment of S aureus infections, Ruhe and colleagues[132] found that among nine separate studies, published between 1971 and 1990, a total of 85 patients with S aureus infections were treated with the long-acting tetracyclines (either as monotherapy or in conjunction with rifampin). The overall cure rate in this population was 85%. SSTI represented the most common treatment indication (53 [62%] of 85 patients). There were too few patients with other treatment indications (pneumonia, osteomyelitis, septic thrombophlebitis, urinary tract infection, endocarditis, and liver abscess) to determine adequately the efficacy of using tetracyclines for infections other than SSTI. These same authors also retrospectively reviewed patients treated at their institution between 1999 and 2004 with either doxycycline or minocycline for culture-proved complicated SSTI (exclusive of folliculitis or other simple skin infection), urinary tract infections, and invasive infections caused by MRSA. Of 24 patients meeting their study criteria, 18 received monotherapy, whereas five patients were treated also with rifampin (four) or TMP-SMX (one). Similar to their literature review findings, 16 patients (67%) had SSTI (cure rates were 91% for individuals treated with doxycycline and 100% for those receiving minocycline) and the overall cure rate for the entire group of 24 patients treated at their institution was 83%.[132] In a larger retrospective cohort study, Ruhe and Menon[133] also evaluated the role of the long-acting tetracyclines for the treatment of CA-MRSA SSTI in patients at their institution between 1999 and 2007. Among 90 cases of MRSA SSTIs treated with doxycycline (97% of cases) or minocycline (3% of cases), the overall cure rate was 96%. Important caveats to this study include the facts that 95% of MRSA isolates identified at the authors' institution during the study period were susceptible to tetracyclines, and most patients (69%) treated with tetracyclines for SSTI underwent surgical drainage of a purulent focus of infection at the time of diagnosis. Finally, in a small prospective study comparing the efficacy of incision and drainage plus either doxycycline or TMP-SMX for the treatment of SSTI, among 34 enrolled patients (27 of whom had S aureus infection) the cure rate was at least 95% among the 20 patients receiving doxycycline and adequate surgical wound management (one patient with MRSA was lost to follow-up and could not be assessed).[126]

Based on these studies, and contingent on local susceptibility patterns and appropriate surgical drainage, doxycycline and minocycline seem to be effective for the treatment of SSTI caused by S aureus. Although there are case series and reviews describing the use of the tetracycline-class in the treatment of other types of staphylococcal infections, including pneumonia, osteomyelitis, prosthetic joint infections, and endocarditis,[132,134] in the absence of more detailed investigations it is difficult to recommend this class of antibiotic as first-line therapy in these settings.

Tigecycline

Tigecycline is a glycylcycline, a modification of the minocycline molecule that was designed to circumvent known mechanisms of resistance to the tetracycline class of antibiotics, including ribosomal modification and efflux pump mediated resistance.[131,135] The drug has an extremely broad spectrum of activity, and the MIC of tigecycline for nearly 600 S aureus clinical isolates (including both MSSA and MRSA), collected from four phase 3 clinical trials, was low and ranged between 0.06 and 1 µg/mL with an MIC_{90} of 0.25 µg/mL. Also of note, the tigecycline MIC was less than or equal to 0.5 µg/mL for 11 minocycline-resistant S aureus isolates.[136] The pharmacokinetics of tigecycline are notable in that the drug has a very large volume of distribution and the maximum serum concentration using the FDA-approved 50-mg dose was a fairly modest 0.62 µg/mL after multiple 50-mg doses.[137]

Tigecycline has been approved by the FDA for the treatment of adults with complex skin and soft tissue structure infections and complex intra-abdominal infections. In a pooled analysis of two studies comparing the efficacy of tigecycline in the treatment of complicated SSTI with that of the combination of vancomycin and aztreonam, the microbiologic cure rates were equivalent for infection caused by both MSSA (approximately 90% in both arms) and MRSA (approximately 75% in both arms).[138]

Although there are case series reports describing the use of tigecycline in the treatment of other invasive staphylococcal infections,[139,140] clinicians must exercise care and give consideration to the modest serum concentration achievable with standard dosing schedules of tigecycline before extrapolating the use of this agent for the treatment of S aureus infections that are beyond its currently approved treatment indications.

AMINOGLYCOSIDES

Aminoglycosides are bactericidal agents that disrupt protein synthesis by binding to the bacterial ribosome. Class-specific side effects include nephrotoxicity and ototoxicity.[141] In the treatment of staphylococcal infections, aminoglycosides function as a component of multidrug treatment regimens and serve to achieve synergistic bacterial killing or to prevent the emergence of bacterial resistance. S aureus endocarditis is the treatment indication for which the addition of an aminoglycoside is most often considered.

In vitro and animal model studies from the 1970s demonstrated the addition of gentamicin to nafcillin afforded synergistic killing of S aureus compared with nafcillin alone.[142] In a randomized trial comparing 4 weeks of β-lactam monotherapy with 2 weeks of gentamicin plus 4 weeks of β-lactam in 25 patients with S aureus native-valve endocarditis related to IV drug use, however, there were no differences in the two treatment groups in terms of time to defervesence, rates of bacteriologic failure, or mortality.[143] Similarly, in a study evaluating patients with either right- or left-sided MSSA endocarditis (with or without a history of IV drug use), although the addition of 2 weeks of gentamicin to a 6-week course of nafcillin resulted in decreased duration of bacteremia (by 1–1.5 days), there was no overall mortality benefit and there was increased nephrotoxicity observed in the non–IV drug use patients with predominantly left-sided endocarditis.[144] When specifically evaluating native-valve, right-sided S aureus endocarditis in the IV drug use population, a 2-week course of low-dose tobramycin plus β-lactam therapy was found to achieve high cure rates (94%).[145] Subsequent data revealed, however, that the addition of the aminoglycoside to 2 weeks of β-lactam (cloxacillin) did not improve treatment success rates (86% for combination therapy versus 89% for cloxacillin alone).[146] Several of these studies[143–146] have also been evaluated as part of a recent meta-analysis, which confirmed that addition of aminoglycosides failed to improve treatment success rates or mortality of S aureus native-valve endocarditis.[147] Guidelines for the treatment of endocarditis issued by the American Heart Association are reflective of the lack of clear efficacy of aminoglycosides in the management of either left-sided or non–IV drug use–associated, right-sided native-valve endocarditis caused by MSSA, and state that the addition of gentamicin (3 mg/kg IV or intramuscularly daily in divided doses) to a β-lactam is an optional consideration and should not be continued beyond the first 3 to 5 days of therapy. Furthermore, in the setting of uncomplicated, IV drug use–associated right-sided MSSA endocarditis, these guidelines note that treatment with 2 weeks of β-lactam therapy, irrespective of the addition of aminoglycoside, seems to be sufficient.[21] The role of aminoglycosides in the treatment of native-valve endocarditis caused by MRSA is limited because of higher rates of aminoglycoside resistance among MRSA; the potential for synergistic nephrotoxicity and ototoxicity when combining an aminoglycoside with vancomycin;[60,141] and high clinical failure rates when used in short-course (2-week) therapy with vancomycin for the treatment of right-sided endocarditis.[148]

The use of aminoglycosides for the treatment of S aureus PVE derives from studies of coagulase-negative staphylococcal PVE. In a study comparing a 6-week regimen of vancomycin plus rifampin with a 6-week regimen of these two agents plus 2 weeks of gentamicin, the cure rates were similar in the two arms. A total of 37% of patients receiving the dual antibiotic regimen developed rifampin-resistant staphylococci, however, necessitating adjustment of the antibiotic regimen (addition of a prolonged course of gentamicin to vancomycin). No patients in the triple antibiotic arm developed rifampin resistance.[149] Extrapolating from these data, American Heart Association guidelines recommend the addition of an initial 2 weeks of gentamicin (3 mg/kg/d in divided doses) to 6 weeks of rifampin plus a semisynthetic penicillin (or vancomycin for methicillin-resistant staphylococci) in the treatment of adult or pediatric PVE caused by gentamicin-susceptible staphylococci, including S aureus.[21] Gentamicin dosing should be adjusted (interval and dose) as necessary to achieve a peak serum concentration of approximately 3 µg/mL and a trough concentration of less than 1 µg/mL.

FLUOROQUINOLONES

Fluoroquinolones are bactericidal agents that inhibit bacterial DNA gyrase and topoisomerase IV. Side effects that may be associated with this class include gastrointestinal distress, neuropsychiatric changes, cardiac conduction disturbances, abnormalities in liver enzymes, hypoglycemia or hyperglycemia, and drug rashes.[150] A recent report noted that more than other frequently used fluoroquinolones (including ciprofloxacin and levofloxacin), moxifloxacin was associated with one of the highest frequency of estimated emergency department visits (per prescription visit) for antibiotic-associated adverse drug reactions.[120] A recent FDA-issued alert focused on the risk of fluoroquinolone-associated tendonitis and tendon rupture, with increased risk among older patients (greater than 60); recipients of corticosteroids; or patients status-post kidney, heart, or lung transplant.[151] Based on studies in juvenile animals, fluoroquinolones may result theoretically in cartilage damage in children and are not presently FDA-approved agents in pediatric populations except in specified cases, which are general exclusive of staphylococcal infections.[152]

Clinically available fluoroquinolones in the United States include norfloxacin, ofloxacin, ciprofloxacin, levofloxacin, moxifloxacin, and gemifloxacin. Against MSSA and MRSA, the MIC_{90} for ciprofloxacin and ofloxacin are lower than that of norfloxacin.[153,154] Time-kill assays have demonstrated bactericidal activity (>3 log killing at 24 hours), however, for all three agents at concentrations $5 \times MIC$.[154] Of note, rapid development of ciprofloxacin resistance has been demonstrated among clinical S aureus, particularly in MRSA.[155] Although in vitro data suggest improved staphylococcal activity for levofloxacin, moxifloxacin, and gemifloxacin compared with that of ciprofloxacin, the presence of ciprofloxacin resistance in S aureus does seem to confer some cross-resistance to even these newer generation fluoroquinolones.[156–159]

In a study evaluating ciprofloxacin for the treatment of either MRSA SSTI or colonization (750 mg ciprofloxacin orally twice daily for 5, 10–14, or 21 days, with the 21-day course being coadministered with rifampin), treatment with ciprofloxacin resulted in clinical improvement in all treatment arms. Among patients treated with 5 or 10 to 14 days of ciprofloxacin, however, MRSA eradication was achieved in only 50% of patients at the end of treatment and all patients subsequently became recolonized. Among the patients treated with the combination of ciprofloxacin and rifampin, all five patients infected with fluoroquinolone- and rifampin-susceptible MRSA demonstrated clinical improvement and eradication of MRSA at the end of therapy and 1 month posttherapy.[160] Comparing moxifloxacin with piperacillin-tazobactam (with the option of transitioning to oral amoxicillin-clavulanate) for the treatment of diabetic foot infections, Lipsky and colleagues[161] demonstrated that among the microbiologically evaluable cases of S aureus infection, moxifloxacin eradicated 81% of S aureus infection (13 of 16 cases) compared with 67% (12 of 18 cases) for the β-lactam comparator. This trial allowed for the use of narrow-spectrum agents, however, such as vancomycin to treat resistant gram-positive pathogens, such as MRSA, and the authors note that because of its lack of consistent activity against MRSA, the role for moxifloxacin in the treatment of diabetic foot infections is limited.[161] As a corollary to these reports, the role of fluoroquinolone monotherapy for the treatment of contemporary SSTI may be continuing to shrink given the rising rates of community-associated MRSA infections, which in some ambulatory populations has been also associated with high rates of ciprofloxacin resistance (>75%).[127]

Multiple other investigators have further evaluated the efficacy of combining a fluoroquinolone with rifampin for the treatment of S aureus infections, including orthopedic infections and endocarditis (see also the section on rifampin).[26,30,162,163] In a prospective, randomized trial comparing a 28-day oral course of ciprofloxacin (750 mg twice daily) plus rifampin (300 mg twice daily) with oxacillin (2 g IV every 4 hours) or vancomycin (1 g every 12 hours) plus 5 days of gentamicin (2 mg/kg IV every 8 hours) for right-sided S aureus endocarditis in injection dug users, Heldman and colleagues[26] demonstrated equivalent microbiologic cure rates in both study arms (95% versus 88%) using test-of-cure blood cultures obtained approximately 1 week after discontinuation of antibiotic therapy. It is important also to note that there was approximately a 50% attrition rate in this study, however, with only 19 of 40 patients available for test-of-cure analysis in the oral treatment group and 25 of 45 patients evaluable in the parenteral treatment group. Schrenzel and colleagues[163] conducted the largest clinical trial to date studying the combination of a fluoroquinolone and rifampin. These investigators compared the efficacy of the oral fluoroquinolone, fleroxacin (not available in the United States), plus rifampin with parenteral flucloxacillin (or vancomycin) for the treatment of S aureus bacteremia or deep-seated infection (including bone and joint infection, pneumonia, right-sided endocarditis, or urinary tract infection). Cure rates were equivalent for both treatment arms among clinically evaluable patients (79% for the fluoroquinolone-rifampin combination and 76% for parenteral therapy) and among the microbiologically evaluable cases (84% for oral combination and 82% for parenteral therapy arm). Of note, although patients receiving the oral regimen had significantly shorter median length of stay (12 versus 23 days), they also had significantly more adverse drug effects compared with the patients receiving parenteral antibiotics therapy.

With rising rates of MRSA in both the community and hospital setting, the role for fluoroquinolone monotherapy in S aureus infections may be decreasing. Combination therapy with a fluoroquinolone and rifampin may be appropriate in certain infections caused by susceptible S aureus, however, particularly when attempting to salvage an infected orthopedic device or in cases of right-sided endocarditis when a transition from parenteral to oral therapy is necessary.

RIFAMPIN

Rifampin is a potent, bactericidal antistaphylococcal agent with data from the early 1980s establishing a rifampin MIC_{90} of 0.015 µg/mL for S aureus.[164,165] Although there are no recent publications reporting the susceptibility of large collections of clinical isolates, the drug seems to be maintaining reliable in vitro activity against target isolates including CA-MRSA.[1] Rifampin acts by inhibiting the bacterial RNA polymerase.[166] Because it is highly bioavailable, rifampin can be administered orally. Rapid resistance can emerge among S aureus on exposure to this drug, however, at frequency of approximately 10^{-8}.[167] In most clinical applications rifampin is used in conjunction with another antibiotic agent to prevent the development of resistance and may be best reserved for situations when the organism burden has already been reduced by prior treatment or surgery. Rifampin is associated with a wide spectrum of side effects and clinicians must also be cognizant of the potential risk for drug-drug interactions caused by rifampin-associated induction of the hepatic cytochrome P-450 system.[168]

Rifampin has been shown to be highly effective in eradicating staphylococcal infections associated with foreign bodies.[169] As such, it is used in the treatment of staphylococcal PVE and orthopedic hardware-related infections.

In patients being treated for Staphylococcus epidermidis PVE, the addition of rifampin to vancomycin increased serum bactericidal activity by more than eightfold compared with serum bactericidal activity of patients treated with vancomycin alone.[170] The clinical correlate of these data was the finding that among patients with S epidermidis PVE the addition of rifampin, an aminoglycoside, or both rifampin and an aminoglycoside to vancomycin therapy resulted in significantly greater cure rates than among patients receiving vancomycin monotherapy.[171] Extrapolating from these data, treatment with rifampin (900 mg/d for adults or 20 mg/kg/d for pediatric patients, in three equally divided doses, and administered either orally or parenterally) in combination with a β-lactam or vancomycin is now recommended for the entire 6-week duration of therapy for staphylococcal PVE, including that caused by S aureus (with an aminoglycoside administered during the initial 2-week period).[21]

Rifampin in combination with a fluoroquinolone[30,172–174] has been efficacious in the treatment of staphylococcal orthopedic hardware-related infections. Zimmerli and colleagues[30] conducted a randomized, controlled trial comparing outcomes in patients with hardware-associated orthopedic infections treated with an antistaphylococcal β-lactam (or vancomycin) plus either rifampin (orally dosed at 450 mg twice daily) or placebo for 2 weeks followed by ciprofloxacin plus either rifampin or placebo for 3 to 6 months. Enrollment criteria included early onset infection, absence of prosthesis loosening, and adequate initial surgical debridement before antibiotic therapy. With follow-up extending to nearly 3 years, all 12 patients receiving rifampin were cured (based on clinical, radiographic, and laboratory parameters) compared with only 58% of the placebo arm (7 of 12 patients).

The use of rifampin plus a fluoroquinolone has been investigated by multiple investigators for other staphylococcal infections (see the section on fluoroquinolones).[26,162,163] Caution must be used, however, in extrapolating from the aforementioned studies to other drug combinations with rifampin and other clinical scenarios. For example, there was no benefit to the addition of rifampin to vancomycin in treatment of primarily right-sided MRSA native-valve endocarditis in a small randomized trial by Levine and colleagues.[62] A more recent retrospective cohort analysis of cases of S aureus native-valve endocarditis (predominantly right-sided and MRSA) found that in addition to hepatoxicity and drug interactions, there was more prolonged bacteremia and increased mortality in patients treated with rifampin in addition to standard therapy.[175] Overall, the role of rifampin in the treatment of staphylococcal infections other than staphylococcal PVE or orthopedic hardware infection remains less well defined by clinical trials. Although some data may support a rifampin-based antibiotic regimen in these settings, other considerations that may weigh against the use of rifampin include risk of adverse drug reaction, possible drug-drug interactions, and the potential development of drug resistance.

Because of the ability to attain high nasopharyngeal drug levels, rifampin has also been used to eradicate S aureus nasal colonization. Oral rifampin has been shown to achieve nasal secretion concentrations exceeding 20 times the MIC_{90} for MRSA[176] in healthy volunteers. Rifampin monotherapy, however, fails to achieve a durable S aureus decolonization response.[177] Other investigators have evaluated the efficacy of staphylococcal decolonization when combining rifampin with TMP-SMX,[178] ciprofloxacin,[160,179] or minocycline[180] and have demonstrated mixed results. More recently, Simor and colleagues[181] showed that MRSA-colonized patients who received 7-day combined regimen of intranasal mupriocin, topical chlorhexidine, plus oral rifampin plus doxycycline were significantly more likely to remain free of MRSA colonization (64 [74%] of 87 treated patients) at 3 months follow-up compared with patients who did not receive this treatment (8 [32%] of 25 patients). Side effects attributable to treatment were noted in 25% of cases, but were reported to be mild in nature. The authors noted that 54% of patients available for follow-up 8 months after the decolonization treatment remained MRSA-free. Of note, because this study included multiple interventions it is difficult to determine the contribution of the rifampin plus doxycycline. Based on these data, if the decision is made to use rifampin in a staphylococcal decolonization regimen, consideration should be given to including an additional antistaphylococcal antibiotic and a topical antibiotic and antiseptic agent maximally to ensure eradication. Irrespective of the regimen used, there seems to be a time-dependent risk for reacquisition of nasal colonization.

MACROLIDES, KETOLIDES, CLINDAMYCIN, QUINUPRISTIN-DALFOPRISTIN

The macrolides-lincosamide-streptogramin (MLS) antibiotics currently in clinical use for staphylococcal infections include several macrolides (erythromycin, clarithromycin, and the azalide azithromycin), the lincosamide drug clindamycin, and streptogramin B antibiotic quinupristin, which is combined with the streptogramin A antibiotic dalfopristin in the drug Synercid. The MLS group of drugs shares a common mechanism of action (ie, they bind to the bacterial ribosome and block protein elongation). Acquired resistance to the MLS drugs in staphylococci is typically conferred by target alteration, specifically *erm*-mediated methylation of the ribosomal target, but drug efflux is also prominent. The *erm*-mediated resistance may be constitutively or inducibly expressed. Constitutive expression results in cross-resistance to all macrolides, lincosamides, and type B streptogramins (MLS$_B$ phenotype). When inducibly expressed in staphylococci, *erm*-mediated macrolide resistance is induced by erythromycin, but not by clindamycin or streptogramin B antibiotics, which retain in vitro activity. In isolates that are resistant to erythromycin, inducible resistance to clindamycin may be detected in the clinical microbiology laboratory by the "D-test."[182] Isolates that show inducible resistance to clindamycin may develop resistance to that drug on treatment; hence, CLSI's suggested cautionary notice for reporting of these isolates, "This *S aureus* is presumed to be resistant based on detection of inducible clindamycin resistance. Clindamycin may still be effective in some patients."[182,183] This phenotype is fairly common and was found in 39% of erythromycin-resistant clindamycin-susceptible *S aureus* isolates in a recent large survey.[90] The in vitro susceptibility of *S aureus* and coagulase-negative staphylococci to macrolides and clindamycin is often correlated with methicillin susceptibility. For example, in a large recent survey including *S aureus* isolates, 66% and 93% of MSSA were susceptible to erythromycin and clindamycin, whereas only 5% and 55% of MRSA were susceptible to these drugs.[184] Most CA-MRSA are resistant to the macrolides, and although clindamycin has been used successfully against CA-MRSA in some populations, isolates from the highly successful USA300 clone are often resistant.[1,184] After *erm*-encoded methylation, the most common mechanism of resistance to macrolides in staphylococci is the Msr ATP-binding cassette pumps that confer resistance to 14-membered ring macrolides (eg, erythromycin and clarithromycin) and type B streptogramins,[185,186] although the prevalence and relative proportion of these resistance determinants varies depending on the isolates sampled.

This group of drugs is generally bacteriostatic against staphylococci, with the noted exception of quinupristin-dalfopristin, which offers the potential for bactericidal activity against staphylococci that are not constitutively resistant to quinupristin.[187,188] Unfortunately, such resistance is fairly common, particularly among MRSA isolates.[188]

Macrolides

Macrolides available for oral treatment of minor SSTI caused by susceptible *S aureus* include erythromycin, clarithromycin, and azithromycin. The available parenteral agents in the United States are IV erythromycin and azithromycin, but these are rarely used for treatment of staphylococcal infection. Because of the prevalence of resistance in MRSA and many MSSA (as noted previously),[184] currently available macrolides are rarely if ever appropriate empiric agents. Given their relatively limited role, dosing for the variety of available macrolides is beyond the scope of this article, but can be found elsewhere.[189] Renal failure that is moderate to severe warrants a dose reduction of clarithromycin.[190] These drugs share some degree of gastrointestinal toxicity, primarily abdominal cramping, nausea, vomiting, and diarrhea, which is a less prominent side effect of the newer agents than for erythromycin.[190] A wide range of significant drug interactions result from the effects of erythromycin, and to a lesser extent clarithromycin on the hepatic cytochrome P-450 system, more precisely inhibition of CYP 3A4.[190,191] Azithromycin, however, has only limited hepatic metabolism and few drug interactions.

Clindamycin

As compared with the macrolides, clindamycin is more widely used to treat staphylococcal infections. It has specific use in patients with β-lactam hypersensitivity, in the treatment of infections caused by isolates resistant to alternative agents, and in the treatment of staphylococcal toxin-mediated disease. Although most nosocomial and many CA-MRSA are clindamycin-resistant, clindamycin has activity against most methicillin-susceptible isolates.[184] Many coagulase-negative staphylococci, particularly nosocomial isolates, are resistant to clindamycin.[184]

Clindamycin (along with sulfonamides and moxifloxacin) was one of the drugs associated with the highest frequency of estimated emergency department visits (per prescription visit) in a recent study.[120] The most common adverse reactions caused by clindamycin involve the gastrointestinal system.[192] Antibiotic-associated diarrhea is not uncommon in patients receiving clindamycin, and in a subset of those patients is caused by the overgrowth of toxogenic *Clostridium difficile*, resulting in antibiotic-associated colitis with pseudomembrane formation. Clindamycin is one of many antimicrobial drugs that have been found to be risk factors for *C difficile*–associated diarrhea, but despite being often invoked as a high-risk agent, some recent studies have not found it to be a greater risk factor than numerous other agents.[193] Clindamycin causes relatively few significant drug interactions, but may potentiate neuromuscular blocking agents and may reduce the levels of cyclosporine.[194,195]

Clindamycin may be administered orally, intramuscularly, or parenterally.[189,190,192] The standard oral preparation is clindamycin hydrochloride, which may be given in doses ranging from 150 to 450 mg every 6 hours. Another oral preparation of clindamycin is a palmitate ester suspension. Oral preparations are absorbed rapidly and have approximately 90% bioavailability. For intravenous delivery, 600 to 900 mg of clindamycin phosphate is infused every 6 to 8 hours. This preparation may also be administered intramuscularly in doses as high as 600 mg. This agent penetrates into most tissues and fluids except cerebrospinal fluid. Like the macrolides, although not to the same extent as azithromycin, it is concentrated in polymorphonuclear neutrophils and macrophages, but the clinical significance of this property is unclear.[189,190,192] Because the metabolites of clindamycin are cleared through the urine and feces, significant dose reduction is recommended only for patients with severe hepatic failure or combined renal and hepatic dysfunction. Clindamycin levels are not reduced by either hemodialysis or peritoneal dialysis.[189,190,192]

Clindamycin is an agent with several well-defined niches in antimicrobial chemotherapy. SSTI caused by *S aureus* are often treatable with clindamycin. Because of its activity against predominant clones of CA-MRSA in some geographic locales, clindamycin has been used for empiric and directed treatment of SSTI, particularly in pediatric patients,[72] but this strategy is ill-advised in other areas where circulating clones of CA-MRSA, particularly multidrug-resistant USA-300, are prevalent.[1] Close attention to the local antibiogram is critical to this consideration. Because of its good penetration into bone, clindamycin is sometimes used in the treatment of osteomyelitis caused by staphylococci or streptococci or may be combined with other agents for polymicrobial osteomyelitis, such as diabetic foot infections or decubitus ulcers.[196] Clindamycin is also included in some surgical antibiotic prophylaxis regimens for β-lactam–allergic patients. Because it inhibits ribosomal protein synthesis clindamycin has been used, in practice often combined with a cell-wall active agent, to stop toxin production in patients with infections caused by toxin-producing *S aureus* (eg, staphylococcal toxic shock syndrome).[197,198] Clindamycin has additional theoretic advantages over β-lactams in that it is less affected by the large inoculum of organisms present in serious infections, such as necrotizing fasciitis; is active against slowly growing organisms; and may also have beneficial immunomodulatory effects.[199]

Quinupristin-Dalfopristin

Quinupristin-dalfopristin is a combination of two semisynthetic derivatives of pristinamycin (pristinamycin streptogramin A and B drugs), providing the potential for synergistic bactericidal activity against staphylococci. Quinupristin, the streptogramin B component, is derived from pristinamycin I, and the streptogramin A antibiotic dalfopristin is derived from pristinamycin IIa. The binding of the type A streptogramin induces a conformational change in the ribosome that increases the affinity of the ribosome for type B drugs.[200] Synercid has in vitro activity against gram-positive organisms including MSSA and MRSA and *S epidermidis*. It is available only as an intravenous drug, and has significant toxicity liabilities including phlebitis (42% of patients in comparative clinical trials had inflammation at the IV site) and the not uncommon occurrence of moderate or severe arthralgias and myalgias.[201] It causes a plethora of potential drug interactions because of its inhibition of cytochrome P-450 3A4. At the dose of 7.5 mg/kg every 12 hours, this drug is approved for treatment of complicated SSTI caused by *S aureus*, although the indication is limited to MSSA, and also for *S pyogenes* for the same indication. Clinically, the relative toxicity of this drug limits its use, but Synercid may be considered as an option for patients with resistance to second-line drugs or multiple drug hypersensitivities.

Telithromycin

The ketolide drug telithromycin has good activity against *S aureus* that are not constitutively resistant to MLS$_B$ drugs, and one global survey of community respiratory tract isolates of *S aureus* from 1999 to 2000 found that 95% of MSSA, but only 18% of MRSA, were susceptible to telithromycin.[202] In addition to significant toxicity liabilities, such as hepatotoxicity (including rare cases of fulminant hepatitis) and QTc prolongation, the drug carries the sole indication of treatment of mild to moderate community-acquired pneumonia caused by organisms other than *S aureus*.[190,203,204]

MLS drugs continue to have a role in the treatment of *S aureus* infections, often when β-lactam agents cannot be used because of methicillin resistance or hypersensitivity; however, this role is increasingly limited by unfavorable trends in antimicrobial drug resistance. Clindamycin remains a potentially useful drug for MSSA and CA-MRSA SSTI in settings where local antibiograms show susceptibility (including attention to D-testing for erythromycin-clindamycin discordant results).

SUMMARY

The treatment of staphylococcal infections continues to vex clinicians, in no small part because of the constantly evolving drug resistance of this virulent and durable pathogen. Additional research may help to understand how best to preserve the existing drugs, including recycling some older drugs for which there are currently only limited clinical data for the treatment of staphylococcal infections. Clinicians can look forward to additional studies of newer FDA-approved agents to understand better their place in treatment algorithms versus currently existing standards of care, and to approval of additional drugs with activity against MRSA that are in late-stage clinical trials.

REFERENCES

1. Diep BA, Chambers HF, Graber CJ, et al. Emergence of multidrug-resistant, community-associated, methicillin-resistant *Staphylococcus aureus* clone usa300 in men who have sex with men. Ann Intern Med 2008;148(4):249–57.
2. Deresinski S. Counterpoint: vancomycin and *Staphylococcus aureus*–an antibiotic enters obsolescence. Clin Infect Dis 2007;44(12):1543–8.
3. Mohr JF, Murray BE. Point: vancomycin is not obsolete for the treatment of infection caused by methicillin-resistant *Staphylococcus aureus*. Clin Infect Dis 2007; 44(12):1536–42.
4. Tenover FC, Moellering RC Jr. The rationale for revising the Clinical and Laboratory Standards Institute vancomycin minimal inhibitory concentration interpretive criteria for *Staphylococcus aureus*. Clin Infect Dis 2007;44(9):1208–15.
5. Jones RN. Microbiological features of vancomycin in the 21st century: minimum inhibitory concentration creep, bactericidal/static activity, and applied breakpoints to predict clinical outcomes or detect resistant strains. Clin Infect Dis 2006;42(Suppl 1):S13–24.
6. Wang G, Hindler JF, Ward KW, et al. Increased vancomycin mics for *Staphylococcus aureus* clinical isolates from a university hospital during a 5-year period. J Clin Microbiol 2006;44(11):3883–6.
7. Sakoulas G, Moise-Broder PA, Schentag J, et al. Relationship of MIC and bactericidal activity to efficacy of vancomycin for treatment of methicillin-resistant *Staphylococcus aureus* bacteremia. J Clin Microbiol 2004;42(6):2398–402.
8. Soriano A, Marco F, Martinez JA, et al. Influence of vancomycin minimum inhibitory concentration on the treatment of methicillin-resistant *Staphylococcus aureus* bacteremia. Clin Infect Dis 2008;46(2):193–200.
9. Hidayat LK, Hsu DI, Quist R, et al. High-dose vancomycin therapy for methicillin-resistant *Staphylococcus aureus* infections: efficacy and toxicity. Arch Intern Med 2006;166(19):2138–44.
10. Andres DFaWA C. Cephalosporins. In: Mandell GL, Dolin R, editors. Mandell, Douglas, and Bennett's principles and practice of infectious diseases, 6th edition, vol. 1. Philadelphia: Elsevier Churchill Livingstone 2005. p. 294–310.
11. Chambers HF. Penicillins. In: Mandell GL, Dolin R, editors. Mandell, Douglas, and Bennett's principles and practice of infectious diseases, 6th edition, vol. 1. Philadelphia: Elsevier Churchill Livingstone 2005. p. 281–93.
12. Chambers HF. Other beta-lactams. In: Mandell GL, Dolin R, editors. Mandell, Douglas, and Bennett's principles and practice of infectious diseases, 6th edition, volumes 1 and 2, vol. 1. Philadelphia: Elsevier Churchill Livingstone 2005. p. 311–17.
13. Gilbert Dn MR, Ellopoulos GM, Sande MA. The Sanford guide to antimicrobial therapy 2008. (38th edition). Sperryville (VA): Antimicrobial Therapy; 2008.
14. Craig WA. Basic pharmacodynamics of antibacterials with clinical applications to the use of beta-lactams, glycopeptides, and linezolid. Infect Dis Clin North Am 2003;17(3):479–501.
15. Glasheen JJ, Fugit RV, Prochazka AV. The risk of overanticoagulation with antibiotic use in outpatients on stable warfarin regimens. J Gen Intern Med 2005; 20(7):653–6.
16. Kim KY, Frey RJ, Epplen K, et al. Interaction between warfarin and nafcillin: case report and review of the literature. Pharmacotherapy 2007;27(10):1467–70.
17. Schito GC, Debbia EA, Pesce A. Susceptibility of respiratory strains of *Staphylococcus aureus* to fifteen antibiotics: results of a collaborative surveillance

study (1992–1993). The Alexander Project Collaborative Group. J Antimicrob Chemother 1996;38(Suppl A):97–106.

18. Lacey CS. Interaction of dicloxacillin with warfarin. Ann Pharmacother 2004; 38(5):898.

19. Maraqa NF, Gomez MM, Rathore MH, et al. Higher occurrence of hepatotoxicity and rash in patients treated with oxacillin, compared with those treated with nafcillin and other commonly used antimicrobials. Clin Infect Dis 2002;34(1):50–4.

20. Fromm LA, Graham DL. Oxacillin-induced tissue necrosis. Ann Pharmacother 1999;33(10):1060–2.

21. Baddour LM, Wilson WR, Bayer AS, et al. Infective endocarditis: diagnosis, antimicrobial therapy, and management of complications: a statement for healthcare professionals from the committee on rheumatic fever, endocarditis, and Kawasaki disease, council on cardiovascular disease in the young, and the councils on clinical cardiology, stroke, and cardiovascular surgery and anesthesia, American heart association. Endorsed by the infectious diseases society of America. Circulation 2005;111(23):e394–434.

22. Mandell LA, Wunderink RG, Anzueto A, et al. Infectious Diseases Society of America/American Thoracic Society consensus guidelines on the management of community-acquired pneumonia in adults. Clin Infect Dis 2007;44(Suppl 2):S27–72.

23. Tunkel AR, Hartman BJ, Kaplan SL, et al. Practice guidelines for the management of bacterial meningitis. Clin Infect Dis 2004;39(9):1267–84.

24. Stevens DL, Smith LG, Bruss JB, et al. Randomized comparison of linezolid (pnu-100766) versus oxacillin-dicloxacillin for treatment of complicated skin and soft tissue infections. Antimicrobial Agents Chemother 2000;44(12):3408–13.

25. Tack K, Wilcox MH, Bouza E, et al. Linezolid vs. Vancomycin or oxacillin/dicloxacillin for the treatment of catheter-related bloodstream infections (crbsi). Conference abstracts of the 47th Interscience Conference on Antimicrobial Agents and Chemotherapy. Chicago, IL. September 17–20 2007. K-1748.

26. Heldman AW, Hartert TV, Ray SC, et al. Oral antibiotic treatment of right-sided staphylococcal endocarditis in injection drug users: prospective randomized comparison with parenteral therapy. Am J Med 1996;101(1):68–76.

27. Arbeit RD, Maki D, Tally FP, et al. The safety and efficacy of daptomycin for the treatment of complicated skin and skin-structure infections. Clin Infect Dis 2004; 38(12):1673–81.

28. Fowler VG Jr, Boucher HW, Corey GR, et al. Daptomycin versus standard therapy for bacteremia and endocarditis caused by Staphylococcus aureus. N Engl J Med 2006;355(7):653–65.

29. Lalani T, Boucher HW, Cosgrove SE, et al. Outcomes with daptomycin versus standard therapy for osteoarticular infections associated with Staphylococcus aureus bacteraemia. J Antimicrob Chemother 2008;61(1):177–82.

30. Zimmerli W, Widmer AF, Blatter M, et al. Role of rifampin for treatment of orthopedic implant-related staphylococcal infections: a randomized controlled trial. Foreign-body infection (FBI) study group. JAMA 1998;279(19):1537–41.

31. Grayson ML, Gibbons GW, Habershaw GM, et al. Use of ampicillin/sulbactam versus imipenem/cilastatin in the treatment of limb-threatening foot infections in diabetic patients. Clin Infect Dis 1994;18(5):683–93.

32. Jones RN, Huynh HK, Biedenbach DJ, et al. Doripenem (s-4661), a novel carbapenem: comparative activity against contemporary pathogens including bactericidal action and preliminary in vitro methods evaluations. J Antimicrob Chemother 2004;54(1):144–54.

33. Acar JF. Therapy for lower respiratory tract infections with imipenem/cilastatin: a review of worldwide experience. Rev Infect Dis 1985;7(Suppl 3):S513–7.
34. Kager L, Nord CE. Imipenem/cilastatin in the treatment of intraabdominal infections: a review of worldwide experience. Rev Infect Dis 1985;7(Suppl 3):S518–21.
35. Colardyn F, Faulkner KL. Intravenous meropenem versus imipenem/cilastatin in the treatment of serious bacterial infections in hospitalized patients. meropenem serious infection study group. J Antimicrob Chemother 1996;38(3):523–37.
36. Graham DR, Lucasti C, Malafaia O, et al. Ertapenem once daily versus piperacillin-tazobactam 4 times per day for treatment of complicated skin and skin-structure infections in adults: results of a prospective, randomized, double-blind multicenter study. Clin Infect Dis 2002;34(11):1460–8.
37. Lipsky BA, Armstrong DG, Citron DM, et al. Ertapenem versus piperacillin/tazobactam for diabetic foot infections (sidestep): prospective, randomised, controlled, double-blinded, multicentre trial. Lancet 2005;366(9498):1695–703.
38. Ortiz-Ruiz G, Vetter N, Isaacs R, et al. Ertapenem versus ceftriaxone for the treatment of community-acquired pneumonia in adults: combined analysis of two multicentre randomized, double-blind studies. J Antimicrob Chemother 2004;53(Suppl 2):ii59–66.
39. Chastre J, Wunderink R, Prokocimer P, et al. Efficacy and safety of intravenous infusion of doripenem versus imipenem in ventilator-associated pneumonia: a multicenter, randomized study. Crit Care Med 2008;36(4):1089–96.
40. Primaxin label information. Food and Drug Administration. Availabe at: http://www.fda.gov/cder/foi/label/2008/050587s065,050630s028lbl.pdf. Accessed August 21, 2008.
41. Merrem label information. Food and Drug Administration. Availabe at: http://www.fda.gov/cder/foi/label/2008/050706s022lbl.pdf. Accessed August 21, 2008.
42. Invanz label information. Food and Drug Administration. Availabe at: http://www.fda.gov/cder/foi/label/2008/021337s028lbl.pdf. Accessed August 21, 2008.
43. Doribax label information. Food and Drug Administration. Availabe at: http://www.fda.gov/cder/foi/label/2007/022106lbl.pdf. Accessed August 21, 2008.
44. Levine DP. Vancomycin: a history. Clin Infect Dis 2006;42(Suppl 1):S5–12.
45. Sakoulas G, Eliopoulos GM, Fowler VG Jr, et al. Reduced susceptibility of Staphylococcus aureus to vancomycin and platelet microbicidal protein correlates with defective autolysis and loss of accessory gene regulator (AGR) function. Antimicrobial Agents Chemother 2005;49(7):2687–92.
46. Tsuji BT, Rybak MJ, Lau KL, et al. Evaluation of accessory gene regulator (AGR) group and function in the proclivity towards vancomycin intermediate resistance in Staphylococcus aureus. Antimicrobial Agents Chemother 2007;51(3):1089–91.
47. Small PM, Chambers HF. Vancomycin for Staphylococcus aureus endocarditis in intravenous drug users. Antimicrobial Agents Chemother 1990;34(6):1227–31.
48. Van Bambeke F, Van Laethem Y, Courvalin P, et al. Glycopeptide antibiotics: from conventional molecules to new derivatives. Drugs 2004;64(9):913–36.
49. Reduced susceptibility of Staphylococcus aureus to vancomycin: Japan, 1996. MMWR Morb Mortal Wkly Rep 1997;46(27):624–6.
50. Sieradzki K, Roberts RB, Haber SW, et al. The development of vancomycin resistance in a patient with methicillin-resistant Staphylococcus aureus infection. N Engl J Med 1999;340(7):517–23.
51. Hiramatsu K. Vancomycin-resistant Staphylococcus aureus: a new model of antibiotic resistance. Lancet Infect Dis 2001;1(3):147–55.

52. Fridkin SK, Hageman J, McDougal LK, et al. Epidemiological and microbiological characterization of infections caused by *Staphylococcus aureus* with reduced susceptibility to vancomycin, United States, 1997–2001. Clin Infect Dis 2003;36(4):429–39.

53. Liu C, Chambers HF. *Staphylococcus aureus* with heterogeneous resistance to vancomycin: epidemiology, clinical significance, and critical assessment of diagnostic methods. Antimicrobial Agents Chemother 2003;47(10):3040–5.

54. Charles PG, Ward PB, Johnson PD, et al. Clinical features associated with bacteremia due to heterogeneous vancomycin-intermediate *Staphylococcus aureus*. Clin Infect Dis 2004;38(3):448–51.

55. Sievert DM, Rudrik JT, Patel JB, et al. Vancomycin-resistant *Staphylococcus aureus* in the United States, 2002–2006. Clin Infect Dis 2008;46(5):668–74.

56. Weigel LM, Clewell DB, Gill SR, et al. Genetic analysis of a high-level vancomycin-resistant isolate of *Staphylococcus aureus*. Science 2003;302(5650):1569–71.

57. Holliman R. Red man syndrome associated with rapid vancomycin infusion. Lancet 1985;1(8442):1399–400.

58. Valero R, Gomar C, Fita G, et al. Adverse reactions to vancomycin prophylaxis in cardiac surgery. J Cardiothorac Vasc Anesth 1991;5(6):574–6.

59. Rybak MJ, Bailey EM, Warbasse LH. Absence of red man syndrome in patients being treated with vancomycin or high-dose teicoplanin. Antimicrobial Agents Chemother 1992;36(6):1204–7.

60. Rybak MJ, Albrecht LM, Boike SC, et al. Nephrotoxicity of vancomycin, alone and with an aminoglycoside. J Antimicrob Chemother 1990;25(4):679–87.

61. Label for vancomycin injection, USP in galaxy plastic container (pl 2040) for intravenous use only. Available at: http://www.fda.gov/cder/foi/label/2008/050671s012lbl.pdf. Accessed September 22, 2008.

62. Levine DP, Fromm BS, Reddy BR. Slow response to vancomycin or vancomycin plus rifampin in methicillin-resistant *Staphylococcus aureus* endocarditis. Ann Intern Med 1991;115(9):674–80.

63. Stryjewski ME, Szczech LA, Benjamin DK Jr, et al. Use of vancomycin or first-generation cephalosporins for the treatment of hemodialysis-dependent patients with methicillin-susceptible *Staphylococcus aureus* bacteremia. Clin Infect Dis 2007;44(2):190–6.

64. Chang FY, Peacock JE Jr, Musher DM, et al. *Staphylococcus aureus* bacteremia: recurrence and the impact of antibiotic treatment in a prospective multicenter study. Medicine (Baltimore) 2003;82(5):333–9.

65. Recommendations for preventing the spread of vancomycin resistance. Recommendations of the Hospital Infection Control Practices Advisory Committee (HICPAC). MMWR Recomm Rep 1995;44(RR-12):1–13.

66. Guidelines for the management of adults with hospital-acquired, ventilator-associated, and healthcare-associated pneumonia. Am J Respir Crit Care Med 2005;171(4):388–416.

67. Moise PA, Forrest A, Bhavnani SM, et al. Area under the inhibitory curve and a pneumonia scoring system for predicting outcomes of vancomycin therapy for respiratory infections by *Staphylococcus aureus*. Am J Health Syst Pharm 2000;57(Suppl 2):S4–9.

68. Lamer C, de Beco V, Soler P, et al. Analysis of vancomycin entry into pulmonary lining fluid by bronchoalveolar lavage in critically ill patients. Antimicrobial Agents Chemother 1993;37(2):281–6.

69. Wunderink RG, Rello J, Cammarata SK, et al. Linezolid vs vancomycin: analysis of two double-blind studies of patients with methicillin-resistant *Staphylococcus aureus* nosocomial pneumonia. Chest 2003;124(5):1789–97.
70. Boselli E, Breilh D, Rimmele T, et al. Pharmacokinetics and intrapulmonary concentrations of linezolid administered to critically ill patients with ventilator-associated pneumonia. Crit Care Med 2005;33(7):1529–33.
71. Stevens DL, Bisno AL, Chambers HF, et al. Practice guidelines for the diagnosis and management of skin and soft-tissue infections. Clin Infect Dis 2005;41(10): 1373–406.
72. Stryjewski ME, Chambers HF. Skin and soft-tissue infections caused by community-acquired methicillin-resistant *Staphylococcus aureus*. Clin Infect Dis 2008; 46(Suppl 5):S368–77.
73. Lew DP, Waldvogel FA. Osteomyelitis. N Engl J Med 1997;336(14):999–1007.
74. Rybak MJ. The pharmacokinetic and pharmacodynamic properties of vancomycin. Clin Infect Dis 2006;42(Suppl 1):S35–9.
75. Steenbergen JN, Alder J, Thorne GM, et al. Daptomycin: a lipopeptide antibiotic for the treatment of serious gram-positive infections. J Antimicrob Chemother 2005;55(3):283–8.
76. Silverman JA, Perlmutter NG, Shapiro HM. Correlation of daptomycin bactericidal activity and membrane depolarization in *Staphylococcus aureus*. Antimicrobial Agents Chemother 2003;47(8):2538–44.
77. Streit JM, Jones RN, Sader HS. Daptomycin activity and spectrum: a worldwide sample of 6737 clinical gram-positive organisms. J Antimicrob Chemother 2004; 53(4):669–74.
78. Cubicin label information. Food and Drug Administration. Availabe at: http://www. fda.gov/cder/foi/label/2007/021572s014lbl.pdf. Accessed August 20, 2008.
79. Pertel PE, Bernardo P, Fogarty C, et al. Effects of prior effective therapy on the efficacy of daptomycin and ceftriaxone for the treatment of community-acquired pneumonia. Clin Infect Dis 2008;46(8):1142–51.
80. Silverman JA, Mortin LI, Vanpraagh AD, et al. Inhibition of daptomycin by pulmonary surfactant: in vitro modeling and clinical impact. J Infect Dis 2005;191(12): 2149–52.
81. Silverman JA, Oliver N, Andrew T, et al. Resistance studies with daptomycin. Antimicrobial Agents Chemother 2001;45(6):1799–802.
82. Hayden MK, Rezai K, Hayes RA, et al. Development of daptomycin resistance in vivo in methicillin-resistant *Staphylococcus aureus*. J Clin Microbiol 2005;43(10): 5285–7.
83. Marty FM, Yeh WW, Wennersten CB, et al. Emergence of a clinical daptomycin-resistant *Staphylococcus aureus* isolate during treatment of methicillin-resistant *Staphylococcus aureus* bacteremia and osteomyelitis. J Clin Microbiol 2006; 44(2):595–7.
84. Cui L, Tominaga E, Neoh HM, et al. Correlation between reduced daptomycin susceptibility and vancomycin resistance in vancomycin-intermediate *Staphylococcus aureus*. Antimicrobial Agents Chemother 2006;50(3):1079–82.
85. Sakoulas G, Alder J, Thauvin-Eliopoulos C, et al. Induction of daptomycin heterogeneous susceptibility in *Staphylococcus aureus* by exposure to vancomycin. Antimicrobial Agents Chemother 2006;50(4):1581–5.
86. First data bank blue book AWP. Available at: http://www.cardinal.com. Accessed September 23, 2008.

87. Kaatz GW, Seo SM. In vitro activities of oxazolidinone compounds u100592 and u100766 against *Staphylococcus aureus* and *Staphylococcus epidermidis*. Antimicrobial Agents Chemother 1996;40(3):799–801.

88. Fines M, Leclercq R. Activity of linezolid against gram-positive cocci possessing genes conferring resistance to protein synthesis inhibitors. J Antimicrob Chemother 2000;45(6):797–802.

89. Long KS, Poehlsgaard J, Kehrenberg C, et al. The Cfr rRNA methyltransferase confers resistance to phenicols, lincosamides, oxazolidinones, pleuromutilins, and streptogramin a antibiotics. Antimicrobial Agents Chemother 2006;50(7): 2500–5.

90. Jones RN, Fritsche TR, Sader HS, et al. LEADER surveillance program results for 2006: an activity and spectrum analysis of linezolid using clinical isolates from the united states (50 medical centers). Diagn Microbiol Infect Dis 2007;59(3):309–17.

91. Jones RN, Fritsche TR, Sader HS, et al. Zyvox annual appraisal of potency and spectrum program results for 2006: an activity and spectrum analysis of linezolid using clinical isolates from 16 countries. Diagn Microbiol Infect Dis 2007;59(2): 199–209.

92. Zyvox label. Available at: http://www.fda.gov/cder/foi/label/2008/021130s016,021131s013,021132s014lbl.pdf.

93. Brier ME, Stalker DJ, Aronoff GR, et al. Pharmacokinetics of linezolid in subjects with renal dysfunction. Antimicrobial Agents Chemother 2003;47(9):2775–80.

94. Lawrence KR, Adra M, Gillman PK. Serotonin toxicity associated with the use of linezolid: a review of postmarketing data. Clin Infect Dis 2006;42(11):1578–83.

95. Hendershot PE, Antal EJ, Welshman IR, et al. Linezolid: pharmacokinetic and pharmacodynamic evaluation of coadministration with pseudoephedrine hcl, phenylpropanolamine hcl, and dextromethorpan hbr. J Clin Pharmacol 2001; 41(5):563–72.

96. Taylor JJ, Wilson JW, Estes LL. Linezolid and serotonergic drug interactions: a retrospective survey. Clin Infect Dis 2006;43(2):180–7.

97. Antal EJ, Hendershot PE, Batts DH, et al. Linezolid, a novel oxazolidinone antibiotic: assessment of monoamine oxidase inhibition using pressor response to oral tyramine. J Clin Pharmacol 2001;41(5):552–62.

98. French G. Safety and tolerability of linezolid. J Antimicrob Chemother 2003; 51(Suppl 2):ii45–53.

99. Lee E, Burger S, Shah J, et al. Linezolid-associated toxic optic neuropathy: a report of 2 cases. Clin Infect Dis 2003;37(10):1389–91.

100. Bressler AM, Zimmer SM, Gilmore JL, et al. Peripheral neuropathy associated with prolonged use of linezolid. Lancet Infect Dis 2004;4(8):528–31.

101. Apodaca AA, Rakita RM. Linezolid-induced lactic acidosis. N Engl J Med 2003; 348(1):86–7.

102. Weigelt J, Itani K, Stevens D, et al. Linezolid versus vancomycin in treatment of complicated skin and soft tissue infections. Antimicrobial Agents Chemother 2005;49(6):2260–6.

103. Rubinstein E, Cammarata S, Oliphant T, et al. Linezolid (pnu-100766) versus vancomycin in the treatment of hospitalized patients with nosocomial pneumonia: a randomized, double-blind, multicenter study. Clin Infect Dis 2001;32(3):402–12.

104. Wunderink RG, Cammarata SK, Oliphant TH, et al. Continuation of a randomized, double-blind, multicenter study of linezolid versus vancomycin in the treatment of patients with nosocomial pneumonia. Clin Ther 2003;25(3):980–92.

105. Powers JH, Ross DB, Lin D, et al. Linezolid and vancomycin for methicillin-resistant *Staphylococcus aureus* nosocomial pneumonia: the subtleties of subgroup analyses. Chest 2004;126(1):314–5, author reply 15–6.
106. Available at: http://clinicaltrials.gov/ct2/show/NCT00084266. Accessed December 1, 2008.
107. Shorr AF, Kunkel MJ, Kollef M. Linezolid versus vancomycin for *Staphylococcus aureus* bacteraemia: pooled analysis of randomized studies. J Antimicrob Chemother 2005;56(5):923–9.
108. Information for healthcare professionals linezolid (marketed as Zyvox). Available at: http://www.fda.gov/cder/drug/InfoSheets/HCP/linezolidHCP.pdf. Accessed September 19, 2008.
109. Falagas ME, Manta KG, Ntziora F, et al. Linezolid for the treatment of patients with endocarditis: a systematic review of the published evidence. J Antimicrob Chemother 2006;58(2):273–80.
110. Bernardo K, Pakulat N, Fleer S, et al. Subinhibitory concentrations of linezolid reduce *Staphylococcus aureus* virulence factor expression. Antimicrobial Agents Chemother 2004;48(2):546–55.
111. Stevens DL, Wallace RJ, Hamilton SM, et al. Successful treatment of staphylococcal toxic shock syndrome with linezolid: a case report and in vitro evaluation of the production of toxic shock syndrome toxin type 1 in the presence of antibiotics. Clin Infect Dis 2006;42(5):729–30.
112. Dumitrescu O, Badiou C, Bes M, et al. Effect of antibiotics, alone and in combination, on Panton-Valentine leukocidin production by a *Staphylococcus aureus* reference strain. Clin Microbiol Infect 2008;14(4):384–8.
113. Jungbluth GL, Welshman IR, Hopkins NK. Linezolid pharmacokinetics in pediatric patients: an overview. Pediatr Infect Dis J 2003;22(9 Suppl):S153–7.
114. Kaplan SL, Deville JG, Yogev R, et al. Linezolid versus vancomycin for treatment of resistant gram-positive infections in children. Pediatr Infect Dis J 2003;22(8): 677–86.
115. Wible K, Tregnaghi M, Bruss J, et al. Linezolid versus cefadroxil in the treatment of skin and skin structure infections in children. Pediatr Infect Dis J 2003;22(4):315–23.
116. Li Z, Willke RJ, Pinto LA, et al. Comparison of length of hospital stay for patients with known or suspected methicillin-resistant staphylococcus species infections treated with linezolid or vancomycin: a randomized, multicenter trial. Pharmacotherapy 2001;21(3):263–74.
117. Falagas ME, Siempos II, Vardakas KZ. Linezolid versus glycopeptide or beta-lactam for treatment of gram-positive bacterial infections: meta-analysis of randomised controlled trials. Lancet Infect Dis 2008;8(1):53–66.
118. Proctor RA. Role of folate antagonists in the treatment of methicillin-resistant *Staphylococcus aureus* infection. Clin Infect Dis 2008;46(4):584–93.
119. Zinner SH, Mayer KH. Sulfonamides and trimethoprim. In: Mandell GL, Douglas RG, Bennett JE, et al, editors. Mandell, Douglas, and Bennett's principles and practice of infectious diseases, 6th edition, vol. 1. New York: Elsevier/Churchill Livingstone; 2005. p. 440–50.
120. Shehab N, Patel PR, Srinivasan A, et al. Emergency department visits for antibiotic-associated adverse events. Clin Infect Dis 2008;47(6):735–43.
121. Lawson DH, Paice BJ. Adverse reactions to trimethoprim-sulfamethoxazole. Rev Infect Dis 1982;4(2):429–33.
122. Scheld WM, Keeley JM, Field MR, et al. Co-trimoxazole versus nafcillin in the therapy of experimental meningitis due to *Staphylococcus aureus*. J Antimicrob Chemother 1987;19(5):647–58.

123. Elwell LP, Wilson HR, Knick VB, et al. In vitro and in vivo efficacy of the combination trimethoprim-sulfamethoxazole against clinical isolates of methicillin-resistant *Staphylococcus aureus*. Antimicrobial Agents Chemother 1986;29(6): 1092–4.

124. Yeldandi V, Strodtman R, Lentino JR. In-vitro and in-vivo studies of trimethoprim-sulphamethoxazole against multiple resistant *Staphylococcus aureus*. J Antimicrob Chemother 1988;22(6):873–80.

125. Kaka AS, Rueda AM, Shelburne SA III, et al. Bactericidal activity of orally available agents against methicillin-resistant *Staphylococcus aureus*. J Antimicrob Chemother 2006;58(3):680–3.

126. Cenizal MJ, Skiest D, Luber S, et al. Prospective randomized trial of empiric therapy with trimethoprim-sulfamethoxazole or doxycycline for outpatient skin and soft tissue infections in an area of high prevalence of methicillin-resistant *Staphylococcus aureus*. Antimicrobial Agents Chemother 2007;51(7):2628–30.

127. Szumowski JD, Cohen DE, Kanaya F, et al. Treatment and outcomes of infections by methicillin-resistant *Staphylococcus aureus* at an ambulatory clinic. Antimicrobial Agents Chemother 2007;51(2):423–8.

128. Markowitz N, Quinn EL, Saravolatz LD. Trimethoprim-sulfamethoxazole compared with vancomycin for the treatment of *Staphylococcus aureus* infection. Ann Intern Med 1992;117(5):390–8.

129. Minuth JN, Holmes TM, Musher DM. Activity of tetracycline, doxycycline, and minocycline against methicillin-susceptible and -resistant staphylococci. Antimicrobial Agents Chemother 1974;6(4):411–4.

130. Meyers B, Salvatore M. Tetracyclines and chloramphenicol. In: Mandell GL, Douglas RG, Bennett JE, et al, editors. Mandell, Douglas, and Bennett's principles and practice of infectious diseases, 6th edition, vol. 1. New York: Elsevier/ Churchill Livingstone; 2005. p. 356–73.

131. Zhanel GG, Homenuik K, Nichol K, et al. The glycylcyclines: a comparative review with the tetracyclines. Drugs 2004;64(1):63–88.

132. Ruhe JJ, Monson T, Bradsher RW, et al. Use of long-acting tetracyclines for methicillin-resistant *Staphylococcus aureus* infections: case series and review of the literature. Clin Infect Dis 2005;40(10):1429–34.

133. Ruhe JJ, Menon A. Tetracyclines as an oral treatment option for patients with community onset skin and soft tissue infections caused by methicillin-resistant *Staphylococcus aureus*. Antimicrobial Agents Chemother 2007;51(9):3298–303.

134. Pavoni GL, Giannella M, Falcone M, et al. Conservative medical therapy of prosthetic joint infections: retrospective analysis of an 8-year experience. Clin Microbiol Infect 2004;10(9):831–7.

135. Noskin GA. Tigecycline: a new glycylcycline for treatment of serious infections. Clin Infect Dis 2005;41(Suppl 5):S303–14.

136. Bradford PA, Weaver-Sands DT, Petersen PJ. In vitro activity of tigecycline against isolates from patients enrolled in phase 3 clinical trials of treatment for complicated skin and skin-structure infections and complicated intra-abdominal infections. Clin Infect Dis 2005;41(Suppl 5):S315–32.

137. Meagher AK, Ambrose PG, Grasela TH, et al. Pharmacokinetic/pharmacodynamic profile for tigecycline-a new glycylcycline antimicrobial agent. Diagn Microbiol Infect Dis 2005;52(3):165–71.

138. Ellis-Grosse EJ, Babinchak T, Dartois N, et al. The efficacy and safety of tigecycline in the treatment of skin and skin-structure infections: results of 2 double-blind phase 3 comparison studies with vancomycin-aztreonam. Clin Infect Dis 2005;41(Suppl 5):S341–53.

139. Saner FH, Heuer M, Rath PM, et al. Successful salvage therapy with tigecycline after linezolid failure in a liver transplant recipient with MRSA pneumonia. Liver Transpl 2006;12(11):1689–92.

140. Munoz-Price LS, Lolans K, Quinn JP. Four cases of invasive methicillin-resistant *Staphylococcus aureus* (MRSA) infections treated with tigecycline. Scand J Infect Dis 2006;38(11–12):1081–4.

141. Gilbert DN. Aminoglycosides. In: Mandell GL, Douglas RG, Bennett JE, et al, editors. Mandell, Douglas, and Bennett's principles and practice of infectious diseases, 6th edition, vol. 1. New York: Elsevier/Churchill Livingstone; 2005. p. 328–55.

142. Sande MA, Courtney KB. Nafcillin-gentamicin synergism in experimental staphylococcal endocarditis. J Lab Clin Med 1976;88(1):118–24.

143. Abrams B, Sklaver A, Hoffman T, et al. Single or combination therapy of staphylococcal endocarditis in intravenous drug abusers. Ann Intern Med 1979;90(5):789–91.

144. Korzeniowski O, Sande MA. Combination antimicrobial therapy for *Staphylococcus aureus* endocarditis in patients addicted to parenteral drugs and in nonaddicts: a prospective study. Ann Intern Med 1982;97(4):496–503.

145. Chambers HF, Miller RT, Newman MD. Right-sided *Staphylococcus aureus* endocarditis in intravenous drug abusers: two-week combination therapy. Ann Intern Med 1988;109(8):619–24.

146. Ribera E, Gomez-Jimenez J, Cortes E, et al. Effectiveness of cloxacillin with and without gentamicin in short-term therapy for right-sided *Staphylococcus aureus* endocarditis: a randomized, controlled trial. Ann Intern Med 1996;125(12):969–74.

147. Falagas ME, Matthaiou DK, Bliziotis IA. The role of aminoglycosides in combination with a beta-lactam for the treatment of bacterial endocarditis: a meta-analysis of comparative trials. J Antimicrob Chemother 2006;57(4):639–47.

148. Fortun J, Navas E, Martinez-Beltran J, et al. Short-course therapy for rightside endocarditis due to *Staphylococcus aureus* in drug abusers: cloxacillin versus glycopeptides in combination with gentamicin. Clin Infect Dis 2001; 33(1):120–5.

149. Karchmer AW. Infections associated with indwelling medical devices. In: Waldvogel FA, Bisno AL, editors, Washington, DC: ASM Press; 2000. p. 145–72.

150. Hooper DC. Quinolones. In: Mandell GL, Douglas RG, Bennett JE, et al, editors. Mandell, Douglas, and Bennett's principles and practice of infectious diseases, 6th edition, vol. 1. New York: Elsevier/Churchill Livingstone; 2005. p. 451–72.

151. Information for healthcare professionals. Fluoroquinolone antimicrobial drugs. Food and Drug Administration. Available at: http://www.fda.gov/cder/drug/InfoSheets/HCP/fluoroquinolonesHCP.htm. Accessed August 20, 2008.

152. The use of systemic fluoroquinolones. Pediatrics 2006;118(3):1287–92.

153. Akaniro JC, Vidaurre CE, Stutman HR, et al. Comparative in vitro activity of a new quinolone, fleroxacin, against respiratory pathogens from patients with cystic fibrosis. Antimicrobial Agents Chemother 1990;34(10):1880–4.

154. Smith SM. In vitro comparison of a-56619, a-56620, amifloxacin, ciprofloxacin, enoxacin, norfloxacin, and ofloxacin against methicillin-resistant *Staphylococcus aureus*. Antimicrobial Agents Chemother 1986;29(2):325–6.

155. Blumberg HM, Rimland D, Carroll DJ, et al. Rapid development of ciprofloxacin resistance in methicillin-susceptible and -resistant *Staphylococcus aureus*. J Infect Dis 1991;163(6):1279–85.

156. Entenza JM, Vouillamoz J, Glauser MP, et al. Levofloxacin versus ciprofloxacin, flucloxacillin, or vancomycin for treatment of experimental endocarditis due to

methicillin-susceptible or -resistant *Staphylococcus aureus*. Antimicrobial Agents Chemother 1997;41(8):1662–7.

157. Jones ME, Visser MR, Klootwijk M, et al. Comparative activities of clinafloxacin, grepafloxacin, levofloxacin, moxifloxacin, ofloxacin, sparfloxacin, and trovafloxacin and nonquinolones linozelid, quinupristin-dalfopristin, gentamicin, and vancomycin against clinical isolates of ciprofloxacin-resistant and -susceptible *Staphylococcus aureus* strains. Antimicrobial Agents Chemother 1999;43(2): 421–3.

158. Hoogkamp-Korstanje JA, Roelofs-Willemse J. Comparative in vitro activity of moxifloxacin against gram-positive clinical isolates. J Antimicrob Chemother 2000;45(1):31–9.

159. Hoban DJ, Bouchillon SK, Johnson JL, et al. Comparative in vitro activity of gemifloxacin, ciprofloxacin, levofloxacin and ofloxacin in a North American surveillance study. Diagn Microbiol Infect Dis 2001;40(1–2):51–7.

160. Smith SM, Eng RH, Tecson-Tumang F. Ciprofloxacin therapy for methicillin-resistant *Staphylococcus aureus* infections or colonizations. Antimicrobial Agents Chemother 1989;33(2):181–4.

161. Lipsky BA, Giordano P, Choudhri S, et al. Treating diabetic foot infections with sequential intravenous to oral moxifloxacin compared with piperacillin-tazobactam/amoxicillin-clavulanate. J Antimicrob Chemother 2007;60(2):370–6.

162. Dworkin RJ, Lee BL, Sande MA, et al. Treatment of right-sided *Staphylococcus aureus* endocarditis in intravenous drug users with ciprofloxacin and rifampicin. Lancet 1989;2(8671):1071–3.

163. Schrenzel J, Harbarth S, Schockmel G, et al. A randomized clinical trial to compare fleroxacin-rifampicin with flucloxacillin or vancomycin for the treatment of staphylococcal infection. Clin Infect Dis 2004;39(9):1285–92.

164. Lobo MC, Mandell GL. Treatment of experimental staphylococcal infection with rifampin. Antimicrobial Agents Chemother 1972;2(3):195–200.

165. Thornsberry C, Hill BC, Swenson JM, et al. Rifampin: spectrum of antibacterial activity. Rev Infect Dis 1983;5(Suppl 3):S412–7.

166. Wehrli W. Rifampin: mechanisms of action and resistance. Rev Infect Dis 1983; 5(Suppl 3):S407–11.

167. O'Neill AJ, Cove JH, Chopra I. Mutation frequencies for resistance to fusidic acid and rifampicin in *Staphylococcus aureus*. J Antimicrob Chemother 2001; 47(5):647–50.

168. Calfee DP. Rifamycins. In: Mandell GL, Douglas RG, Bennett JE, et al. editors. Mandell, Douglas, and Bennett's principles and practice of infectious diseases, 6th edition, vol. 1. New York: Elsevier/Churchill Livingstone; 2005. p. 374–87.

169. Widmer AF, Frei R, Rajacic Z, et al. Correlation between in vivo and in vitro efficacy of antimicrobial agents against foreign body infections. J Infect Dis 1990; 162(1):96–102.

170. Karchmer AW, Archer GL, Dismukes WE. Rifampin treatment of prosthetic valve endocarditis due to *Staphylococcus epidermidis*. Rev Infect Dis 1983;5(Suppl 3): S543–8.

171. Karchmer AW, Archer GL, Dismukes WE. *Staphylococcus epidermidis* causing prosthetic valve endocarditis: microbiologic and clinical observations as guides to therapy. Ann Intern Med 1983;98(4):447–55.

172. Drancourt M, Stein A, Argenson JN, et al. Oral rifampin plus ofloxacin for treatment of staphylococcus-infected orthopedic implants. Antimicrobial Agents Chemother 1993;37(6):1214–8.

173. Widmer AF, Gaechter A, Ochsner PE, et al. Antimicrobial treatment of orthopedic implant-related infections with rifampin combinations. Clin Infect Dis 1992; 14(6):1251–3.
174. Berdal JE, Skramm I, Mowinckel P, et al. Use of rifampicin and ciprofloxacin combination therapy after surgical debridement in the treatment of early manifestation prosthetic joint infections. Clin Microbiol Infect 2005;11(10):843–5.
175. Riedel DJ, Weekes E, Forrest GN. Addition of rifampin to standard therapy for treatment of native valve infective endocarditis caused by *Staphylococcus aureus*. Antimicrobial Agents Chemother 2008;52(7):2463–7.
176. Darouiche R, Perkins B, Musher D, et al. Levels of rifampin and ciprofloxacin in nasal secretions: correlation with mic90 and eradication of nasopharyngeal carriage of bacteria. J Infect Dis 1990;162(5):1124–7.
177. Yu VL, Goetz A, Wagener M, et al. *Staphylococcus aureus* nasal carriage and infection in patients on hemodialysis: efficacy of antibiotic prophylaxis. N Engl J Med 1986;315(2):91–6.
178. Roccaforte JS, Bittner MJ, Stumpf CA, et al. Attempts to eradicate methicillin-resistant *Staphylococcus aureus* colonization with the use of trimethoprim-sulfamethoxazole, rifampin, and bacitracin. Am J Infect Control 1988; 16(4):141–6.
179. Peterson LR, Quick JN, Jensen B, et al. Emergence of ciprofloxacin resistance in nosocomial methicillin-resistant *Staphylococcus aureus* isolates: resistance during ciprofloxacin plus rifampin therapy for methicillin-resistant s aureus colonization. Arch Intern Med 1990;150(10):2151–5.
180. Darouiche R, Wright C, Hamill R, et al. Eradication of colonization by methicillin-resistant *Staphylococcus aureus* by using oral minocycline-rifampin and topical mupirocin. Antimicrobial Agents Chemother 1991; 35(8):1612–5.
181. Simor AE, Phillips E, McGeer A, et al. Randomized controlled trial of chlorhexidine gluconate for washing, intranasal mupirocin, and rifampin and doxycycline versus no treatment for the eradication of methicillin-resistant *Staphylococcus aureus* colonization. Clin Infect Dis 2007;44(2):178–85.
182. Lewis JS II, Jorgensen JH. Inducible clindamycin resistance in staphylococci: should clinicians and microbiologists be concerned? Clin Infect Dis 2005; 40(2):280–5.
183. CLSI. Performance standards for antimicrobial susceptibility testing; eighteenth informational supplement M100-S18. Wayne, PA: Clinical and Laboratory Standards Institute; 2008.
184. Biedenbach DJ, Ross JE, Fritsche TR, et al. Activity of dalbavancin tested against *Staphylococcus* spp. And beta-hemolytic *Streptococcus* spp. isolated from 52 geographically diverse medical centers in the united states. J Clin Microbiol 2007;45(3):998–1004.
185. Lina G, Quaglia A, Reverdy ME, et al. Distribution of genes encoding resistance to macrolides, lincosamides, and streptogramins among staphylococci. Antimicrobial Agents Chemother 1999;43(5):1062–6.
186. Schmitz FJ, Sadurski R, Kray A, et al. Prevalence of macrolide-resistance genes in *Staphylococcus aureus* and enterococcus faecium isolates from 24 European university hospitals. J Antimicrob Chemother 2000;45(6):891–4.
187. Low DE, Nadler HL. A review of in-vitro antibacterial activity of quinupristin/dalfopristin against methicillin-susceptible and -resistant *Staphylococcus aureus*. J Antimicrob Chemother 1997;39(Suppl A):53–8.

188. Lin G, Appelbaum PC. Activity of ceftobiprole compared with those of other agents against *Staphylococcus aureus* strains with different resistotypes by time-kill analysis. Diagn Microbiol Infect Dis 2008;60(2):233–5.

189. Gold Hs MRJ. Macrolides and clindamycin. In: Root RK, Corey L, Waldvogel F, editors. Clinical infectious diseases: a practical approach. New York: Oxford University Press; 1999. p. 291–7.

190. Zuckerman JM. Macrolides and ketolides: azithromycin, clarithromycin, telithromycin. Infect Dis Clin North Am 2004;18(3):621–49.

191. Westphal JF. Macrolide—induced clinically relevant drug interactions with cytochrome p-450a (cyp) 3a4: an update focused on clarithromycin, azithromycin and dirithromycin. Br J Clin Pharmacol 2000;50(4):285–95.

192. Kasten MJ. Clindamycin, metronidazole, and chloramphenicol. Mayo Clin Proc 1999;74(8):825–33.

193. Owens RC Jr, Donskey CJ, Gaynes RP, et al. Antimicrobial-associated risk factors for *Clostridium difficile* infection. Clin Infect Dis 2008;46(Suppl 1): S19–31.

194. al Ahdal O, Bevan DR. Clindamycin-induced neuromuscular blockade. Can J Anaesth 1995;42(7):614–7.

195. Thurnheer R, Laube I, Speich R. Possible interaction between clindamycin and cyclosporin. BMJ 1999;319(7203):163.

196. Duckworth C, Fisher JF, Carter SA, et al. Tissue penetration of clindamycin in diabetic foot infections. J Antimicrob Chemother 1993;31(4):581–4.

197. Dann EJ, Weinberger M, Gillis S, et al. Bacterial laryngotracheitis associated with toxic shock syndrome in an adult. Clin Infect Dis 1994;18(3):437–9.

198. Coyle EA. Targeting bacterial virulence: the role of protein synthesis inhibitors in severe infections. Insights from the Society of Infectious Diseases Pharmacists. Pharmacotherapy 2003;23(5):638–42.

199. Stevens DL, Yan S, Bryant AE. Penicillin-binding protein expression at different growth stages determines penicillin efficacy in vitro and in vivo: an explanation for the inoculum effect. J Infect Dis 1993;167(6):1401–5.

200. Cocito C, Di Giambattista M, Nyssen E, et al. Inhibition of protein synthesis by streptogramins and related antibiotics. J Antimicrob Chemother 1997;39 (Suppl A):7–13.

201. Synercid IV package insert June 2008. Available at: http://www.fda.gov/cder/foi/label/2008/050748s008,050747s008lbl.pdf. Accessed September 19, 2008.

202. Canton R, Loza E, Morosini MI, et al. Antimicrobial resistance amongst isolates of *Streptococcus pyogenes* and *Staphylococcus aureus* in the Protekt Antimicrobial Surveillance Programme during 1999–2000. J Antimicrob Chemother 2002;50(Suppl S1):9–24.

203. Ketek Label Information. Food and Drug Administration. Available at: http://www.fda.gov/cder/foi/label/2007/021144s012lbl.pdf. Accessed August 25, 2008.

204. Clay KD, Hanson JS, Pope SD, et al. Brief communication. Severe hepatotoxicity of telithromycin: three case reports and literature review. Ann Intern Med 2006; 144(6):415–20.

Staphylococcus aureus Decolonization as a Prevention Strategy

Andrew E. Simor, MD[a,b,c,*], Nick Daneman, MD[a,c]

KEYWORDS

- *Staphylococcus aureus* • MRSA • Decolonization
- Mupirocin • Prophylaxis • Prevention

Staphylococcus aureus is one of the most successful human pathogens, with a world-wide distribution and the ability to cause serious and life-threatening disease. The importance of nasal carriage of *S aureus* in the development of nosocomial staphylococcal infections has been recognized for decades.[1] Staphylococcal decolonization therefore is among the various strategies that have been employed to reduce the risk of these infections occurring. Decolonization may be defined as treatment (using topical or systemic antimicrobials) to eradicate staphylococcal colonization or carriage. Despite uncertainty regarding the efficacy of this approach, recommendations to consider the use of decolonization often are made.[2–4] Indeed, a recent survey of Infectious Diseases Society of America (IDSA) members determined that decolonization is used as a strategy in various health care settings, most commonly in patients who have recurrent furunculosis caused by community-associated strains of methicillin-resistant *S aureus* (CA-MRSA).[5] This article reviews available data regarding the effectiveness of decolonization for preventing *S aureus* infections, and examines its potential role as an infection control measure to limit the transmission of MRSA.

THE RATIONALE FOR DECOLONIZATION

Asymptomatic colonization with *S aureus* is common, and appears to be a prerequisite for developing infection. In cross-sectional studies, approximately 30% of healthy

[a] Department of Medicine, University of Toronto, Toronto, ON, Canada M4N 3M5
[b] Department of Laboratory Medicine and Pathobiology, University of Toronto, Toronto, ON, Canada M4N 3M5
[c] Department of Microbiology and the Division of Infectious Diseases, Sunnybrook Health Sciences Centre, B103-2075 Bayview Avenue, Toronto, ON, Canada M4N 3M5
* Corresponding author. Department of Microbiology and the Division of Infectious Diseases, Sunnybrook Health Sciences Centre, B103-2075 Bayview Avenue, Toronto, ON, Canada M4N 3M5.
E-mail address: andrew.simor@sunnybrook.ca (A.E. Simor).

Infect Dis Clin N Am 23 (2009) 133–151
doi:10.1016/j.idc.2008.10.006
0891-5520/08/$ – see front matter © 2009 Elsevier Inc. All rights reserved.

id.theclinics.com

adults have been found to be colonized with S aureus at any point in time.[1,6,7] In a recent large United States population-based survey, 28.6% of subjects had nasal colonization with S aureus, and 1.5% were colonized with MRSA.[8] Higher rates of colonization may be seen in hospitalized patients and other high-risk groups. The major site of staphylococcal colonization in people is the anterior nares,[1,6] although throat, perineal, or gastrointestinal (GI) colonization also may occur relatively frequently.[9–11] Other cutaneous sites, surgical wounds, decubitus ulcers, and medical device exit sites also may be colonized.

Most S aureus infections appear to arise from an endogenous source (the patient's own colonizing strain of S aureus), although exogenous sources, including colonized health care workers, also may be an important source of infection in hospitalized patients. The relationship between staphylococcal colonization and the development of infection is complex and recently was reviewed by Wertheim and colleagues.[12] It is evident, however, that nasal carriage of S aureus is a predominant risk factor for subsequent staphylococcal infection, especially during hospitalization.[13–15] The risk of infection in nasal carriers is estimated to increase from two- to 12-fold as compared with non-carriers.[6,16] Nasal S aureus carriers are more likely than noncarriers to develop nosocomial S aureus bacteremia, dialysis-associated infections, or postoperative staphylococcal surgical site infections, and these infections are generally with the same strain as that colonizing the nose.[14,17–21] Colonization with MRSA appears to pose an even greater risk of subsequent infection; nasal carriers of MRSA were 3.9 times more likely to develop nosocomial staphylococcal bacteremia than were nasal carriers of susceptible strains of S aureus.[22] Between 20% and 30% of adults who have newly identified MRSA colonization are at risk of developing MRSA infection in the subsequent 12 to 18 months.[13,15]

Therefore, elimination of S aureus or MRSA nasal colonization would seem to be a reasonable approach to preventing staphylococcal infections. There are at least two reasons to consider staphylococcal decolonization: (1) to prevent the subsequent development of infection in a colonized patient, and (2) to prevent transmission of the organism (primarily MRSA) to others. An additional benefit of MRSA decolonization, if effective, would be to eliminate the need for use of isolation or contact precautions. In certain situations (eg, preoperative prophylaxis), transient suppression of the organism may suffice. There may be other circumstances, however, in which the goal of decolonization would be long-term eradication of MRSA carriage.

ERADICATION OF NASAL *STAPHYLOCOCCUS AUREUS*

For decolonization to prevent staphylococcal infection or transmission, it first must be capable of eradicating S aureus carriage. Numerous approaches and agents have been used in an attempt to accomplish this (**Table 1**). Unfortunately, many of these regimens were found to be ineffective, resulted in only short-term decolonization, or were associated with adverse effects or development of resistance to the agent used.[16,23] A strategy that had been used in the past was bacterial interference, attempting to replace the colonizing strain of S aureus with another strain (502A) that was considered to be minimally pathogenic. This approach was not always effective, and resulted in infection caused by the implanted strain of S aureus 502A in some patients.[24]

Randomized controlled trials of the efficacy of decolonization for the eradication of S aureus carriage in patients are summarized in **Table 2**.[25–36] These investigations exhibit significant heterogeneity in that diverse patient populations have been studied, using various topical or systemic decolonizing agents, and with variable lengths of

Table 1
Agents used for *Staphylococcus aureus* decolonization

Topical Agents	Systemic Agents	Other Strategies
Bacitracin	Ciprofloxacin	Aerosolized/nebulized solutions
Chlorhexidine	Cloxacillin	Bacterial interference (*S aureus* 502a)
Chlortetracycline	Doxycycline	*S aureus* phage therapy
Fusidic acid	Fusidic acid	*S aureus* vaccine
Gentamicin	Minocycline	
Hexachlorophene	Novobiocin	
Lysostaphin	Rifampin	
Mersacidin	Sulphathiazole	
Mupirocin	Trimethoprim-sulfamethoxazole	
Neomycin	Vancomycin	
Polymyxin B		
Sulfonamides		
Tea tree oil		
Vancomycin		

follow-up. Most of the studies have involved hospitalized patients colonized with MRSA, although inpatients and outpatients with susceptible strains of *S aureus* were included in some investigations. Many studies only considered nasal sites of staphylococcal colonization and did not investigate extranasal carriage of the organism. Some of the studies also had methodological flaws such as small sample size, or lack of blinding. Nevertheless, a review of these studies provides useful information regarding the efficacy of decolonization.

Among the topical agents that have been used, the one that has been evaluated most extensively, and that has shown the greatest potential for efficacy has been mupirocin calcium, formulated as an ointment or cream. When applied intranasally as directed, mupirocin has been safe and well tolerated. Treatment with mupirocin was found to be more effective than bacitracin,[37] and was able to eradicate nasal *S aureus* colonization in hospital staff for at least 4 weeks.[38,39] Moreover, intranasal application of mupirocin also eliminated hand carriage of *S aureus* in health care workers.[40] Mupirocin has been effective in eradicating nasal carriage in select patient populations, such as those who have HIV, and those undergoing long-term hemodialysis or ambulatory peritoneal dialysis.[32,41,42] The drug has been used successfully to decolonize nursing home residents who have nasal carriage of either methicillin-susceptible or methicillin-resistant strains of *S aureus*.[30,43] Mupirocin, however, appears to be less effective in decolonizing extranasal sites of carriage, as compared with nasal colonization.[44] There is also concern about the emergence of mupirocin resistance with extensive or prolonged use of this drug.[45–47] As a result, there has been interest in the use of other topical agents, such as tea tree oil, mersacidin (a lanthionine-containing antibiotic), and lysostaphin, but larger clinical trials are needed to determine their efficacy.[35,48,49]

As topical intranasal therapy may not be effective for eradicating extranasal sites of colonization, several systemic antimicrobial agents, used alone or in combination with topical therapy, have been evaluated (see **Tables 1** and **2**). Among the oral agents that have been used, rifampin appears to have had the greatest success.[25,50] In a recent

Table 2
Randomized controlled trials evaluating decolonization regimens for eradication of *Staphylococcus aureus* carriage in various patient populations

Reference (Number of Patients)	MSSA, MRSA, or Both	Follow-up (Weeks)	Treatment(s) versus Comparator	Eradication Rate (%)	Relative Risk (95% CI)
Wheat[25] (80)	Both	12	Rifampin Cloxacillin Rifampin + cloxacillin No treatment	65 0 60 0	Rifampin 0 (undefined) Cloxacillin 0.96 (0.72–1.30)
Peterson[26] (21)	MRSA	24	Rifampin + ciprofloxacin Rifampin + TMP-SMX	27 40	1.33 (0.39–4.6)
Walsh[27] (94)	MRSA	2	Rifampin + novobiocin Rifampin + TMP-SMX	67 53	0.80 (0.57–1.11)
Muder[28] (35)	MRSA	12	Rifampin Minocycline Rifampin + minocycline No treatment	70 38 50 14	Rifampin 0.44 (0.18–1.11) Minocycline 1.06 (0.52–2.18)
Parras[29] (84)	MRSA	12	Mupirocin Fusidic acid + TMP-SMX	78 71	0.92 (0.71–1.20)
Watanakunokorn[30] (59)	Both	12	Chlorhexidine Chlorhexidine + mupirocin	76 85	0.89 (0.68–1.17)
Harbarth[31] (102)	MRSA	4	Chlorhexidine + mupirocin Chlorhexidine + placebo	25 18	0.57 (0.31–1.04)
Martin[32] (76)	Both	10	Mupirocin Placebo	29 3	0.09 (0.01–0.67)
Chang[33] (23)	MRSA	2	Fusidic acid No treatment	33 50	3.5 (0.51–23.8)
Mody[34] (127)	Both	12	Mupirocin Placebo	61 15	0.22 (0.07–0.67)
Dryden[35] (224)	MRSA	2	Chlorhexidine + mupirocin + silver sulfadiazine Tea tree oil	49 41	1.17 (0.88–1.57)
Simor[36] (146)	MRSA	12	Chlorhexidine + mupirocin + rifampin + doxycycline No treatment	74 32	0.44 (0.24–0.78)

Abbreviations: MRSA, methicillin-resistant *Staphylococcus aureus*; MSSA, methicillin-susceptible *S aureus*; TMP-SMX, trimethoprim-sulfamethoxazole.

review of comparative studies, treatment with rifampin was found to be effective for eradicating *S aureus* carriage, although the development of rifampin resistance during and after treatment occurred in a significant proportion of patients.[50]

Long-term eradication of MRSA carriage has been more difficult to achieve than decolonization of susceptible strains of *S aureus*. In a systematic review done in 2003,[51] six randomized controlled trials of topical or systemic agents used for MRSA decolonization in hospitalized or long-term care facility patients were identified (included in **Table 2**).[26–29,31,33] No statistically significant difference in MRSA eradication was identified in any of these studies, although most were small and not adequately powered. The duration of follow-up in many of these studies was also relatively brief. Variables that have been associated with persistence of MRSA or recolonization following attempts to eradicate carriage with mupirocin have included the recovery of MRSA from multiple anatomic sites, prior exposure to fluoroquinolones, and MRSA isolates with mupirocin resistance.[36,52] Failure of decolonization may have occurred with certain drugs, such as ciprofloxacin and fusidic acid, because of the development of resistance during therapy.[26,33]

In contrast to these findings, treatment with mupirocin was found to be effective in eradicating *S aureus*, including MRSA, colonization for up to 3 months in a randomized controlled trial involving long-term care facility residents.[34] In a more recent investigation, treatment with intranasal mupirocin ointment, 2% chlorhexidine gluconate washes, oral rifampin, and doxycycline for 7 days was found to be safe and effective in long-term eradication of MRSA colonization in hospitalized patients (see **Table 2**).[36] At 3 months of follow-up, 74% of those treated had negative cultures for MRSA, as compared with only 32% of those not treated (*P*=.0001). The difference remained significant at 8 months of follow-up, at which time 54% of those treated had negative culture results. Mupirocin resistance emerged in 5% of follow-up isolates.

Although studies with topical or oral agents provide evidence that elimination of staphylococcal carriage may be feasible in various patient populations, most of these investigations do not address the question of whether such an approach reduces the risk of infection.

DECOLONIZATION AS SURGICAL PROPHYLAXIS

In theory, transient or short-term eradication of *S aureus* carriage at the time of surgery should reduce the risk of postoperative staphylococcal infections. Several studies have suggested the potential efficacy of staphylococcal decolonization as a strategy to prevent surgical site infections.[53–56] Some investigations have focused on decolonization to prevent infection in surgical patients colonized with MRSA.[57–59] Each of these studies used preoperative intranasal mupirocin for decolonization, but unfortunately, most were uncontrolled case series, or used historical controls. Randomized controlled trials thus far have failed to confirm the results obtained in these studies using less rigorous methods.

There have been four randomized controlled trials of preoperative mupirocin decolonization, and one study used perioperative chlorhexidine gluconate (**Table 3**).[60–64] In a large double-blind, randomized controlled trial, more than 4000 patients undergoing various elective surgical procedures were allocated to receive either intranasal mupirocin or placebo for up to 5 days.[60] There was no difference in overall surgical site infection rates, or in the rate of surgical site infections caused by *S aureus*. In a secondary analysis of the 891 patients who had preoperative nasal *S aureus* carriage, however, there were significantly fewer nosocomial staphylococcal infections in those who were treated with mupirocin as compared with those who received placebo

Table 3
Randomized controlled trials of *Staphylococcus aureus* decolonization for surgical infection prophylaxis

Reference; Surgery (Number of Patients)	Nosocomial Infections (%)		RR (95% CI)	Surgical Site Infections (%)		RR (95% CI)	S aureus Surgical Site Infections (%)		RR (95% CI)
	Mupirocin	Placebo		Mupirocin	Placebo		Mupirocin	Placebo	
Elective;[60] (3864)	11.3	11.4	1.0 (0.98–1.02)	7.9	8.5	0.99 (0.97–1.01)	2.3	2.4	1.0 (0.99–1.0)
Orthopedic;[61] (614)				3.8	4.7	0.99 (0.96–1.02)	1.6	2.7	1.0 (0.97–1.01)
Gastrointestinal;[62] (395)				14.5	10.9	1.04 (0.97–1.12)	2.1	2.5	1.0 (0.97–1.03)
Cardiac;[63] (263)[a]				13.8	8.6	1.06 (0.97–1.16)	3.8	3.2	1.0 (0.96–1.06)
	Chlorhexidine Gluconate	Placebo		Chlorhexidine Gluconate	Placebo		Chlorhexidine Gluconate	Placebo	
Cardiac;[64] (954)	19.8	26.2	0.92 (0.86–0.99)	9.9	10.9	0.99 (0.95–1.03)	1.9	5.1	1.0 (0.96–1.01)

Abbreviation: RR, Relative risk.
[a] All S aureus carriers.

(4.0% as compared with 7.7%; odds ratio [OR] for infection, 0.49; 95% CI, 0.25–0.92; $P = .02$). Unfortunately, smaller randomized controlled trials in GI, orthopedic, and cardiac surgery patients failed to detect a protective effect of preoperative treatment with intranasal mupirocin.[61–63] Even the study that targeted only those patients who had documented preoperative colonization with S aureus did not identify a reduction in the overall rate of surgical site infections, or of infections caused by S aureus.[63]

Although not designed to be a study of decolonization, the efficacy of perioperative nasopharyngeal and oropharyngeal decontamination with 0.12% chlorhexidine gluconate was investigated in patients undergoing cardiac surgery (see **Table 3**).[64] A significant reduction (58%) in S aureus carriage was found in the chlorhexidine gluconate-treated group, and this appeared to be associated with a decreased incidence of nosocomial infection in chlorhexidine gluconate recipients (20%) as compared with the infection rate in the placebo recipients (26.2%) (absolute risk reduction [ARR], 6.4%; 95% CI, 1.1% to 11.7%; $P = .002$). In particular, lower respiratory tract infections (ARR, 6.5%; 95% CI, 2.3% to 10.7%; $P = .002$) and deep surgical site infections (ARR, 3.2%; 95% CI, 0.9% to 5.5%; $P = .002$) were less common in the chlorhexidine group than in the placebo group.

DECOLONIZATION TO PREVENT INFECTION IN NONSURGICAL PATIENTS

Hospitalized medical patients and residents of long-term care facilities who are colonized with S aureus are at increased risk of developing a nosocomial staphylococcal infection. Consequently, there has been interest in determining the potential for decolonization to reduce the risk of these infections. Whereas short-term or transient elimination of S aureus carriage may suffice to reduce risks of infection in surgical patients who are at-risk for a brief period of time, long-term decolonization may be required if this strategy is contemplated in nonsurgical patients who are in a health care facility or nursing home for prolonged periods of time. An observational study was conducted in France over 55 months in a gastroenterology unit with many long-term patients who had chronic liver diseases to determine the effect of intranasal mupirocin decolonization of MRSA carriers.[65] Decolonization treatment was associated with decreased nosocomial MRSA carriage rates (10.2% versus 14.3%; $P = .006$), and importantly decreased MRSA infection rates (2.4% versus 5.5%; $P = .002$), as compared with rates at the outset of the study. No changes in mupirocin susceptibility were noted during this study.

Two randomized controlled trials of decolonization have been conducted involving nonsurgical hospital inpatients (**Table 4**).[31,66] In a study in Geneva, Switzerland, hospitalized patients colonized with MRSA who were generally elderly and had multiple comorbidities were randomized to treatment with either intranasal mupirocin or a placebo ointment.[31] Mupirocin was not more effective than the placebo for the primary outcome measure, eradication of MRSA carriage (25% in the mupirocin group versus 18% in placebo recipients; RR 1.39, 95% CI, 0.64–2.99; $P = .40$). Nor was a significant decrease in MRSA infection rates detected (1.48 infections per 1000 days versus 2.82 infections per 1000 days; RR 0.52, 95% CI, 0.14–2.02; $P = .53$). A study involving 1627 hospitalized patients was done on medical units of four Dutch hospitals with low rates of MRSA.[66] S aureus carriers were randomized to receive treatment with intranasal mupirocin or with a placebo ointment. Subsequent nosocomial S aureus infection rates were not significantly different (2.6% in mupirocin recipients versus 2.8% in placebo recipients; risk difference: 0.2%, 95% CI, –1.5% to 1.9%; OR 0.93, 95% CI, 0.5–1.7).

One study was conducted in elderly residents of two United States long-term care facilities.[34] Those who persistently were colonized with S aureus (50% with MRSA) were randomized to treatment with either mupirocin or a placebo ointment. Most

Table 4
Randomized controlled trials of *Staphylococcus aureus* decolonization in nonsurgical patients or residents of long-term care facilities

Reference; Patient Population (Number of Patients)	Nosocomial *S aureus* Infection Rate (%)		
	Mupirocin	Placebo	RR (95% CI)
MRSA colonized inpatients;[31] (98)	6 (1.48 infections/ 1000 days)	14 (2.82 infections/ 1000 days)	0.92 (0.80–1.05)
S aureus colonized inpatients;[66] (1,627)	2.6	2.8	1.00 (0.98–1.01)
S aureus colonized long-term care facility residents;[34] (127; 50% with MRSA)	5	15	0.90 (0.79–1.03)

Abbreviations: MRSA, methicillin-resistant *S aureus*; RR, relative risk.

mupirocin recipients were decolonized successfully even up to 90 days after treatment, and there was a trend (albeit not statistically significant) toward a reduced infection rate in those who were treated as compared with placebo recipients (5% versus 15% respectively; $P = .10$).

DECOLONIZATION OF DIALYSIS PATIENTS

Patients receiving long-term hemodialysis or continuous ambulatory peritoneal dialysis are at particularly high risk of developing serious staphylococcal infections, and the risk of infection appears to be related to the duration of staphylococcal carriage. A randomized controlled trial involving 44 hemodialysis patients colonized with *S aureus* compared decolonization with oral rifampin and topical bacitracin administered every 3 months with no treatment (**Table 5**).[67] After 3 years of follow-up, fewer infections occurred in those receiving decolonization (11.1% infection rate compared with 46.2%; $P = .02$), although rifampin resistance emerged in a small number of isolates.

Ten studies evaluating infection prophylaxis with topical mupirocin in hemodialysis and peritoneal dialysis patients were reviewed systematically in a meta-analysis.[68] The review concluded that mupirocin prophylaxis substantially reduces the rate of *S aureus* infections in dialysis patients (**Fig. 1**). Risk reductions were 80% (95% CI, 65% to 89%) among patients undergoing hemodialysis, and 63% (95% CI, 50% to 73%) among patients undergoing peritoneal dialysis. When the data were stratified by type of infection, there was an approximately 78% reduction in *S aureus* bloodstream infections in hemodialysis patients, a 66% reduction in peritoneal dialysis-associated peritonitis, and a 62% reduction in peritoneal dialysis catheter-related *S aureus* exit site infections. Unfortunately only three of the studies included in the meta-analysis were randomized controlled trials. Most of the studies used historical controls, and many were biased, because there was a shorter period of follow-up in mupirocin-treated subjects.

Two randomized controlled trials with mupirocin have been conducted in hemodialysis patients (see **Table 5**).[69,70] These studies involved small numbers of study subjects followed for relatively short periods of time. In both trials, however, repeated courses of treatment with mupirocin reduced the rates of *S aureus* infections. The one randomized placebo-controlled trial of mupirocin in peritoneal dialysis patients involved 267 *S aureus* carriers in nine European centers.[71] In up to 18 months of

Table 5
Randomized controlled trials of *Staphylococcus aureus* decolonization in dialysis patients

Study; (Number of Patients)		Infection Rates			
Hemodialysis	*S aureus* infections	No treatment	RR (95% CI)		
67 (44)	Rifampin and bacitracin	No treatment	0.61 (0.41–0.90)		
	• 11.1%	• 46.2%			
69 (34)	Mupirocin	Placebo	0.24 (0.03–1.9)		
	• 1.0/100 mo	• 4.1/100 mo			
		S aureus bloodstream infections	RR (95% CI)		
70 (36)		Mupirocin	No treatment	0.86 (0.78–0.96)	
		• 1.4%	• 14.9%		
		• 0.35/1000 patient days	• 5.95/1000 patient days	0.06 (0.01–0.46)	
Peritoneal dialysis	Exit site infections (per 100 patient months)	RR (95% CI)	*S aureus* exit site infections (per 100 patient months)	RR (95% CI)	*S aureus* peritonitis (per 100 patient months)	RR (95% CI)
71 (267)	Mupirocin	Placebo	0.53 (0.35–0.82)	Mupirocin	Placebo	0.28 (0.16–0.52)	Mupirocin	Placebo	0.66 (0.47–0.92)
	• 2.4	• 4.4		• 1.0	• 3.6		• 0.1	• 0.2	

Abbreviation: RR = Relative risk or incident rate ratio where applicable.

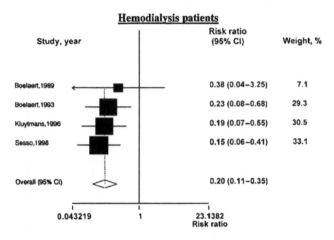

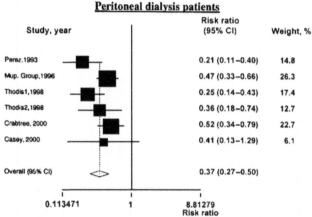

Fig. 1. Risk ratios and 95% CIs for mupirocin versus placebo or no prophylaxis in clinical trials of prevention of *Staphylococcus aureus* infection in the dialysis population. (*From* Tacconelli E, Carmeli Y, Aizer A, et al. Mupirocin prophylaxis to prevent Staphylococcus aureus infection in patients undergoing dialysis: a meta-analysis. Clin Infect Dis 2003;37:1634; with permission.)

follow-up, the mupirocin-treated subjects were more likely to have had eradication of staphylococcal carriage, and were less likely to develop *S aureus* exit site infections. There was no significant reduction in overall exit site infections, or in peritonitis rates, however (see **Table 5**). A randomized, double-blind trial comparing exit site application of topical mupirocin ointment with gentamicin cream found reduced incidence of exit site infections and peritonitis with gentamicin, largely because of a reduction in infections caused by gram-negative organisms.[72]

For decolonization to be effective in dialysis patients, it appears that repeated courses of treatment need to be administered to prevent recolonization.[41,67,71,72] In short-term follow-up, emergence of resistance to the decolonizing agent was observed infrequently. In a peritoneal dialysis unit that had used prophylactic mupirocin for approximately 10 years, however, mupirocin resistance in *S aureus* isolates increased, and this was associated with an increased rate of *S aureus* exit site infections.[47] This observation raises concerns about the long-term effect of mupirocin decolonization in dialysis patients.

DECOLONIZATION TO PREVENT RECURRENT SKIN AND SOFT TISSUE INFECTIONS

Skin and soft tissue infections are among the most common manifestations of disease caused by *S aureus*. Cutaneous infections, particularly furunculosis and abscesses, are also the major sites of infection caused by CA-MRSA. Nasal colonization with CA-MRSA strains has been associated with an increased risk of subsequent skin and soft tissue infection, and recurrence rates of at least 10% have been reported.[73,74] Recurrent furunculosis may signal the presence of an underlying immune defect, but this more commonly is caused by autoinoculation from persistent or recurrent *S aureus* colonization.[75,76] Consequently, decolonization as a preventive strategy has been employed, although data regarding the effectiveness of this treatment are lacking, particularly with regards to the management of recurrent skin and soft tissue infections caused by CA-MRSA. Open-label, noncomparative studies with topical or systemic agents have suggested that decolonization or long-term suppressive therapy is effective in treating and preventing recurrent staphylococcal furunculosis caused by methicillin-susceptible strains.[77,78] In an observational study in Germany, the use of topical mupirocin for decolonization of carriers appeared to prevent recurrent infections and to interrupt transmission in a community outbreak of Panton-Valentine leukocidin (PVL)-positive methicillin-susceptible *S aureus* furunculosis.[79]

Two randomized placebo-controlled trials have been conducted to determine the efficacy of decolonization with mupirocin for preventing recurrent staphylococcal skin and soft tissue infections.[80,81] The first study involved 34 otherwise healthy adults who had recurrent skin infections caused by methicillin-susceptible strains of *S aureus*.[80] Study subjects were treated monthly for 1 year with a 5-day course of either intranasal mupirocin or a placebo ointment. Those treated with mupirocin had reduced *S aureus* nasal colonization rates, and also experienced significantly lower rates of recurrent skin and soft tissue infections. The second study involved 134 military recruits colonized with CA-MRSA who received a single 5-day course of either intranasal mupirocin or placebo, and who then were monitored for 16 weeks for the development of infection.[81] Although CA-MRSA was eradicated successfully in most of the mupirocin-treated group, there was no difference in the subsequent skin or soft tissue infection rates (7.7% in placebo recipients versus 10.6% in mupirocin recipients). The failure to demonstrate efficacy of a single course of therapy with mupirocin was attributed to a lower than expected infection rate in the placebo recipients. Frequent recolonization with CA-MRSA during the study follow-up also occurred. Similarly, in a retrospective study, mupirocin treatment of a small number of patients who had recurrent skin and skin structure infections caused by CA-MRSA had little effect on recurrent infection rates.[82]

DECOLONIZATION AS AN INFECTION CONTROL MEASURE

Eradication of MRSA carriage has been an important component of search-and-destroy strategies used in several European countries that have maintained low endemic rates of nosocomial MRSA.[83] In addition, many studies have reported successful use of decolonization in the termination of staphylococcal outbreaks, or in reducing MRSA transmission rates in hospitals and other health care facilities.[84–94] The decolonization strategies employed in these reports were highly variable. In some outbreaks, decolonization was targeted at only colonized health care workers, and in other studies decolonization treatment was provided only to colonized patients. Occasionally, decolonization was attempted in both patients and health care workers. Regardless of the decolonization strategy implemented, reported staphylococcal eradication rates were generally high (at least in short-term follow-up), and outbreaks often terminated, or there was a reduction in endemic MRSA rates. It is, however, important to note that in these reports decolonization was almost always part of a broader infection control program, with implementation of multiple interventions along with attempts to eradicate staphylococcal carriage. Two recent studies employed universal MRSA admission screening using rapid molecular (multiplex polymerase chain reaction) assays, implementation of contact isolation, and routine decolonization of MRSA carriers.[94,95] In one study using historic controls, there was a substantial decrease in nosocomial MRSA infections.[94] In the other investigation using a cross-over study design, however, there was no reduction in MRSA acquisition or infection rates.[95] Consequently, it is not possible to determine the role, if any, that decolonization has in preventing subsequent staphylococcal transmission.

A causal link between decolonization and successful infection control was suggested in some studies by a temporal association with the addition of decolonization to an otherwise failing infection control strategy, or by the recurrence of MRSA transmission after decolonization with mupirocin was discontinued.[84,86] Somewhat stronger evidence is provided by quasi-experimental before-and-after studies, in which the only new intervention associated with termination of the outbreak appeared to be decolonization.[90–92] Selective use of intranasal mupirocin with daily chlorhexidine bathing for ICU patients who had MRSA were used in two studies.[90,92] In one, there was a 48% decrease in the incidence of MRSA in the unit beyond that seen with an active surveillance culture program that was in place before implementation of decolonization.[92] Similarly, in a Brazilian ICU that introduced active surveillance cultures and decolonization of carriers, there was a significant decrease in the incidence of nosocomial MRSA infection that persisted over 5 years without any increase in mupirocin resistance.[90] The use of enteric vancomycin prescribed to colonized mechanically ventilated patients appeared to reduce the incidence of MRSA acquisition and infection in two ICUs.[88,91] There is, however, concern that using oral vancomycin for decolonization may promote the emergence of glycopeptide resistance in staphylococci and enterococci.[3]

A few studies have described treatment with topical mupirocin alone, or in combination with oral antimicrobial agents (such as rifampin and minocycline) to successfully terminate transmission of CA-MRSA and prevent recurrent infections in outbreak settings among military recruits, in a daycare facility, and in a neonatal ICU.[96–98] In contrast, decolonization with mupirocin was ineffective for managing CA-MRSA infections occurring in two football teams, possibly because of poor compliance with the recommended treatment in one of the outbreaks.[99,100]

SUMMARY AND FUTURE RESEARCH NEEDS

Eradication of S aureus carriage appears to be feasible, especially if mupirocin or rifampin is included as part of the treatment. There is little evidence, however, that decolonization reduces the risk of more meaningful endpoints such as staphylococcal infection or transmission. Therefore, there is currently no indication for routine decolonization preoperatively or in hospitalized nonsurgical patients. Decolonization with mupirocin or rifampin may be considered in those undergoing dialysis, although there is a risk of resistance emerging with long-term use of either of these drugs. Decolonization also may be useful in patients who have recurrent staphylococcal skin or soft tissue infection. Eradication of MRSA carriage in colonized health care workers or patients may be considered as a component of outbreak management in health care facilities. Mupirocin susceptibility testing should be done before using this agent for decolonization.

Although S aureus and MRSA decolonization may be achieved, at least in certain patient populations, further studies are required to identify more effective agents for long-term eradication of nasal and extra-nasal sites of colonization, to evaluate the efficacy of this strategy for preventing infection in various clinical situations, and to determine whether it has any significant role to play as an infection control measure. For example, adequately powered, randomized controlled trials of decolonization for preventing postoperative infections in surgical patients known to be colonized with S aureus should be done. Outcome measures should include overall infection rates and staphylococcal infection rates. Decolonization to prevent recurrent infections in patients who have CA-MRSA needs to be evaluated. The role of decolonization as an infection control intervention to reduce MRSA transmission needs to be defined. Ongoing surveillance of mupirocin resistance should be conducted, especially in settings with repeated or long-term mupirocin use, such as dialysis units. The effectiveness of novel agents, particularly those less likely to induce antimicrobial resistance, should be determined. Other strategies, such as developing a safe and effective staphylococcal vaccine, also need to be evaluated.

REFERENCES

1. Williams REO. Healthy carriage of *Staphylococcus aureus*: its prevalence and importance. Bacteriol Rev 1963;27:56–71.
2. Arnold MS, Dempsey JM, Fishman M, et al. The best hospital practices for controlling methicillin-resistant *Staphylococcus aureus*: on the cutting edge. Infect Control Hosp Epidemiol 2002;23:69–76.
3. Muto CA, Jernigan JA, Ostrowsky BE, et al. SHEA guideline for preventing nosocomial transmission of multidrug-resistant strains of *Staphylococcus aureus* and *Enterococcus*. Infect Control Hosp Epidemiol 2003;24:362–86.
4. Kallen AJ, Wilson CT, Larson RJ. Perioperative intranasal mupirocin for the prevention of surgical site infections: systematic review of the literature and meta-analysis. Infect Control Hosp Epidemiol 2005;26:916–22.
5. West SK, Plantenga MS, Strausbaugh LJ, et al. Use of decolonization to prevent staphylococcal infections in various healthcare settings: results of an Emerging Infections Network survey. Infect Control Hosp Epidemiol 2007;28:1111–3.
6. Kluytmans J, van Belkum A, Verbrugh H. Nasal carriage of *Staphylococcus aureus*: epidemiology, underlying mechanisms, and associated risks. Clin Microbiol Rev 1997;10:505–20.
7. Graham PL III, Lin SX, Larson EL. A US population-based survey of *Staphylococcus aureus* colonization. Ann Intern Med 2006;144:318–25.
8. Gorwitz RJ, Kruszon-Moran D, McAllister SK, et al. Changes in the prevalence of nasal colonization with *Staphylococcus aureus* in the United States, 2001–2004. J Infect Dis 2008;197:1226–34.
9. Boe J, Solberg CO, Vogelsang TM, et al. Perineal carriers of staphylococci. Br Med J 1964;5404:280–1.
10. Boyce JM, Havill NL, Maria B. Frequency and possible infection control implications of gastrointestinal colonization with methicillin-resistant *Staphylococcus aureus*. J Clin Microbiol 2005;43:5992–5.
11. Nilsson P, Ripa T. *Staphylococcus aureus* throat colonization is more frequent than colonization in the anterior nares. J Clin Microbiol 2006;44:3334–9.

12. Wertheim HFL, Melles DC, Vos MC, et al. The role of nasal carriage in *Staphylococcus aureus* infections. Lancet Infect Dis 2005;5:751–62.
13. Davis KA, Stewart JJ, Crouch HK, et al. Methicillin-resistant *Staphylococcus aureus* (MRSA) nares colonization at hospital admission and its effect on subsequent MRSA infection. Clin Infect Dis 2004;39:776–82.
14. von Eiff C, Becker K, Machka K, et al. Nasal carriage as a source of *Staphylococcus aureus* bacteremia. N Engl J Med 2001;344:11–6.
15. Huang SS, Platt R. Risk of methicillin-resistant *Staphylococcus aureus* infection after previous infection or colonization. Clin Infect Dis 2003;36:281–5.
16. Perl TM, Golub JE. New approaches to reduce *Staphylococcus aureus* nosocomial infection rates: treating *S. aureus* nasal carriage. Ann. Pharmacother 1998; 32:S7–16.
17. Wertheim HFL, Vos MC, Ott A, et al. Risk and outcome of nosocomial *Staphylococcus aureus* bacteraemia in nasal carriers versus non-carriers. Lancet 2004; 364:703–5.
18. Luzar MA, Coles GA, Faller B, et al. *Staphylococcus aureus* nasal carriage and infection in patients on continuous ambulatory peritoneal dialysis. N Engl J Med 1990;322:505–9.
19. Wenzel RP, Perl TM. The significance of nasal carriage of *Staphylococcus aureus* and the incidence of postoperative wound infection. J Hosp Infect 1995;31:13–24.
20. Kluytmans JAJW, Mouton JW, Ijzerman EPF, et al. Nasal carriage of *Staphylococcus aureus* as a major risk factor for wound infections after cardiac surgery. J Infect Dis 1995;171:216–9.
21. Kalmeijer MD, van Nieuwland-Bollen E, Bogaers-Hofman D, et al. Nasal carriage of *Staphylococcus aureus* is a major risk factor for surgical site infections in orthopedic surgery. Infect Control Hosp Epidemiol 2000;21:319–23.
22. Pujol M, Peña C, Pallares R, et al. Nosocomial *Staphylococcus aureus* bacteremia among nasal carriers of methicillin-resistant and methicillin-susceptible strains. Am J Med 1996;100:509–16.
23. Boyce JM. Preventing staphylococcal infections by eradicating nasal carriage of *Staphylococcus aureus*: proceeding with caution. Infect Control Hosp Epidemiol 1996;17:775–9.
24. Houck PW, Nelson JD, Kay JL. Fatal septicemia due to *S aureus* 502A. Report of a case and review of the infectious complications of bacterial interference programs. Am J Dis Child 1972;123:45–8.
25. Wheat LJ, Kohler RB, Luft FC, et al. Long-term effect of rifampin on nasal carriage of coagulase-positive staphylococci. Rev Infect Dis 1983;5(Suppl 3):S459–62.
26. Peterson LR, Quick JN, Jensen B, et al. Emergence of ciprofloxacin resistance in nosocomial methicillin-resistant *Staphylococcus aureus* isolates. Resistance during ciprofloxacin plus rifampin therapy for methicillin-resistant *S. aureus* colonization. Arch Intern Med 1990;150:2151–5.
27. Walsh TJ, Standiford HC, Reboli AC, et al. Randomized double-blinded trial of rifampin with either novobiocin or trimethoprim-sulfamethoxazole against methicillin-resistant *Staphylococcus aureus* colonization: prevention of antimicrobial resistance and effect of host factors on outcome. Antimicrob Agents Chemother 1993;37:1134–42.
28. Muder RR, Boldin M, Brennen C, et al. A controlled trial of rifampicin, minocycline, and rifampicin plus minocycline for eradication of methicillin-resistant *Staphylococcus aureus* in long-term care patients. J Antimicrob Chemother 1994;34:189–90.

29. Parras F, del Carmen Guerrero M, Bouza E, et al. Comparative study of mupirocin and oral cotrimoxazole plus topical fusidic acid in eradication of nasal carriage of methicillin-resistant *Staphylococcus aureus*. Antimicrob Agents Chemother 1995; 39:175–9.

30. Watanakunakorn C, Axelson C, Bota B, et al. Mupirocin ointment with and without chlorhexidine baths in the eradication of *Staphylococcus aureus* nasal carriage in nursing home residents. Am J Infect Control 1995;23:306–9.

31. Harbarth S, Dharan S, Liassine N, et al. Randomized, placebo-controlled, double-blind trial to evaluate the efficacy of mupirocin for eradicating carriage of methicillin-resistant *Staphylococcus aureus*. Antimicrob Agents Chemother 1999;43:1412–6.

32. Martin JN, Perdreau-Remington F, Kartalija M, et al. A randomized clinical trial of mupirocin in the eradication of *Staphylococcus aureus* nasal carriage in human immunodeficiency virus disease. J Infect Dis 1999;180:896–9.

33. Chang S-C, Hsieh S-M, Chen M-L, et al. Oral fusidic acid fails to eradicate methicillin-resistant *Staphylococcus aureus* colonization and results in emergence of fusidic acid-resistant strains. Diagn Microbiol Infect Dis 2000;36:131–6.

34. Mody L, Kauffman CA, McNeil SA, et al. Mupirocin-based decolonization of *Staphylococcus aureus* carriers in residents of 2 long-term care facilities: a randomized, double-blind, placebo-controlled trial. Clin Infect Dis 2003;37:1467–74.

35. Dryden MS, Dailly S, Crouch M. A randomized, controlled trial of tea tree topical preparations versus a standard topical regimen for the clearance of MRSA colonization. J Hosp Infect 2004;56:283–6.

36. Simor AE, Phillips E, McGeer A, et al. Randomized controlled trial of chlorhexidine gluconate for washing, intranasal mupirocin, and rifampin and doxycycline versus no treatment for the eradication of methicillin-resistant *Staphylococcus aureus* colonization. Clin Infect Dis 2007;44:178–85.

37. Soto NE, Vaghjimal A, Stahl-Avicolli A, et al. Bacitracin versus mupirocin for *Staphylococcus aureus* nasal colonization. Infect Control Hosp Epidemiol 1999;20:351–3.

38. Doebbeling BN, Breneman DL, Neu HC, et al. Elimination of *Staphylococcus aureus* nasal carriage in health care workers: analysis of six clinical trials with calcium mupirocin ointment. Clin Infect Dis 1993;17:466–74.

39. Fernandez C, Gaspar C, Torrellas A, et al. A double-blind, randomized, placebo-controlled trial to evaluate the safety and efficacy of mupirocin calcium ointment for eliminating nasal carriage of *Staphylococcus aureus* among hospital personnel. J Antimicrob Chemother 1995;35:399–408.

40. Reagan DR, Doebbeling BN, Pfaller MA, et al. Elimination of coincident *Staphylococcus aureus* nasal and hand carriage with intranasal application of mupirocin calcium ointment. Ann Intern Med 1991;114:101–6.

41. Pérez-Fontán M, García-Falcón T, Rosales M, et al. Treatment of *Staphylococcus aureus* nasal carriers in continuous ambulatory peritoneal dialysis with mupirocin: long-term results. Am J Kidney Dis 1993;22:708–12.

42. Laupland KB, Conly JM. Treatment of *Staphylococcus aureus* colonization and prophylaxis for infection with topical intranasal mupirocin: an evidence-based review. Clin Infect Dis 2003;37:933–8.

43. Cederna JE, Terpenning MS, Ensberg M, et al. *Staphylococcus aureus* nasal colonization in a nursing home: eradication with mupirocin. Infect Control Hosp Epidemiol 1990;11:13–6.

44. Wertheim HFL, Verveer J, Boelens HAM, et al. Effect of mupirocin treatment on nasal, pharyngeal, and perineal carriage of *Staphylococcus aureus* in healthy adults. Antimicrob Agents Chemother 2005;49:1465–7.

45. Miller MA, Dascal A, Portnoy J, et al. Development of mupirocin resistance among methicillin-resistant *Staphylococcus aureus* after widespread use of nasal mupirocin ointment. Infect Control Hosp Epidemiol 1996;17:811–3.
46. Vasquez JE, Walker ES, Franzus BW, et al. The epidemiology of mupirocin resistance among methicillin-resistant *Staphylococcus aureus* at a Veterans Affairs hospital. Infect Control Hosp Epidemiol 2000;21:459–64.
47. Pérez-Fontán M, Rosales M, Rodríguez-Carmona A, et al. Mupirocin resistance after long-term use for *Staphylococcus aureus* colonization in patients undergoing chronic peritoneal dialysis. Am J Kidney Dis 2002;39:337–41.
48. Kruszewska D, Sahl H-G, Bierbaum G, et al. Mersacidin eradicates methicillin-resistant *Staphylococcus aureus* (MRSA) in a mouse rhinitis model. J Antimicrob Chemother 2004;54:648–53.
49. Kokai-Kun JF, Walsh SM, Chanturiya T, et al. Lysostaphin cream eradicates *Staphylococcus aureus* nasal colonization in a cotton rat model. Antimicrob Agents Chemother 2003;47:1589–97.
50. Falagas ME, Bliziotis IA, Fragoulis KN. Oral rifampin for eradication of *Staphylococcus aureus* carriage from healthy and sick populations: a systematic review of the evidence from comparative trials. Am J Infect Control 2007;35:106–14.
51. Loeb M, Main C, Walker-Dilks C, et al. Antimicrobial agents for treating methicillin-resistant *Staphylococcus aureus*. Cochrane Database Syst Rev 2003;4: CD003340.
52. Harbarth S, Liassine N, Dharan S, et al. Risk factors for persistent carriage of methicillin-resistant *Staphylococcus aureus*. Clin Infect Dis 2000;31:1380–5.
53. Kluytmans JAJW, Mouton JW, VandenBergh MFQ, et al. Reduction of surgical site infections in cardiothoracic surgery by elimination of nasal carriage of *Staphylococcus aureus*. Infect Control Hosp Epidemiol 1996;17:780–5.
54. Gernaat-van der Sluis AJ, Hoogenboom-Verdegaal AM, Edixhoven PJ, et al. Prophylactic mupirocin could reduce orthopedic wound infections: 1044 patients treated with mupirocin compared with 1260 historical controls. Acta Orthop Scand 1998;69:412–4.
55. Yano M, Doki Y, Inoue M, et al. Preoperative intranasal mupirocin ointment significantly reduces postoperative infection with *Staphylococcus aureus* in patients undergoing upper gastrointestinal surgery. Surg Today 2000;30:16–21.
56. Cimochowski GE, Harostock MD, Brown R, et al. Intranasal mupirocin reduces sternal wound infection after open heart surgery in diabetics and nondiabetics. Ann Thorac Surg 2001;71:1572–9.
57. Wilcox MH, Hall J, Pike H, et al. Use of perioperative mupirocin to prevent methicillin-resistant *Staphylococcus aureus* (MRSA) orthopaedic surgical site infections. J Hosp Infect 2003;54:196–201.
58. Horiuchi A, Nakayama Y, Kajiyama M, et al. Nasopharyngeal decolonization of methicillin-resistant *Staphylococcus aureus* can reduce PEG peristomal wound infection. Am J Gastroenterol 2006;101:274–7.
59. Thomas S, Cantrill S, Waghorn DJ, et al. The role of screening and antibiotic prophylaxis in the prevention of percutaneous gastrostomy site infection caused by methicillin-resistant *Staphylococcus aureus*. Aliment Pharmacol Ther 2007;25: 593–7.
60. Perl TM, Cullen JJ, Wenzel RP, et al. Intranasal mupirocin to prevent postoperative *Staphylococcus aureus* infections. N Engl J Med 2002;346:1871–7.
61. Kalmeijer MD, Coertjens H, van Nieuwland-Bollen PM, et al. Surgical site infections in orthopedic surgery: the effect of mupirocin nasal ointment in a double-blind, randomized, placebo-controlled study. Clin Infect Dis 2002;35:353–8.

62. Suzuki Y, Kamigaki T, Fujino Y, et al. Randomized clinical trial of preoperative intranasal mupirocin to reduce surgical-site infection after digestive surgery. Br J Surg 2003;90:1072–5.
63. Konvalinka A, Errett L, Fong IW. Impact of treating *Staphylococcus aureus* nasal carriers on wound infections in cardiac surgery. J Hosp Infect 2006;64: 162–8.
64. Segers P, Speekenbrink RGH, Ubbink DT, et al. Prevention of nosocomial infection in cardiac surgery by decontamination of the nasopharynx and oropharynx with chlorhexidine gluconate: a randomized controlled trial. JAMA 2006;296: 2460–6.
65. Dupeyron C, Campillo B, Richardet J-P, et al. Long-term efficacy of mupirocin in the prevention of infections with methicillin-resistant *Staphylococcus aureus* in a gastroenterology unit. J Hosp Infect 2006;63:385–92.
66. Wertheim HFL, Vos MC, Ott A, et al. Mupirocin prophylaxis against nosocomial *Staphylococcus aureus* infections in nonsurgical patients. A randomized study. Ann Intern Med 2004;140:419–25.
67. Yu VL, Goetz A, Wagener M, et al. *Staphylococcus aureus* nasal carriage and infection in patients on hemodialysis. Efficacy of antibiotic prophylaxis. N Engl J Med 1986;315:91–6.
68. Tacconelli E, Carmeli Y, Aizer A, et al. Mupirocin prophylaxis to prevent *Staphylococcus aureus* infection in patients undergoing dialysis: a meta-analysis. Clin Infect Dis 2003;37:1629–38.
69. Boelaert JR, De Smedt RA, De Baere YA, et al. The influence of calcium mupirocin nasal ointment on the incidence of *Staphylococcus aureus* infections in haemodialysis patients. Nephrol Dial Transplant 1989;4:278–81.
70. Sesso R, Barbosa D, Leme IL, et al. *Staphylococcus aureus* prophylaxis in hemodialysis patients using central venous catheter: effect of mupirocin ointment. J Am Soc Nephrol 1998;9:1085–92.
71. The Mupirocin Study Group. Nasal mupirocin prevents *Staphylococcus aureus* exit site infection during peritoneal dialysis. J Am Soc Nephrol 1996;7: 2403–8.
72. Bernardini J, Bender F, Florio T, et al. Randomized, double-blind trial of antibiotic exit site cream for prevention of exit site infection in peritoneal dialysis patients. J Am Soc Nephrol 2005;16:539–45.
73. Daum RS. Skin and soft-tissue infections caused by methicillin-resistant *Staphylococcus aureus*. N Engl J Med 2007;357:380–90.
74. Ellis MW, Hospenthal DR, Dooley DP, et al. Natural history of community-acquired methicillin-resistant *Staphylococcus aureus* colonization and infection in soldiers. Clin Infect Dis 2004;39:971–9.
75. Hedström SA. Recurrent staphylococcal furunculosis. Bacteriological findings and epidemiology. Scand J Infect Dis 1981;13:115–9.
76. Tuazon CU. Skin and skin structure infections in the patient at risk: carrier state of *Staphylococcus aureus*. Am J Med 1984;75:166–71.
77. Hedström SA. Treatment and prevention of recurrent staphylococcal furunculosis: clinical and bacteriological follow-up. Scand J Infect Dis 1985;17:55–8.
78. Aminzadeh A, Demircay Z, Ocak K, et al. Prevention of chronic furunculosis with low-dose azithromycin. J Dermotolog Treat 2007;18:105–8.
79. Wiese-Posselt M, Heuck D, Draeger A, et al. Successful termination of a furunculosis outbreak due to lukS-lukF-positive, methicillin-susceptible *Staphylococcus aureus* in a German village by stringent decolonization, 2002–2005. Clin Infect Dis 2007;44:e88–95.

80. Raz R, Miron D, Colodner R, et al. A 1-year trial of nasal mupirocin in the prevention of recurrent staphylococcal nasal colonization and skin infection. Arch Intern Med 1996;156:1109–12.
81. Ellis MW, Griffith ME, Dooley DP, et al. Targeted intranasal mupirocin to prevent colonization and infection by community-associated methicillin-resistant *Staphylococcus aureus* strains in soldiers: a cluster randomized controlled trial. Antimicrob Agents Chemother 2007;51:3591–8.
82. Rahimian J, Khan R, LaScalea KA. Does nasal colonization or mupirocin treatment affect recurrence of methicillin-resistant *Staphylococcus aureus* skin and skin structure infections? Infect Control Hosp Epidemiol 2007;28:1415–6.
83. Verhoef J, Beaujean D, Blok H, et al. A Dutch approach to methicillin-resistant *Staphylococcus aureus*. Eur J Clin Microbiol Infect Dis 1999;18:461–6.
84. Hill RLR, Duckworth GJ, Casewell MW. Elimination of nasal carriage of methicillin-resistant *Staphylococcus aureus* with mupirocin during a hospital outbreak. J Antimicrob Chemother 1988;22:377–84.
85. Girou E, Pujade G, Legrand P, et al. Selective screening of carriers for control of methicillin-resistant *Staphylococcus aureus* (MRSA) in high-risk hospital areas with a high level of endemic MRSA. Clin Infect Dis 1998;27:543–50.
86. Hitomi S, Kubota M, Mori N, et al. Control of a methicillin-resistant *Staphylococcus aureus* outbreak in a neonatal intensive care unit by unselective use of nasal mupirocin ointment. J Hosp Infect 2000;46:123–9.
87. Koitilainen P, Routamaa M, Peltonen R, et al. Eradication of methicillin-resistant *Staphylococcus aureus* from a health center ward and associated nursing home. Arch Intern Med 2001;161:859–63.
88. Silvestri L, Milanese M, Oblach L, et al. Enteral vancomycin to control methicillin-resistant *Staphylococcus aureus* outbreak in mechanically ventilated patients. Am J Infect Control 2002;30:391–9.
89. Tomic V, Svetina SP, Trinkaus D, et al. Comprehensive strategy to prevent nosocomial spread of methicillin-resistant *Staphylococcus aureus* in a highly endemic setting. Arch Intern Med 2004;164:2038–43.
90. Sandri AM, Dalarosa MG, Ruschel de Alcântara L, et al. Reduction in incidence of nosocomial methicillin-resistant *Staphylococcus aureus* (MRSA) infection in an intensive care unit: role of treatment with mupirocin ointment and chlorhexidine baths for nasal carriers of MRSA. Infect Control Hosp Epidemiol 2006;27: 185–7.
91. Cerdá E, Abella A, de la Cal MA, et al. Enteral vancomycin controls methicillin-resistant *Staphylococcus aureus* endemicity in an intensive care burn unit. A 9-year prospective study. Ann Surg 2007;245:397–407.
92. Ridenour G, Lampen R, Federspiel J, et al. Selective use of intranasal mupirocin and chlorhexidine bathing and the incidence of methicillin-resistant *Staphylococcus aureus* colonization and infection among intensive care unit patients. Infect Control Hosp Epidemiol 2007;28:1155–61.
93. Raineri E, Crema L, De Silvestri A, et al. Methicillin-resistant *Staphylococcus aureus* control in an intensive care unit: a 10-year analysis. J Hosp Infect 2007;67:308–15.
94. Robiscek A, Beaumont JL, Paule SM, et al. Universal surveillance for methicillin-resistant *Staphylococcus aureus* in 3 affiliated hospitals. Ann Intern Med 2008; 148:409–18.
95. Harbarth S, Frankhauser C, Schrenzel J, et al. Universal screening for methicillin-resistant *Staphylococcus aureus* at hospital admission and nosocomial infection in surgical patients. JAMA 2008;299:1149–57.

96. Zinderman CE, Conner B, Malakooti MA, et al. Community-acquired methicillin-resistant *Staphylococcus aureus* among military recruits. Emerg Infect Dis 2004; 10:941–4.

97. Shahin R, Johnson IL, Jamieson F, et al. Methicillin-resistant *Staphylococcus aureus* carriage in a child care center following a case of disease. Arch Pediatr Adolesc Med 1999;153:864–8.

98. Regev-Yochay G, Rubinstein E, Barzilai A, et al. Methicillin-resistant *Staphylococcus aureus* in neonatal intensive care unit. Emerg Infect Dis 2005;11:453–6.

99. Nguyen DM, Mascola L, Bancroft E. Recurring methicillin-resistant *Staphylococcus aureus* infections in a football team. Emerg Infect Dis 2005;11:526–32.

100. Rihn JA, Posfay-Barbe K, Harner CD, et al. Community-acquired methicillin-resistant *Staphylococcus aureus* outbreak in a local high school football team. Unsuccessful interventions. Pediatr Infect Dis J 2005;24:841–3.

Staphylococcal Vaccines and Immunotherapies

Adam C. Schaffer, MD[a], Jean C. Lee, PhD[b],*

KEYWORDS

- *Staphylococcus aureus* • Vaccine • Active immunization
- Passive immunization

Staphylococcus aureus is an important bacterial pathogen that causes various human infections, which can be life-threatening.[1,2] Methicillin-resistant *S aureus* (MRSA) strains are responsible for 40% to 60% of nosocomial staphylococcal infections in the United States, and many of these isolates are multidrug-resistant.[2] The emergence of community-associated MRSA infections has heightened concern about this microbe[3–5] and has lent a new urgency to efforts to control the spread of MRSA. Although new antimicrobial agents are under investigation, there is little doubt that *S aureus* ultimately will devise resistance mechanisms to circumvent the effectiveness of antibiotics.[6] Not only has resistance to methicillin among *S aureus* isolates become more common,[2] but MRSA strains with reduced susceptibility to vancomycin also have been reported.[7–9] Given the emergence of multidrug-resistant strains, including some with resistance to vancomycin, there is a pressing need for nonantimicrobial approaches, such as vaccines, to combat the spread of *S aureus*.

An *S aureus* vaccine offers a mechanism to boost the immune system so that effector molecules are elicited by the host to contain and eradicate the infecting microbe. Because many of the individuals most susceptible to staphylococcal infections are the least competent to mount an effective immune response, both passive and active immunization strategies need to be considered. This article discusses recent work in the development of *S aureus* vaccines and immunotherapies. Older research in this area has been summarized in other reviews.[10–12]

This work is supported by NIH Grant AI29040 and *Adapted from* Schaffer AC, Lee JC. Vaccination and passive immunisation against *Staphylococcus aureus*. Int J Antimicrob Agents 2008;32:S71–8; and Schaffer AC, Lee JC. Vaccine based strategies for prevention of staphylococcal infection. In: Crossley KB, Archer GL, Fowler VG Jr, Jefferson KK, editors. The staphylococci in human disease. Oxford (England): Blackwell Publishing Limited; with permission.
[a] Department of Medicine, Brigham and Women's Hospital and Harvard Medical School, PBB-B-422, 75 Francis street, Boston, MA 02115, USA
[b] Channing Laboratory, Department of Medicine, Brigham and Women's Hospital and Harvard Medical School, 181 Longwood Avenue, Boston, MA 02115, USA
* Corresponding author.
E-mail address: jclee@rics.bwh.harvard.edu (J.C. Lee).

Infect Dis Clin N Am 23 (2009) 153–171
doi:10.1016/j.idc.2008.10.005
0891-5520/08/$ – see front matter © 2009 Published by Elsevier Inc.

id.theclinics.com

IS AN EFFECTIVE *STAPHYLOCOCCUS AUREUS* VACCINE FEASIBLE?

Controversy has existed for years over whether it was possible to develop an *S aureus* vaccine. Successful vaccine design relies on an understanding of how the pathogen relates to the host. Although the understanding of *S aureus* pathogenesis has increased dramatically in recent years, the protean clinical manifestations of staphylococcal infections still leave many gaps in our understanding of the interactions between the host and this versatile microbe. Importantly, little evidence supports the premise that immunity to *S aureus* infection exists, at least for the unimmunized host. Recovery from an *S aureus* infection does not appear to confer immunity against subsequent infections.

S aureus produces various molecules with seemingly redundant functions, such that if one is eliminated (or targeted by a vaccine), other staphylococcal products may compensate for that loss of function. Other challenges to vaccine development include the diverse strategies that *S aureus* has developed to avoid human innate immunity,[13] and its ability to persist in biofilms[14,15] and as small colony variants.[16,17] Moreover, current animal models in which to test candidate vaccines are imperfect, generally requiring large inocula of *S aureus* to establish an infection. Laboratory mice, in which candidate vaccines often are tested, also do not have pre-existing antibodies to *S aureus* antigens, which may be present in people, and could affect the efficacy of a vaccine or the outcome in a control group.

TARGET POPULATIONS

A crucial question faced by researchers designing a staphylococcal vaccine is who would be the appropriate target population for such a vaccine. There are certain groups, listed in **Box 1**, that are obvious candidates for vaccination against *S aureus*. Hemodialysis patients are at elevated risk for *S aureus* infection, because their vascular compartment is accessed frequently. Additionally, they spend many hours a week in health care facilities; they have numerous comorbidities, and the uremia accompanying their renal failure itself may suppress the immune system.[18] Similarly, peritoneal dialysis patients, military personnel, firefighters, policemen, and individuals undergoing elective major surgery are prime vaccine candidates. Other groups, such as health care providers, intravenous drug abusers, and men who have sex with men, also might benefit from an *S aureus* vaccine.

Passive immunoprophylaxis against staphylococcal infections is indicated for people who are unable to respond to active immunization because they are immunocompromised (see **Box 1**). This group would include patients undergoing chemotherapy and patients who have immune disorders. Likewise, passive immunotherapy would be appropriate for individuals who are at immediate risk of infection and for whom time constraints prohibit an active immunization approach. Patients undergoing emergency surgeries and premature neonates are examples of populations that would benefit from passive immunotherapy.

ACTIVE IMMUNIZATION APPROACHES IN CLINICAL TRIALS

Active immunization approaches in clinical trials are summarized in **Table 1**.

StaphVAX

Most *S aureus* strains are encapsulated, with strains producing either capsular polysaccharides serotype 5 (CP5) or serotype 8 (CP8) (**Fig. 1**) being the most common among clinical isolates.[19] Capsular antigens are obvious targets for vaccine

> **Box 1**
> **Target populations for a *Staphylococcus aureus* vaccine**
>
> *Active immunization*
>
>   Hemodialysis patients
>
>   Residents of nursing homes and other long-term care facilities
>
>   Men who have sex with men
>
>   Military personnel
>
>   Prisoners
>
>   Patients undergoing elective surgery
>
>   Diabetic individuals
>
>   HIV patients
>
>   Intravenous drug users
>
>   Heath care providers
>
>   Athletes
>
>   School children
>
> *Passive immunization*
>
>   Patients undergoing emergency surgery
>
>   Patients implanted with intravascular or prosthetic devices
>
>   Trauma victims
>
>   Immunocompromised individuals
>
>   Low-birth-weight neonates
>
>   Patients in intensive care units

development, because capsule-based vaccines directed against other encapsulated bacterial pathogens have been successful.[20–25]

Fattom and colleagues[26] were the first to conjugate CP5 and CP8 to protein (recombinant *Pseudomonas aeruginosa* exotoxoid A). The conjugate vaccines were highly immunogenic in mice and people, and antibodies elicited by immunization opsonized encapsulated *S aureus* for phagocytosis.[26,27] Passive immunization with antibodies to CP5 was protective in a mouse model of *S aureus* lethality and disseminated infection.[28] Similarly, administration of antibodies to the *S aureus* CP5 conjugate vaccine protected rats against infection in a catheter-induced model of staphylococcal endocarditis, if the animals were challenged by the intraperitoneal (IP) route.[29]

Nabi Biopharmaceuticals combined the CP5- and CP8-conjugate vaccines into a bivalent vaccine called StaphVAX for immunization of people at elevated risk for *S aureus* infection. The vaccine was composed of *S aureus* type 5 and 8 CPs conjugated to recombinant pseudomonal exoprotein A. A phase 3 clinical trial of the vaccine, conducted between April 1998 and April 2000, enrolled 1804 hemodialysis patients.[30] Subjects were randomized to receive either a single intramuscular injection of the vaccine or a placebo injection.

The primary hypothesis of the study was that the vaccine would prevent *S aureus* bacteremia during the period from week 3 to week 54 after immunization. At week 54, however, the vaccine efficacy was only 26%, which was not statistically significant (**Fig. 2**). When earlier time intervals were analyzed, the vaccine was found to

Table 1
Staphylococcus aureus vaccines in clinical trials

Product	Corporate Sponsor	Composition	Status
Active immunization			
StaphVAX	Nabi	CP5 and CP8	Phase 3 failed
V710 (0657 nl)	Merck	IsdB	Phase 2 in progress
Passive immunization			
INH-A21 (Veronate)	Inhibitex	Clumping factor A (ClfA, selected IVIG)	Phase 3 failed
Tefibazumab (Aurexis)	Inhibitex	ClfA (mAb)	Phase 2 completed
Altastaph	Nabi	Antibodies to CP5 and CP8	Phase 2 completed
Aurograb	NeuTec	Antibodies to ATP-binding cassette transporter	Phase 3 completed
Pagibaximab (BSYX-A110)	Biosynexus	Lipoteichoic acid (mAb)	Phase 2 completed

significantly reduce the incidence of *S aureus* bacteremia between weeks 3 and 40. During this period, *S aureus* bacteremia occurred in 11 of the 892 patients who received the vaccine, compared with 26 of the 906 control patients. The vaccine efficacy up to 40 weeks after immunization was 57% ($P = .02$).

A confirmatory phase 3 clinical trial was performed involving 3600 hemodialysis patients who were evaluated for bacteremia from 3 to 35 weeks after receiving StaphVAX. Following a booster dose of StaphVAX, the patients were followed for an additional 6 months. Results from the second trial, announced in November 2005, showed that StaphVAX offered no significant protection against bacteremia over the placebo control. These results led Nabi to halt further development of StaphVAX. Although Nabi attributed the clinical failure of the vaccine to the immunocompromised status of the patients in the trial and a manufacturing problem in vaccine production, these data suggest that a conjugate vaccine that targets the *S aureus* CPs alone is insufficient to protect against staphylococcal bacteremia. Nabi's newest

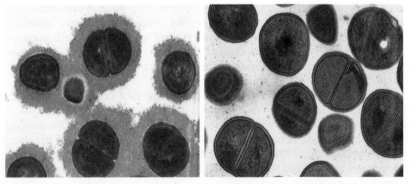

Fig. 1. Transmission electron micrographs of stationary-phase *Staphylococcus aureus* cells. Before fixation, the bacteria were incubated with CP5-specific antibodies to stabilize and visualize the capsule. *Left,* CP5-producing strain Reynolds. *Right,* nonencapsulated *S aureus* mutant. (*From* O'Riordan K, Lee JC. *Staphylococcus aureus* capsular polysaccharides. Clin Microbiol Rev 2004;17(1):222; with permission.)

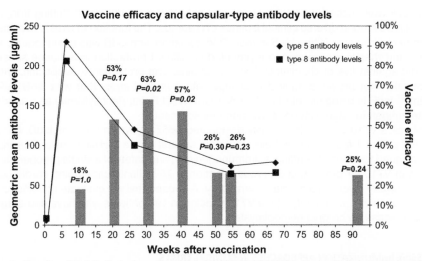

Fig. 2. Results of Nabi's first phase 3 clinical trial of StaphVAX in hemodialysis patients. The graph depicts the temporal relationship between vaccine efficacy and serum antibody levels to CP5 and CP8. Vaccine efficacy was evaluated at weeks 10, 20, 30, 40, 50, 54, and 91. A significant reduction in bacteremia was observed 3 to 40 weeks after immunization, but not at the later time points. The outcome of the second phase 3 trial of StaphVAX failed to confirm these results. (*From* Schaffer AC, Lee JC. Vaccination and passive immunisation against *Staphylococcus aureus*. Int J Antimicrob Agents 2008;32:S73; with permission.)

multicomponent vaccine candidate, PentaStaph, includes protein conjugates of CP5, CP8, and surface polysaccharide 336 (wall teichoic acid), as well as nontoxic mutants of alpha toxin and Panton-Valentine leukocidin.

Why then is a CP-conjugate vaccine protective against pathogens like *Haemophilus influenzae* type b and *Streptococcus pneumoniae*, but not *S aureus*? Indeed, antibodies to CP5 and CP8 have been shown to opsonize *S aureus* for phagocytic killing by human neutrophils.[31] Differences become apparent, however, when one considers experimental animal studies that have examined the effect of CP production on bacterial virulence. The CPs elaborated by *Streptococcus pneumoniae* and *H influenzae* type b play critical roles in the virulence of these invasive pathogens (ie, the bacteria are rendered avirulent in the absence of CP production). In contrast, *S aureus* shows only a modest reduction in virulence in animal models of abscess formation, arthritis, wound infection, and bacteremia in the absence of CP expression.[19] Moreover, capsule-negative mutants are more virulent than the parental isolates in the catheter-induced endocarditis infection model.[32] Only approximately 75% to 80% of *S aureus* clinical isolates are encapsulated by CP5 or CP8; the remaining strains produce no CP because of mutations in the cap5(8) locus or in genes that regulate CP expression.[33] Importantly, serotype 5 and 8 *S aureus* only elaborate CP in vitro during the stationary growth phase; thus actively replicating staphylococci are acapsular.[19,34] Therefore, the CP in *S aureus* is less crucial to its virulence than is the case with bacteria such as *H influenzae* type b, so targeting CP alone may be an inadequate strategy.

Vaccine V710 (IsdB)

Using *S aureus* peptide expression libraries displayed on *Escherichia coli*, which were probed with patient sera, Etz and colleagues[35] identified IsdB as a candidate antigen.

This cell wall-anchored protein, expressed only under conditions of limiting iron, is conserved among diverse clinical isolates of S aureus. The function of IsdB is to assist with heme iron acquisition by S aureus.[36] Vaccination with IsdB was immunogenic in mice and rhesus monkeys, and it provided significant protection in a murine sepsis model against five of six clinical S aureus strains. The protection was specific, with protection not provided against challenge with a mutant strain that was IsdB deficient.[37] IsdB is being targeted by Merck & Co. (West Point, Pennsylvania) as a candidate antigen for staphylococcal vaccine development.

Merck's V710 vaccine (previously designated 0657 nl), which contains IsdB, completed phase 1 testing and is being tested in several phase 2 clinical trials. One trial is designed to assess the efficacy, immunogenicity, and safety of a single preoperative dose of V710 for preventing S aureus infection in 76 patients undergoing cardiothoracic surgery involving a median sternotomy. A second trial will evaluate the efficacy, immunogenicity, and safety of the V710 vaccine in 198 patients who have end-stage renal disease on chronic hemodialysis.

PASSIVE IMMUNIZATION APPROACHES IN CLINICAL TRIALS

Passive immunization approaches in clinical trials are summarized in **Table 1**.

S Aureus Clumping Factor A-Based Products

S aureus adheres to host molecules such as fibrinogen, fibronectin, collagen, and IgG through surface protein adhesins, also referred to as microbial surface components recognizing adhesive matrix molecules, or MSCRAMMs.[38,39] Clumping factor A (ClfA) is an adhesin that mediates S aureus binding to fibrinogen[40] and promotes the attachment of S. aureus to biomaterial surfaces,[41] blood clots,[42] and damaged endothelial surfaces.[42] ClfA also plays an important role in S aureus binding to platelets, an interaction that is critical in animal models of catheter-induced staphylococcal endocarditis.[43]

Based on the protective potential of anti-ClfA antibodies demonstrated in preclinical studies,[44–46] Inhibitex developed INH-A21 (Veronate), a pooled human immunoglobulin preparation from donors with high antibody titers against staphylococcal adhesins that bind fibrinogen and fibrin (S aureus ClfA and S epidermidis SdrG).

A phase 2 trial of INH-A21 showed a trend toward fewer episodes of S aureus sepsis and candidemia, and lower mortality among infants receiving up to four doses of 750 mg/kg of INH-A21, as compared with placebo.[47] A follow-up phase 3 double-blind, placebo-controlled study of INH-A21 was conducted in 1983 infants who received up to four doses of either placebo or 750 mg/kg of INH-A21.[48] The primary outcome measure was the rate of late onset sepsis caused by S aureus, and in this measure there was no significant difference between the 6% rate in the INH-A21 group and the 5% rate in the placebo group ($P = .34$) (**Table 2**). Similarly, there were no differences between the two groups in mortality or in the rates of late-onset sepsis caused by coagulase-negative staphylococci or Candida species. This failure of INH-A21 is striking, because the infants who were given INH-A21 were compared with infants who received placebo, rather than an intravenous immunoglobulin preparation lacking elevated levels of antibodies to ClfA and SdrG. The results were particularly disappointing, because the INH-A21 product, although selected for its antibodies to ClfA and SdrG, likely contained antibodies to many other staphylococcal antigens, and so could be considered multicomponent passive immunotherapy. The INH-A21 product, however, was not elicited by immunization but by natural exposure to

Table 2
Results of failed phase 3 clinical trial of INH-A21 (Veronate) in protection of low-birthweight neonates against late-onset sepsis

Outcome	Placebo N = 989, n (%)	INH-A21, N = 994, n (%)	P Value
Blood infection with			
Staphylococcus aureus	50 (5%)	60 (6%)	0.34
Coagulase-negative staphylococci	227 (23%)	247 (25%)	0.32
Candida species	30 (3%)	33 (3%)	0.72
Mortality	73 (7%)	57 (6%)	0.13

Data from DeJonge M, Burchfield D, Bloom B, et al. Clinical trial of safety and efficacy of INH-A21 for the prevention of nosocomial staphylococcal bloodstream infection in premature infants. J Pediatr 2007;151(3):260–5.

staphylococci, and so the antibodies might have recognized the wrong ClfA epitopes, or may have been of low affinity or avidity toward the target antigens.

Another Inhibitex product in the pipeline is the murine monoclonal antibody (mAb) 12-9 that binds ClfA and inhibits fibrinogen binding to ClfA. A humanized version of mAb 12-9, known as tefibazumab (Aurexis), was produced by Inhibitex. In a rabbit model of endocarditis, two doses of tefibazumab (30 mg/kg), in combination with vancomycin, resulted in fewer animals with bacteremia and a significant reduction in the bacterial counts in the spleens and kidneys compared with animals given vancomycin alone.[49]

A phase 2 study of tefibazumab enrolled hospitalized patients who had documented *S aureus* bacteremia.[50] Subjects were randomized to receive either a single tefibazumab dose of 20 mg/kg plus standard therapy or standard therapy alone. To evaluate efficacy, a composite clinical endpoint was used, consisting of a relapse of *S aureus* bacteremia, a complication related to the *S aureus* bacteremia (such as endocarditis), or death. In the tefibazumab group, 2 of 30 (6.7%) patients reached the composite clinical endpoint, compared with 4 of 30 (13.3%) patients in the placebo group ($P = .455$). Although preliminary clinical trials of tefibazumab in hemodialysis patients[51] and cystic fibrosis patients have been performed, Inhibitex is seeking a partner to support further efforts before proceeding with additional clinical trials of tefibazumab.

AltaStaph

AltaStaph, produced by Nabi, is a hyperimmune polyclonal antibody preparation derived from healthy volunteers immunized with the bivalent StaphVAX preparation. The product contains high levels of vaccine-induced antibodies to the *S aureus* serotypes 5 and 8 CPs. In a phase 2 study designed primarily to assess the safety of AltaStaph, 206 neonates, weighing from 500 to 1500 g, were given an initial 1000 mg/kg intravenous dose of AltaStaph or placebo.[52] A second dose was given 14 days later. No significant difference was seen in the rate of adverse events between the two arms. Although not specifically powered to look for differences in the rates of *S aureus* bacteremia, this was a secondary endpoint of the study, and the rates of *S aureus* bacteremia were nearly identical in both groups, at about 3%.

Another phase 2 trial looking at AltaStaph enrolled 40 patients, age 7 years or older, who had documented *S aureus* bacteremia and persistent fever.[53] Five of 21 patients (24%) who received AltaStaph died, compared with 2 of 18 patients (11%) in the placebo group ($P = .42$). These results provide additional support for the premise that vaccine-induced antibodies to CP5 and CP8 alone are insufficient to significantly reduce *S aureus* bacteremia in at-risk populations.

Aurograb

NeuTec Pharma has identified a S aureus ATP-binding cassette (ABC) transporter as a novel target for passive immunization therapies against staphylococcal infection.[54,55] The company developed Aurograb, which is a single-chain variable antibody fragment against the S aureus ABC transporter. In June 2006, the company completed a double-blind, placebo-controlled phase 3 clinical trial. Performed in six European countries, the study involved the recruitment of 161 adult hospitalized patients who had deep-seated staphylococcal infections. The trial compared the effects of Aurograb (1 mg/kg intravenously twice daily) in combination with vancomycin versus vancomycin alone for treating MRSA infections. The results of this trial were released. In July 2006, NeuTec Pharma was taken over by Novartis, who discontinued development of Aurograb following disappointing results in clinical studies.

Pagibaximab

Lipoteichoic acid (LTA) is a plasma membrane-embedded glycolipid unique to gram-positive bacteria.[56] Like its gram-negative counterpart lipopolysaccharide, purified LTA has immunostimulatory activity.[57–59] Biosynexus has developed a humanized mouse chimeric mAb against LTA called pagibaximab (formerly known as BSYX-A110). The targeted population of this antibody is low birth-weight infants, in whom it is designed to help prevent bloodstream infections by S aureus and coagulase-negative staphylococci, the latter being the leading cause of bloodstream infections among premature neonates.[60] A phase 2 trial in 88 low birth-weight neonates has been conducted. Although preliminary results of this trial have been released and show that infants treated with the 90 mg/kg dose had fewer episodes of S aureus sepsis than either the 60 mg/kg dose or placebo groups,[61] no peer-reviewed reports on this pagibaximab trial have been published. Nonetheless, Biosynexus will proceed to a phase 2b/3 clinical trial in 2009 in which 1550 very low birth-weight neonates will receive up to six infusions of 100 mg/kg pagibaximab in a study to evaluate safety, pharmacokinetics, and efficacy of the product for the prevention of staphylococcal sepsis.

PRECLINICAL DEVELOPMENT—SURFACE-ASSOCIATED STAPHYLOCOCCUS AUREUS ANTIGENS
Poly-N-acetylglucosamine

Poly-N-acetylglucosamine (PNAG), also known as polysaccharide intracellular adhesin,[62] is a surface polymer produced by S aureus and S epidermidis, which promotes biofilm formation.[63] The native form of PNAG is partially de-N-acetylated. Kelly-Quintos and colleagues[64] demonstrated that only antibodies to the partially de-N-acetylated form of PNAG (dPNAG) mediated antibody-dependent opsonophagocytic killing of S aureus by human neutrophils. In a follow-up study, the investigators immunized mice, rabbits, and goats with either native PNAG or dPNAG conjugated to diphtheria toxoid.[65] Mice were passively immunized by the intraperitoneal route with immune or nonimmune serum and challenged intravenously with S aureus 48 hours later. Quantitative blood cultures performed 2 hours after bacterial challenge revealed that mice given dPNAG antibodies had between 54% and 91% fewer S aureus in their blood than mice given control serum. Antibodies to the native PNAG conjugate were ineffective in clearing the bacteremia in mice. These data indicate that antibodies to dPNAG (but not native PNAG) are opsonic and provide significant protection against experimental S aureus infections in mice. Because dPNAG is preferentially retained on the bacterial cell surface, antibodies to dPNAG may be more effective in achieving protection than native PNAG antibodies.[66]

Multicomponent Staphylococcus aureus Adhesin Vaccine

Stranger-Jones and colleagues[67] systematically evaluated 19 cell wall-anchored *S aureus* protein adhesins for their vaccine potential in mice. The animals were immunized, then challenged 21 days later with *S aureus* Newman, and the bacterial burden in the kidneys was evaluated four days later. Four antigens (SdrE, IsdA, SdrD, and IsdB) were conserved among *S aureus* isolates and showed the best protection in a renal infection model. IsdB previously was identified by Merck scientists as a protective staphylococcal antigen.[37] IsdA, a heme-binding surface protein, also is involved in heme iron uptake.[68] SdrD and SdrE are cell wall-anchored proteins that are structurally similar to ClfA, but their molecular functions remain unknown.

Animals that were immunized with the combination of all four surface components and then challenged IP with 2×10^{10} colony-forming-units of strain Newman had 100% survival at 7 days (**Fig. 3**). In comparison, animals immunized with either phosphate buffered saline (PBS, frequently used for placebo injections) or one of the individual components had survival rates of 50% to 70%. Immunization with the multivalent vaccine significantly reduced *S aureus*-induced mortality in mice compared with PBS for four of five *S aureus* clinical isolates.[67]

Heteropolymers

A novel heteropolymer technology is being developed by Elusys Therapeutics to combat *S aureus* bacteremias. The product (ETI-211) consists of a mAb to *S aureus* protein A linked to another mAb directed against the human complement receptor 1 (CR1).[69,70] The concept promoted by Elusys is that blood-borne *S aureus*, bridged by the bispecific mAb complex, binds to CR1 on erythrocytes, and that this complex is taken up and destroyed by tissue macrophages in the liver and spleen.[69-71]

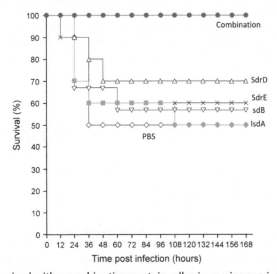

Fig. 3. Mice immunized with a combination protein adhesin vaccine survived challenge with an IP lethal dose of *Staphylococcus aureus* Newman. Animals immunized with individual surface protein antigens (IsdA, IsdB, SdrD, or SdrE) or with PBS showed survival rates of 50% to 70%. (*From* Stranger-Jones YK, Bae T, Schneewind O. Vaccine assembly from surface proteins of *Staphylococcus aureus*. Proc Natl Acad Sci U S A 2006;103(45):16945; with permission. Copyright © 2006, National Academy of Sciences, USA.)

Preclinical studies to demonstrate efficacy used transgenic mice expressing human CR1 on red blood cells. Mice pretreated with the heteropolymers survived a lethal S aureus challenge dose, in contrast to mice pretreated with the protein A mAb alone. Therapeutic administration of the heteropolymer to infected mice resulted in more efficient clearance of the bacteria from the liver, kidneys, and spleen, compared with control mice given PBS. Elusys now has a research collaboration with Pfizer to evaluate heteropolymers targeting S aureus.

EXOTOXIN VACCINES
Alpha-Hemolysin

Alpha-hemolysin (also know as alpha-toxin) is a secreted S aureus protein that can cause pore formation within eukaryotic cells[72] and interfere with S aureus adhesion to epithelial cells.[73] Adlam and colleagues[74] first reported that immunization with a toxoid prepared from alpha-toxin protected rabbits against the lethal gangrenous form of S aureus mastitis but did not prevent abscess formation. Menzies and Kernodle[75] created a nontoxic and nonhemolytic alpha-hemolysin mutant toxin (H35L) by site-directed mutagenesis. Passive immunization with rabbit anti-H35L serum protected mice from lethal challenge with native alpha-hemolysin and against acute lethal challenge with a high-alpha-hemolysin-producing S aureus strain.

In a recent study, the severity of staphylococcal lung infection in mice was shown to correlate with the levels of alpha-hemolysin produced by different S aureus isolates.[76] Wardenburg and Schneewind[76] used the H35L alpha-hemolysin mutant protein to immunize mice and evaluate protection against S aureus in a murine pneumonia model. Compared with animals immunized with PBS, mice immunized with the H35L protein and then challenged intranasally with S aureus showed reduced lethality attributable to S aureus (**Fig. 4**). Similarly, in passive immunization experiments, antibodies to the H35L protein administered IP protected mice after intranasal challenge with either methicillin-resistant or -sensitive S aureus strains. Antibodies to alpha-hemolysin play a role in neutralizing the lethal effects induced by this toxin; their efficacy in modulating other types of staphylococcal infections remains to be determined.

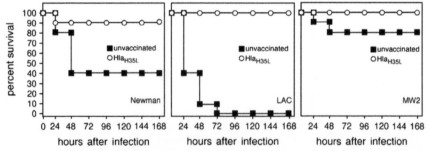

Fig. 4. Survival curves of mice immunized with alpha hemolysin H35L compared with unimmunized mice. The animals were challenged intranasally with Staphylococcus aureus strains Newman (*left*), LAC (*middle*), or MW2 (*right*). Survival in the control mice showed an inverse correlation with the amount of alpha hemolysin produced by each strain. (*From* Wardenburg JB, Schneewind O. Vaccine protection against Staphylococcus aureus pneumonia. J Exp Med 2008;205(2):290; with permission. Copyright © 2008, The Rockefeller University Press.)

Superantigens

S aureus has the capability to secrete various superantigen exoproteins, including toxic shock syndrome toxin-1 (TSST-1) and approximately 15 different enterotoxins, with clinical isolates varying markedly in their production of these proteins. Superantigens act as potent oligoclonal T-cell activators, stimulating a massive release of proinflammatory cytokines.[77,78] Aerosol exposure of nonhuman primates to staphylococcal enterotoxin B (SEB) results in gastrointestinal symptoms, lethargy, shock, and death. Early studies, reviewed previously,[10] have indicated that mutant forms of the superantigenic proteins that are devoid of their biological properties can be used as vaccines to elicit antibodies that neutralize the native toxin molecules. Importantly, when monkeys were immunized actively with a proteasome-SEB toxoid vaccine, all of the animals were protected against severe symptoms and death due to aerosolized SEB intoxication.[79] Passive immunization with antibodies to SEB before or 4 hours after aerosol exposure to SEB provided similar protection to rhesus monkeys.[80] Nontoxic derivatives of the staphylococcal superantigens may be useful vaccine candidates to protect against aerosolized superantigens in biological warfare.

ANTIBODIES TO BLOCK *STAPHYLOCOCCUS AUREUS* VIRULENCE

Vaccines that target bacterial virulence have the potential of weakening the microbe so that the host immune system can eradicate it more easily. The major global regulator of virulence in *S aureus* is the accessory gene regulator (*agr*), which modulates bacterial physiology and virulence factor expression through quorum sensing mediated by the secretion of small cyclic autoinducing peptides (AIPs).[81,82] *S aureus* strains can be classified into four *agr* groups, depending on the amino acid sequence of the exported AIP, and AIPs from the different groups inhibit *agr* expression by members of the heterologous groups. A recent study by Park and colleagues[83] described the preparation of a mAb to AIP-4 that inhibits agr function (ie, the mAb reduced the expression of RNAIII [the effector molecule of the agr locus] and alpha toxin, and it increased protein A expression and biofilm formation in an AIP subgroup-specific manner). The mAb to AIP-4 did not affect bacterial growth in vitro. Importantly, mice passively immunized IP with 1 mg of the AIP-4 mAb were protected from a lethal dose of *S aureus* administered by the IP route; mice given an isotype matched mAb were not protected. Likewise, mice challenged with *S aureus* mixed with cytodex beads and 0.6 mg of the AIP-4 mAb (but not the control mAb) were protected from subcutaneous abscess formation.

Whether disruption of quorum sensing signaling will be beneficial against other *S aureus* strains and other AIP groups will need to be addressed in future studies. Because *agr* negatively regulates staphylococcal biofilm formation and the production of many surface adhesins, it is questionable whether antibodies to AIPs will be beneficial against all manifestations of *S aureus* disease. For example, inhibition of *agr* potentially could enhance staphylococcal infections that are initiated by adherence to traumatized tissue or prosthetic devices and promote chronic infection. Nonetheless, this conceptual approach of targeting *S aureus* virulence factors is intriguing.

A VACCINE TO PREVENT NASAL COLONIZATION

The primary niche for *S aureus* in people is the nares, and nasal carriage is a documented risk factor for staphylococcal infection.[84,85] The source of approximately 80% of *S aureus* bacteremias is endogenous, with the infecting bacteria being identical to organisms recovered from the nasal mucosa.[86,87] These observations support an approach in which systemic S aureus infections are prevented by eliminating or reducing nasal carriage. Although topical treatment with mupirocin is usually effective in decolonizing nasal carriers,[88] the emergence of mupirocin resistance in S aureus potentially limits the effectiveness of this approach.[89] Moreover, recolonization of mupirocin-sensitive strains often occurs from extranasal carriage sites. In a mouse model, intranasal immunization with killed S aureus cells led to reduced nasal colonization compared with control animals. Likewise, mice that were immunized systemically or intranasally with a recombinant vaccine composed of domain A of ClfB demonstrated lower levels of colonization compared with control animals. An anti-ClfB mAb inhibited S aureus binding to mouse cytokeratin 10 and reduced nasal colonization compared with a control mAb.[90]

Using a different approach to identifying candidate antigens for a vaccine against nasal carriage, Clarke and colleagues[91] probed S aureus expression libraries with sera from infected and uninfected patients to identify immunogenic proteins. Eleven proteins identified in their screen were investigated further by measuring antibodies reactive with the recombinant proteins in serum from healthy individuals (S aureus nasal carriers and noncarriers), as well as patient sera. Antibodies to IsdA and IsdH were higher among noncarriers, and so the investigators immunized cotton rats with the recombinant proteins. Rats immunized with IsdA or IsdH and inoculated with S aureus showed reduced nasal colonization compared with control rats.

SUMMARY AND CONSIDERATIONS

Despite the progress made over the past 10 years toward development of an S aureus vaccine, unresolved issues and unanswered questions remain. Unresolved issues in S aureus vaccine development include:

Can S aureus infections be prevented by vaccination?

Who should receive the S aureus vaccine?

What are the measurable correlates of protective immunity?

What are the appropriate antigens for inclusion in a multicomponent staphylococcal vaccine?

Can a multicomponent vaccine address the protean clinical manifestations of S aureus disease?

Can one expect a vaccine to protect against an infection involving a prosthetic device?

Do the animal models chosen for preclinical studies reflect the pathogenesis of human disease?

Will a vaccine that reduces S aureus nasal colonization reduce staphylococcal infections?

Lessons learned from the initially promising results and ultimate failures of the StaphVAX[30] and Veronate[47,48] phase 3 clinical trials are broadly applicable to the development of a vaccine against S aureus. First, a multicomponent vaccine will be essential. It is not surprising that a vaccine based only on a single S aureus virulence determinant would be unsuccessful, given the multifactorial nature of the pathogenesis of staphylococcal infections. Neutralizing one of the myriad staphylococcal virulence factors is not sufficient to protect a susceptible human host.

The second lesson learned focuses on the vaccine target population. The patients most in need of a staphylococcal vaccine comprise a population whose immune systems may not respond adequately to immunization. For example, hemodialysis patients are at persistently elevated risk for S aureus bacteremia, and they are an obvious target population for active immunization. The immune response to vaccination may be suboptimal in this cohort, however.[92–94] Targeting otherwise healthy at-risk individuals, like those undergoing elective surgical procedures, may be the best way to demonstrate vaccine efficacy in clinical trials. Such trials may be essential to demonstrate proof of principle (ie, a protective *S aureus* vaccine can be formulated). Such a trial, however, would not solve the greater problem of protecting compromised hosts from life-threatening *S aureus* infections.

Choosing appropriate antigens to include in a multicomponent vaccine is a major challenge in the development of a staphylococcal vaccine. Candidate antigens should be surface exposed, expressed by most clinical *S aureus* isolates belonging to diverse lineages, and show minimal serologic variability among strains. At least some of the candidate antigens should elicit antibodies that promote opsonophagocytic killing in vitro by human neutrophils. In addition, an ideal vaccine would include antigens that elicit antibodies to block staphylococcal adherence or biofilm formation and neutralize toxic *S aureus* exoproteins. Vaccine efficacy would need to be tested in diverse models of *S aureus* infection, such as endocarditis, bacteremia, surgical wound infection, and pneumonia.

The accessibility of *S aureus* surface antigens has important implications for vaccine development, because optimal targets for immunization should be surface exposed. This does not necessarily translate into recognition by antibodies to the antigen on *S aureus* cells evaluated in flow cytometry experiments, because antibodies to surface proteins can penetrate the *S aureus* CP layer and bind to proteins that are masked by capsule.[95] As an example, ClfA and CP both are expressed by *S aureus* in postexponential growth, but CP production at least partially masks cell wall-associated ClfA and prevents it from binding to fibrinogen.[96] If an antibody to a surface antigen is masked by CP, it will not retain functionality (mediating opsonization or blocking attachment).

Evaluation of the results of the clinical and preclinical studies summarized herein suggests several good candidate vaccine antigens: CP5, CP8, PNAG, cell wall-anchored proteins (ClfA and IsdB), and alpha hemolysin H135A. The authors would argue for developing a multi-component staphylococcal vaccine that includes at least one surface antigen (such a fibronectin-binding protein A or IsdB) that is expressed during the exponential phase of bacterial growth. Antigen expression in vivo and under different growth conditions and media also should be explored.

Ultimately, it is likely that an *S aureus* vaccine will form only part of the antistaphylococcal armamentarium. In developing an *S aureus* vaccine, both active and passive approaches should be pursued, as these are not mutually exclusive, and may turn out to be complementary. For severe *S aureus* infections, such as endocarditis, passive antistaphylococcal immunization could be used in addition to antibiotics. In the past, there was much skepticism about the ability to develop a vaccine against *S aureus*. Some of that skepticism is beginning to abate, as the array of recently discovered proteins and polysaccharides that may be critical targets for protective immunity against *S aureus* raise the possibility that an effective vaccine could be developed. Development of an *S aureus* vaccine that provides the levels of protection seen with other commonly administered vaccines is unlikely to occur in the near future, however.

REFERENCES

1. Lowy FD. *Staphylococcus aureus* infections. N Engl J Med 1998;339(8):520–32.
2. Klein E, Smith DL, Laxminarayan R. Hospitalizations and deaths caused by methicillin-resistant *Staphylococcus aureus*, United States, 1999–2005. Emerging Infect Dis 2007;13(12):1840–6.

3. Chambers HF. The changing epidemiology of *Staphylococcus aureus*? Emerg Infect Dis 2001;7(2):178–82.
4. Shastry L, Rahimian J, Lascher S. Community-associated methicillin-resistant *Staphylococcus aureus* skin and soft tissue infections in men who have sex with men in New York City. Arch Intern Med 2007;167(8):854–7.
5. Daum RS. Clinical practice. Skin and soft-tissue infections caused by methicillin-resistant *Staphylococcus aureus*. N Engl J Med 2007;357(4):380–90.
6. de Lencastre H, Oliveira D, Tomasz A. Antibiotic resistant *Staphylococcus aureus*: a paradigm of adaptive power. Curr Opin Microbiol 2007;10(5):428–35.
7. Graber CJ, Wong MK, Carleton HA, et al. Intermediate vancomycin susceptibility in a community-associated MRSA clone. Emerg Infect Dis 2007;13(3):491–3.
8. Chang S, Sievert DM, Hageman JC, et al. Infection with vancomycin-resistant *Staphylococcus aureus* containing the *vanA* resistance gene. N Engl J Med 2003;348(14):1342–7.
9. Zhu W, Clark NC, McDougal LK, et al. Vancomycin-resistant *Staphylococcus aureus* isolates associated with Inc18-like *vanA* plasmids in Michigan. Antimicrobial Agents Chemother 2008;52(2):452–7.
10. Lee JC. *Staphylococcus aureus* vaccine. In: Ellis RW, Brodeur BR, editors. New bacterial vaccines. New York: Kluwer Academic/Plenum Publishers; 2003. p. 283–93.
11. Deresinski S. Antistaphylococcal vaccines and immunoglobulins: current status and future prospects. Drugs 2006;66(14):1797–806.
12. Projan SJ, Nesin M, Dunman PM. Staphylococcal vaccines and immunotherapy: to dream the impossible dream? Curr Opin Pharmacol 2006;6(5):473–9.
13. Foster TJ. Immune evasion by staphylococci. Nat Rev Microbiol 2005;3(12):948–58.
14. Yarwood JM, Paquette KM, Tikh IB, et al. Generation of virulence factor variants in *Staphylococcus aureus* biofilms. J Bacteriol 2007;189(22):7961–7.
15. Gotz F. *Staphylococcus* and biofilms. Mol Microbiol 2002;43(6):1367–78.
16. Vaudaux P, Kelley WL, Lew DP. *Staphylococcus aureus* small colony variants: difficult to diagnose and difficult to treat. Clin Infect Dis 2006;43(8):968–70.
17. Sendi P, Rohrbach M, Graber P, et al. *Staphylococcus aureus* small colony variants in prosthetic joint infection. Clin Infect Dis 2006;43(8):961–7.
18. Minnaganti VR, Cunha BA. Infections associated with uremia and dialysis. Infect Dis Clin North Am 2001;15(2):385–406.
19. O'Riordan K, Lee JC. *Staphylococcus aureus* capsular polysaccharides. Clin Microbiol Rev 2004;17(1):218–34.
20. Eskola J, Kayhty H, Takala AK, et al. A randomized, prospective field trial of a conjugate vaccine in the protection of infants and young children against invasive *Haemophilus influenzae* type b disease. N Engl J Med 1990;323(20):1381–7.
21. Swingler G, Fransman D, Hussey G. Conjugate vaccines for preventing *Haemophilus influenzae* type B infections. Cochrane Database Syst Rev 2007;(2):CD001729.
22. Gardner P. Clinical practice. Prevention of meningococcal disease. N Engl J Med 2006;355(14):1466–73.
23. Maiden MCJ, Stuart JM. Carriage of serogroup C meningococci 1 year after meningococcal C conjugate polysaccharide vaccination. Lancet 2002;359(9320):1829–31.
24. Rennels MB, Edwards KM, Keyserling HL, et al. Safety and immunogenicity of heptavalent pneumococcal vaccine conjugated to CRM197 in United States infants. Pediatrics 1998;101(4 Pt 1):604–11.

25. Black SB, Shinefield HR, Ling S, et al. Effectiveness of heptavalent pneumococcal conjugate vaccine in children younger than five years of age for prevention of pneumonia. Pediatr Infect Dis J 2002;21(9):810–5.
26. Fattom A, Schneerson R, Szu SC, et al. Synthesis and immunologic properties in mice of vaccines composed of *Staphylococcus aureus* type 5 and type 8 capsular polysaccharides conjugated to *Pseudomonas aeruginosa* exotoxin A. Infect Immun 1990;58(7):2367–74.
27. Fattom A, Schneerson R, Watson DC, et al. Laboratory and clinical evaluation of conjugate vaccines composed of *Staphylococcus aureus* type 5 and type 8 capsular polysaccharides bound to *Pseudomonas aeruginosa* recombinant exoprotein A. Infect Immun 1993;61(3):1023–32.
28. Fattom AI, Sarwar J, Ortiz A, et al. A *Staphylococcus aureus* capsular polysaccharide (CP) vaccine and CP-specific antibodies protect mice against bacterial challenge. Infect Immun 1996;64(5):1659–65.
29. Lee JC, Park JS, Shepherd SE, et al. Protective efficacy of antibodies to the *Staphylococcus aureus* type 5 capsular polysaccharide in a modified model of endocarditis in rats. Infect Immun 1997;65(10):4146–51.
30. Shinefield H, Black S, Fattom A, et al. Use of a *Staphylococcus aureus* conjugate vaccine in patients receiving hemodialysis. N Engl J Med 2002;346(7):491–6.
31. Karakawa WW, Sutton A, Schneerson R, et al. Capsular antibodies induce type-specific phagocytosis of capsulated *Staphylococcus aureus* by human polymorphonuclear leukocytes. Infect Immun 1988;56(5):1090–5.
32. Baddour LM, Lowrance C, Albus A, et al. *Staphylococcus aureus* microcapsule expression attenuates bacterial virulence in a rat model of experimental endocarditis. J Infect Dis 1992;165(4):749–53.
33. Cocchiaro JL, Gomez MI, Risley A, et al. Molecular characterization of the capsule locus from nontypeable *Staphylococcus aureus*. Mol Microbiol 2006;59(3):948–60.
34. Pohlmann-Dietze P, Ulrich M, Kiser KB, et al. Adherence of *Staphylococcus aureus* to endothelial cells: influence of capsular polysaccharide, global regulator *agr*, and bacterial growth phase. Infect Immun 2000;68(9):4865–71.
35. Etz H, Minh DB, Henics T, et al. Identification of in vivo expressed vaccine candidate antigens from *Staphylococcus aureus*. Proc Natl Acad Sci U S A 2002;99(10):6573–8.
36. Torres VJ, Pishchany G, Humayun M, et al. *Staphylococcus aureus* IsdB is a hemoglobin receptor required for heme iron utilization. J Bacteriol 2006;188(24):8421–9.
37. Kuklin NA, Clark DJ, Secore S, et al. A novel *Staphylococcus aureus* vaccine: iron surface determinant B induces rapid antibody responses in rhesus macaques and specific increased survival in a murine *S aureus* sepsis model. Infect Immun 2006;74(4):2215–23.
38. Foster TJ, Hook M. Surface protein adhesins of *Staphylococcus aureus*. Trends Microbiol 1998;6(12):484–8.
39. Clarke SR, Foster SJ. Surface adhesins of *Staphylococcus aureus*. Adv Microb Physiol 2006;51:187–224.
40. McDevitt D, Francois P, Vaudaux P, et al. Molecular characterization of the clumping factor (fibrinogen receptor) of *Staphylococcus aureus*. Mol Microbiol 1994;11(2):237–48.
41. Vaudaux PE, Francois P, Proctor RA, et al. Use of adhesion-defective mutants of *Staphylococcus aureus* to define the role of specific plasma proteins in promoting bacterial adhesion to canine arteriovenous shunts. Infect Immun 1995;63(2):585–90.

42. Moreillon P, Entenza JM, Francioli P, et al. Role of *Staphylococcus aureus* coagulase and clumping factor in pathogenesis of experimental endocarditis. Infect Immun 1995;63(12):4738–43.

43. Sullam PM, Bayer AS, Foss WM, et al. Diminished platelet binding in vitro by *Staphylococcus aureus* is associated with reduced virulence in a rabbit model of infective endocarditis. Infect Immun 1996;64(12):4915–21.

44. Josefsson E, Hartford O, O'Brien L, et al. Protection against experimental *Staphylococcus aureus* arthritis by vaccination with clumping factor A, a novel virulence determinant. J Infect Dis 2001;184(12):1572–80.

45. Vernachio J, Bayer AS, Le T, et al. Anti-clumping factor A immunoglobulin reduces the duration of methicillin-resistant *Staphylococcus aureus* bacteremia in an experimental model of infective endocarditis. Antimicrob Agents Chemother 2003;47(11):3400–6.

46. Vernachio JH, Bayer AS, Ames B, et al. Human immunoglobulin G recognizing fibrinogen-binding surface proteins is protective against both *Staphylococcus aureus* and *Staphylococcus epidermidis* infections in vivo. Antimicrob Agents Chemother 2006;50(2):511–8.

47. Bloom B, Schelonka R, Kueser T, et al. Multicenter study to assess safety and efficacy of INH-A21, a donor-selected human staphylococcal immunoglobulin, for prevention of nosocomial infections in very low birth weight infants. Pediatr Infect Dis J 2005;24(10):858–66.

48. DeJonge M, Burchfield D, Bloom B, et al. Clinical trial of safety and efficacy of INH-A21 for the prevention of nosocomial staphylococcal bloodstream infection in premature infants. J Pediatr 2007;151(3):260–5.

49. Patti JM. A humanized monoclonal antibody targeting *Staphylococcus aureus*. Vaccine 2004;22(Suppl 1):S39–43.

50. Weems JJ Jr, Steinberg JP, Filler S, et al. Phase II, randomized, double-blind, multicenter study comparing the safety and pharmacokinetics of tefibazumab to placebo for treatment of *Staphylococcus aureus* bacteremia. Antimicrob Agents Chemother 2006;50(8):2751–5.

51. Hetherington S, Texter M, Wenzel E, et al. Phase I dose escalation study to evaluate the safety and pharmacokinetic profile of tefibazumab in subjects with end-stage renal disease requiring hemodialysis. Antimicrob Agents Chemother 2006;50(10):3499–500.

52. Benjamin DK, Schelonka R, White R, et al. A blinded, randomized, multicenter study of an intravenous *Staphylococcus aureus* immune globulin. J Perinatol 2006;26(5):290–5.

53. Rupp ME, Holley HP Jr, Lutz J, et al. Phase II, randomized, multicenter, double-blind, placebo-controlled trial of a polyclonal anti-*Staphylococcus aureus* capsular polysaccharide immune globulin in treatment of *Staphylococcus aureus* bacteremia. Antimicrob Agents Chemother 2007;51(12):4249–54.

54. Garmory HS, Titball RW. ATP-binding cassette transporters are targets for the development of antibacterial vaccines and therapies. Infect Immun 2004;72(12):6757–63.

55. Burnie JP, Matthews RC, Carter T, et al. Identification of an immunodominant ABC transporter in methicillin-resistant *Staphylococcus aureus* infections. Infect Immun 2000;68(6):3200–9.

56. Ruhland GJ, Fiedler F. Occurrence and structure of lipoteichoic acids in the genus *Staphylococcus*. Arch Microbiol 1990;154(4):375–9.

57. von Aulock S, Morath S, Hareng L, et al. Lipoteichoic acid from *Staphylococcus aureus* is a potent stimulus for neutrophil recruitment. Immunobiology 2003; 208(4):413–22.
58. Morath S, Geyer A, Hartung T. Structure-function relationship of cytokine induction by lipoteichoic acid from *Staphylococcus aureus*. J Exp Med 2001;193(3): 393–7.
59. Morath S, Stadelmaier A, Geyer A, et al. Synthetic lipoteichoic acid from *Staphylococcus aureus* is a potent stimulus of cytokine release. J Exp Med 2002; 195(12):1635–40.
60. Stoll BJ, Hansen N, Fanaroff AA, et al. Late-onset sepsis in very low birth weight neonates: the experience of the NICHD Neonatal Research Network. Pediatrics 2002;110(2 Pt 1):285–91.
61. Weisman LE. Antibody for the prevention of neonatal noscocomial staphylococcal infection: a review of the literature. Arch Pediatr 2007;14(Suppl 1):S31–4.
62. Maira-Litran T, Kropec A, Joyce J, et al. Immunochemical properties of the staphylococcal poly-N-acetylglucosamine surface polysaccharide. Infect Immun 2002; 70(8):4433–40.
63. Cramton SE, Gerke C, Schnell NF, et al. The intercellular adhesion (*ica*) locus is present in *Staphylococcus aureus* and is required for biofilm formation. Infect Immun 1999;67(10):5427–33.
64. Kelly-Quintos C, Kropec A, Briggs S, et al. The role of epitope specificity in the human opsonic antibody response to the staphylococcal surface polysaccharide poly N-acetyl glucosamine. J Infect Dis 2005;192(11):2012–9.
65. Maira-Litran T, Kropec A, Goldmann DA, et al. Comparative opsonic and protective activities of *Staphylococcus aureus* conjugate vaccines containing native or deacetylated staphylococcal poly-*N*-acetyl-beta-(1-6)-glucosamine. Infect Immun 2005;73(10):6752–62.
66. Cerca N, Jefferson KK, Maira-Litran T, et al. Molecular basis for preferential protective efficacy of antibodies directed to the poorly acetylated form of staphylococcal poly-*N*-acetyl-beta-(1-6)-glucosamine. Infect Immun 2007;75(7): 3406–13.
67. Stranger-Jones YK, Bae T, Schneewind O. Vaccine assembly from surface proteins of *Staphylococcus aureus*. Proc Natl Acad Sci U S A 2006;103(45):16942–7.
68. Mazmanian SK, Skaar EP, Gaspar AH, et al. Passage of heme-iron across the envelope of *Staphylococcus aureus*. Science 2003;299(5608):906–9.
69. Gyimesi E, Bankovich AJ, Schuman TA, et al. *Staphylococcus aureus* bound to complement receptor 1 on human erythrocytes by bispecific monoclonal antibodies is phagocytosed by acceptor macrophages. Immunol Lett 2004;95(2): 185–92.
70. Mohamed N, Jones SM, Casey LS, et al. Heteropolymers: a novel technology against blood-borne infections. Curr Opin Mol Ther 2005;7(2):144–50.
71. Lindorfer MA, Hahn CS, Foley PL, et al. Heteropolymer-mediated clearance of immune complexes via erythrocyte CR1: mechanisms and applications. Immunol Rev 2001;183:10–24.
72. Song L, Hobaugh MR, Shustak C, et al. Structure of staphylococcal alpha-hemolysin, a heptameric transmembrane pore. Science 1996;274(5294):1859–66.
73. Liang X, Ji Y, Liang X, et al. Alpha-toxin interferes with integrin-mediated adhesion and internalization of *Staphylococcus aureus* by epithelial cells. Cell Microbiol 2006;8(10):1656–68.

74. Adlam C, Ward PD, McCartney AC, et al. Effect of immunization with highly puri-fied alpha- and beta-toxins on staphylococcal mastitis in rabbits. Infect Immun 1977;17(2):250–6.
75. Menzies BE, Kernodle DS. Passive immunization with antiserum to a nontoxic alpha-toxin mutant from *Staphylococcus aureus* is protective in a murine model. Infect Immun 1996;64(5):1839–41.
76. Wardenburg JB, Schneewind O. Vaccine protection against *Staphylococcus aureus* pneumonia. J Exp Med 2008;205(2):287–94.
77. Dinges MM, Orwin PM, Schlievert PM. Exotoxins of *Staphylococcus aureus*. Clin Microbiol Rev 2000;13(1):16–34.
78. Murray RJ. Recognition and management of *Staphylococcus aureus* toxin-medi-ated disease. Intern Med J 2005;35(Suppl 2):S106–19.
79. Lowell GH, Colleton C, Frost D, et al. Immunogenicity and efficacy against lethal aerosol staphylococcal enterotoxin B challenge in monkeys by intramuscular and respiratory delivery of proteosome-toxoid vaccines. Infect Immun 1996;64(11): 4686–93.
80. LeClaire RD, Hunt RE, Bavari S, et al. Protection against bacterial superantigen staphylococcal enterotoxin B by passive vaccination. Infect Immun 2002;70(5): 2278–81.
81. George EA, Muir TW. Molecular mechanisms of *agr* quorum sensing in virulent staphylococci. Chembiochem 2007;8(8):847–55.
82. Goerke C, Wolz C. Regulatory and genomic plasticity of *Staphylococcus aureus* during persistent colonization and infection. Int J Med Microbiol 2004;294(2–3): 195–202.
83. Park J, Jagasia R, Kaufmann GF, et al. Infection control by antibody dis-ruption of bacterial quorum sensing signaling. Chem Biol 2007;14(10): 1119–27.
84. Kluytmans J, van Belkum A, Verbrugh H. Nasal carriage of *Staphylococcus au-reus*: epidemiology, underlying mechanisms, and associated risks. Clin Microbiol Rev 1997;10(3):505–20.
85. Wertheim HFL, Melles DC, Vos MC, et al. The role of nasal carriage in *Staphylo-coccus aureus* infections. Lancet Infect Dis 2005;5(12):751–62.
86. Wertheim HF, Vos MC, Ott A, et al. Risk and outcome of nosocomial *Staphylococ-cus aureus* bacteraemia in nasal carriers versus noncarriers. Lancet 2004; 364(9435):703–5.
87. von Eiff C, Becker K, Machka K, et al. Nasal carriage as a source of *Staphylococ-cus aureus* bacteremia. N Engl J Med 2001;344(1):11–6.
88. Kluytmans JA, Wertheim HF. Nasal carriage of *Staphylococcus aureus* and prevention of nosocomial infections. Infection 2005;33(1):3–8.
89. Jones JC, Rogers TJ, Brookmeyer P, et al. Mupirocin resistance in patients colo-nized with methicillin-resistant *Staphylococcus aureus* in a surgical intensive care unit. Clin Infect Dis 2007;45(5):541–7.
90. Schaffer AC, Solinga RM, Cocchiaro J, et al. Immunization with *Staphylococcus aureus* clumping factor B, a major determinant in nasal carriage, reduces nasal colonization in a murine model. Infect Immun 2006;74(4):2145–53.
91. Clarke SR, Brummell KJ, Horsburgh MJ, et al. Identification of in vivo-expressed antigens of *Staphylococcus aureus* and their use in vaccinations for protection against nasal carriage. J Infect Dis 2006;193(8):1098–108.
92. Welch PG, Fattom A, Moore J Jr, et al. Safety and immunogenicity of *Staphylo-coccus aureus* type 5 capsular polysaccharide-*Pseudomonas aeruginosa*

recombinant exoprotein A conjugate vaccine in patients on hemodialysis. J Am Soc Nephrol 1996;7(2):247–53.

93. Tanzi E, Amendola A, Pariani E, et al. Lack of effect of a booster dose of influenza vaccine in hemodialysis patients. J Med Virol 2007;79(8):1176–9.

94. Johnson DW, Fleming SJ. The use of vaccines in renal failure. Clin Pharmacokinet 1992;22(6):434–46.

95. Watts A, Ke D, Wang Q, et al. *Staphylococcus aureus* strains that express serotype 5 or serotype 8 capsular polysaccharides differ in virulence. Infect Immun 2005;73(6):3502–11.

96. Risley AL, Loughman A, Cywes-Bentley C, et al. Capsular polysaccharide masks clumping factor A-mediated adherence of *Staphylococcus aureus* to fibrinogen and platelets. J Infect Dis 2007;196(6):919–27.

Index

Note: Page numbers of article titles are in **boldface** type.

A

Alpha-hemolysin, 162
AltaStaph, 159
Aminoglycoside(s), for *S. aureus* infections, 112–113
Antibiotic(s), for staphylococcal infections, cycle of use and resistance, 5
Antibody(ies), in blocking *S. aureus* virulence, 163
Antimicrobial resistance, in coagulase-negative staphylococci, 88
Antistaphylococcal agents, **99–131**
    aminoglycosides, 112–113
    carbapenems, 102
    cephalosporins, 101–102
    clindamycin, 118–119
    daptomycin, 105–107
    described, 99–100
    doxycycline, 111–112
    fluoroquinolones, 113–115
    glycylcyclines, 111–112
    ß-lactam(s), 100–102
    ß-lactam–ß-lactamase inhibitor combinations, 101
    linezolid, 107–109
    macrolides, 116–117
    minocycline, 111–112
    monobactams, 102
    penicillins, 100–101
    rifampin, 115–116
    telithromycin, 119
    tetracyclines, 111–112
    tigecycline, 112
    TMP-SMX, 109–110
    vancomycin, 102–105
Apoptosis, neutrophil, in *S. aureus* infections, inflammation resolution due to, 22–24
Arginine catabolic mobile element, in *S. aureus* infections, 27
Aurograb, 160

B

Bathing, preoperative, in staphylococcal surgical site infection prevention, 63

C

Carbapenem(s), for *S. aureus* infections, 102
Cardiac devices, infections associated with, coagulase-negative, 76
Central nervous system (CNS) shunt infections, coagulase-negative, 77

Infect Dis Clin N Am 23 (2009) 173–179
doi:10.1016/S0891-5520(08)00101-3
0891-5520/08/$ – see front matter © 2009 Elsevier Inc. All rights reserved.

id.theclinics.com

Moving?

Make sure your subscription moves with you!

To notify us of your new address, find your **Clinics Account Number** (located on your mailing label above your name), and contact customer service at:

E-mail: elspcs@elsevier.com

800-654-2452 (subscribers in the U.S. & Canada)
314-453-7041 (subscribers outside of the U.S. & Canada)

Fax number: 314-523-5170

Elsevier Periodicals Customer Service
11830 Westline Industrial Drive
St. Louis, MO 63146

*To ensure uninterrupted delivery of your subscription, please notify us at least 4 weeks in advance of move.

ELSEVIER

Printed and bound by CPI Group (UK) Ltd, Croydon, CR0 4YY

03/10/2024

01040464-0015